Surgical, Hybrid and Minimally Invasive Structural Cardiac Interventions

Grigore Tinică • Alexandru Burlacu
Editors

Surgical, Hybrid and Minimally Invasive Structural Cardiac Interventions

Springer

Editors
Grigore Tinică
Cardiovascular Surgery
Cardiovascular Diseases Institute, Iaşi &
Grigore T. Popa University of Medicine
and Pharmacy
Iaşi, Romania

Alexandru Burlacu
Interventional Cardiology
Cardiovascular Diseases Institute, Iaşi &
Grigore T. Popa University of Medicine
and Pharmacy
Iaşi, Romania

ISBN 978-3-032-16675-3 ISBN 978-3-032-16676-0 (eBook)
https://doi.org/10.1007/978-3-032-16676-0

This Springer imprint is published by the registered company Springer Nature Switzerland AG
The registered company address is: Gewerbestrasse 11, 6330 Cham, Switzerland

To Professor Ioan Pop de Popa and Professor Francis Robicsek—visionary cardiovascular surgeons, scientists with a deep sense of humanity, and mentors who have shaped generations. This work is humbly dedicated in honor of their legacy.

Grigore Tinică and Alexandru Burlacu

Contents

Introduction

1

Grigore Tinică and Alexandru Burlacu

When, in 1960, the pioneering cardiac surgeon Dr. Dwight Harken performed one of the first successful open-heart procedures using cardiopulmonary bypass, few could have imagined the astonishing trajectory that cardiac surgery would follow in the decades to come. At the time, the very notion of stopping the heart, repairing its inner architecture, and restarting it with precision was a revolutionary step. Who could have foreseen that by 2025, structural heart disease would be approached not only through sternotomy and sutures, but also through catheter-based valve implantation, robot-assisted resections, and hybrid operating rooms where interventional cardiologists and cardiac surgeons collaborate in real time? What once required massive incisions and prolonged recovery is now often performed through mini-thoracotomies, percutaneous routes, or even fully endovascular techniques, delivering life-saving therapy to patients once deemed inoperable. Today, structural cardiac interventions are not just evolving—they are being redefined.

In the early to mid-twentieth century, severe aortic stenosis was often viewed as an irreversible condition with an unfavorable prognosis, particularly among elderly or frail patients. With no effective pharmacological options and surgical aortic valve replacement (SAVR) still emerging as a high-risk procedure, many patients were managed conservatively, with palliation rather than cure. The turning point came with the advent of transcatheter aortic valve replacement (TAVR). This transformative innovation reshaped not only the treatment algorithm but also the very

G. Tinică
Cardiovascular Surgery, Cardiovascular Diseases Institute, Iași & Grigore T. Popa University of Medicine and Pharmacy, Iași, Romania
e-mail: grigore.tinica@umfiasi.ro

A. Burlacu (✉)
Interventional Cardiology, Cardiovascular Diseases Institute, Iași & Grigore T. Popa University of Medicine and Pharmacy, Iași, Romania
e-mail: alexandru.burlacu@umfiasi.ro

G. Tinică, A. Burlacu (eds.), *Surgical, Hybrid and Minimally Invasive Structural Cardiac Interventions*, https://doi.org/10.1007/978-3-032-16676-0_1

philosophy of structural heart care. What was once considered unapproachable surgically is now often treated percutaneously via femoral access, with outcomes that rival—and in selected populations, surpass—those of traditional surgery. TAVR is no longer reserved for the inoperable; it is now a viable, guideline-endorsed option across a spectrum of risk profiles, catalyzing a paradigm shift in how we treat valvular disease.

This volume, *Surgical, Hybrid, and Minimally Invasive Structural Cardiac Interventions*, was conceived to address the urgent need for a comprehensive and cohesive reference that reflects these monumental shifts in clinical practice. While the legacy of classical surgery remains essential, modern structural interventions demand a multidisciplinary mindset, new technical proficiencies, and an openness to technological convergence.

We open in Chap. 1 with a foundational review of cardiovascular anatomy and physiology, emphasizing anatomical nuances with implications for minimally invasive and transcatheter procedures. Chapter 2 explores the evolution of cardiac surgery, tracing the path from traditional open techniques to the refinement of robotic and video-assisted modalities. This historical arc is complemented in Chap. 3 by a detailed exposition of classical surgical techniques, such as coronary artery bypass grafting and surgical valve replacement, establishing the bedrock upon which innovation has been built.

Chapter 4 introduces the conceptual and technical pillars of minimally invasive surgery, offering insights into its rationale, limitations, and integration into modern practice. The following three chapters (Chaps. 5, 6, and 7) focus on valve-specific minimally invasive techniques for the mitral, aortic, and tricuspid valves, highlighting patient selection criteria, procedural planning, and intraoperative nuances that differentiate them from open approaches.

Recognizing the increasingly blurred boundaries between disciplines, Chap. 8 presents the emerging role of hybrid procedures, an area emblematic of the collaborative future of cardiovascular care. The Chaps. 9, 10, and 11 sections expand this discussion with focused content on transcatheter valve interventions, detailing procedural advances and clinical outcomes for the mitral, aortic, tricuspid, and pulmonary positions.

Aortic pathology, long considered the realm of high-risk surgical correction, is revisited in Chap. 12, which presents contemporary approaches to advanced aortic repair, including hybrid and endovascular strategies. In Chap. 13, attention turns to congenital heart disease in adults, a growing and often underrepresented patient population, where individualized and durable interventions are increasingly essential.

Modern cardiac interventions rely not only on operator skill but on the tools that extend and amplify those skills. Chapter 14 explores cutting-edge technologies, including robotic systems, advanced imaging, and intraoperative navigation tools. This is followed by Chap. 16, which reviews innovative biomaterials and devices, such as new-generation prosthetic valves and tissue-engineered constructs, reflecting the convergence between bioengineering and clinical medicine.

The complexity of these interventions necessitates vigilance in complication management. Chapter 17 presents an in-depth review of complications and their solutions, including both procedural and post-procedural challenges. Ethical and medico-legal dimensions, especially relevant in the context of experimental technologies and informed consent, are addressed in Chap. 18.

From a forward-looking perspective, Chap. 19 examines the role of artificial intelligence in cardiac surgery, encompassing intraoperative decision-making, predictive analytics, and personalized therapy. Finally, the same chapter discusses educational tools and the future of surgical training, emphasizing simulation, virtual reality, and case-based learning as pillars of a new pedagogical paradigm.

Ultimately, this book aims to bridge tradition and innovation—to honor the foundational principles of cardiac surgery while equipping clinicians and researchers for the challenges of the next generation. It is a resource designed not only to document the current state of the field but to provoke critical thinking, collaborative models, and technologically informed practice that place the patient at the center of structural cardiac care.

Cardiac Structural Anatomy and Physiology

2

Cristina Furnica, Raluca Ozana Chistol, Elena Sapte, and Grigore Tinică

Cardiac Development

With the first heartbeats starting during the 21st to 23rd days of intrauterine life, the heart is the first functional embryofetal human organ.

Progenitor heart cells originating from the splanchnic layer of the lateral plate mesoderm begin to differentiate in response to endodermic induction signals, mainly the transcription factor BMP4. The newly differentiated cells migrate toward the cephalic end of the embryo to form the cardiac crescent (primitive heart field—origin of the atria, left ventricle (LV), and a part of the right ventricle (RV)), a horseshoe-shaped structure presenting two asymmetric parts connected anteriorly [1].

C. Furnica (✉)
Department of Anatomy, Faculty of Medicine, Grigore T. Popa University of Medicine and Pharmacy, Iasi, Romania

Institute of Forensic Pathology, Iasi, Romania

R. O. Chistol
Department of Anatomy, Faculty of Medicine, Grigore T. Popa University of Medicine and Pharmacy, Iasi, Romania

Department of Medical Imaging, Prof. Dr. George I.M. Georgescu Institute of Cardiovascular Diseases, Iasi, Romania

E. Sapte
Department of Anatomy, Faculty of Medicine, Ovidius University, Constanta, Romania

G. Tinică
Cardiovascular Surgery, Cardiovascular Diseases Institute, Iaşi & Grigore T. Popa University of Medicine and Pharmacy, Iaşi, Romania
e-mail: grigore.tinica@umfiasi.ro

G. Tinică, A. Burlacu (eds.), *Surgical, Hybrid and Minimally Invasive Structural Cardiac Interventions*, https://doi.org/10.1007/978-3-032-16676-0_2

In response to the embryo's cephalo-caudal and lateral folding, the two parts of the cardiac crescent migrate anteriorly and fuse, forming the primitive heart tube.

A second cellular differentiation and migration wave occurs in the splanchnic mesoderm, at the inner part of the cardiac crescent and the origin of the RV and outflow tract (*conus cordis* and *truncus arteriosus*), leading to the formation of the secondary heart field. Under the influence of various genes (Nk2, MEF2, GATA, Tbx, and Hand), the cardiac cells differentiate into cardiomyocytes (atrial, ventricular, conduction tissue) and endocardial cells [2].

The primitive heart tube is a highly regionalized structure, organized along anteroposterior, craniocaudal, and right-left axes. The ventricles derive from anterior precursor cells, while the atria derive from posterior cells. In each segment, the inner and outer cellular layers differentiate to form the endocardium and myocardium, respectively. Between these two layers lies the extracellular matrix, also named *cardiac jelly*.

As the heart tube elongates, four regions begin to dilate, forming in cephalon-caudal direction four cavities: *bulbus cordis*, primitive ventricle, primitive atrium, and *sinus venosus*. The primitive heart tube remains connected at its cranial end (arterial pole) to the aortic sac and aortic arches and at its caudal end (venous pole), through two horns, with the vitelline, umbilical, and cardinal veins.

The development of the cardiac loop between the 23rd and the 28th day of intrauterine life involves simultaneous bending and rotation: the heart tube curves to the right (D-loop), initially in a C-shape structure while adopting afterwards an S-shaped structure. These looping processes place the future RV ventrally and to the right, the future LV dorsally and to the left, and the atria in a superior and posterior position, with the left atrium (LA) as the most posterior heart chamber. The right-left patterning is controlled by genes such as lefty 1 and 2, Pitx2 [1].

In this stage, the cardiovascular system involves an "*in series*" circulation. Cardiac septation begins alongside the development of the right and left ventricles, the narrow atrioventricular canal connecting initially only the left part of the common atrium to the future LV (common ventricle). This developmental stage heralds the formation of systemic veins and the aortic arches. The outflow tract (*conotruncus*, the distal part of *bulbus cordis*) is entirely located above the future RV (proximal part of *bulbus cordis*) right side to the inflow tract. Cardiac septation begins with the development on the 28th day of the *septum primum* in the atria and of *septum muscularis* in the ventricles. During this developmental stage, the heart's apex is oriented to the right (dextrocardia) [2].

During the following embryofetal period, from the 29th to the 35th day of intrauterine life, ventricular development and differentiation of the atrioventricular valves continues, heralding the future atrioventricular septation. The subaortic conus disappears, while the great vessels define their definitive relationships with each other and with the corresponding ventricles and atrioventricular valves. The aorta and the pulmonary arteries separate, semilunar valves appear, and the development of pharyngeal arches continues toward establishing the definitive thoracic aorta and supra-aortic trunks. The heart's apex shifts to the left (levocardia), establishing the "*in parallel*" circulation. Cardiac septation is now almost complete, with the *septum secundum* developing during the 33rd day, and the *septum muscularis* mostly defined during the 35th day of embryonic life.

During the S6-S7, definitive ventricular septation and development of the aortic arches are achieved.

The final stage of cardiogenesis consists of epicardium development (originating from the proepicardium) and the modeling of the coronary vessel architecture.

Cardiac Anatomy

General Features

Covered by the pericardium, the heart is a valvular, muscular, four-chambered structure located in the middle compartment of the inferior mediastinum, superior to the diaphragm, between the two pleuropulmonary regions.

Morphologically, the heart consists of four cavities: two atria and two ventricles. The atria, located cranially, are considered the heart's inflow (injection) chambers, and present prolongations, the so-called auricles, while the ventricles, located caudally, pump blood to the tissues and represent the outflow (ejection) chambers.

Functionally, the heart is a pressure-propulsion pump (6000 liters/day) divided into two halves: the right heart and the left heart [3].

The right atrium (RA) communicates with the right ventricle (RV) through the right atrioventricular valve, forming a morphofunctional complex referred to in medical and surgical terms as *the right heart*. The right heart is adapted to the low-pressure venous system and ensures the circulation of venous blood, injected into the RA through the two *venae cavae* and ejected from the RV through the pulmonary trunk.

The left atrium (LA) communicates with the left ventricle (LV) through the left atrioventricular orifice, forming a morphofunctional complex similarly referred to as *the left heart*. The left heart is adapted to the high-pressure arterial system, receiving oxygenated blood from the pulmonary gas exchange through the pulmonary veins, which open into the LA. Blood passes from the LA to the LV, from where it is then pumped into the aorta.

Superficially, the boundaries between the atria and ventricles are marked by fat-filled grooves (sulci): the interatrial and interventricular grooves, running along the long axis of the pyramidal-shaped heart, and the atrioventricular grooves, oriented perpendicular to the long axis of the heart. The main trunks of the coronary arteries and their main branches run within these grooves, surrounded by epicardial fat, thus explaining their accessibility during coronary bypass surgery at this level (Fig. 2.1).

The blood flow through the heart is unidirectional, regulated by the synergistic action of a quadrivalvular complex consisting of the atrioventricular valves (tricuspid and mitral), which allow blood to flow from the atria to the ventricles, and the semilunar valves (pulmonary and aortic), which facilitate blood flow from the ventricles to the great arteries, the aorta, and the pulmonary trunk.

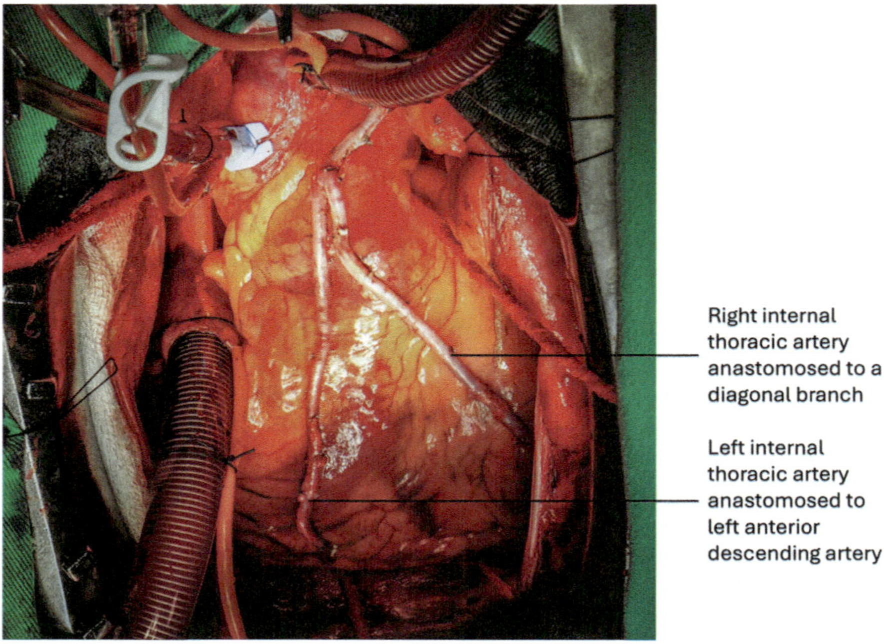

Fig. 2.1 Coronary artery bypass with a composite LITA-RITA-Y graft (LITA—left internal thoracic artery, RITA—right internal thoracic artery): LITA anastomosed to the left anterior descending artery and RITA anastomosed to a diagonal branch. (Cardiac surgery image, collection of the Institute of Cardiovascular Diseases, Iasi, Romania)

Orientation and Heart Relations

Inside the pericardial sac, the human heart is situated obliquely, with 1/3 to the right and 2/3 to the left of the midsagittal line, in a plane connecting the right shoulder to the left nipple. Its long axis is oriented forward, leftward, and slightly downward, revealing anatomical variations upon the thorax morphology: more vertical in patients with a narrow thorax or more horizontal in those with a wide thorax. Typically, the apex of the heart is oriented to the left of the midsagittal line, anteriorly and inferiorly, while its base is oriented posterosuperiorly, to the right. Clinically, the apex can be palpated in the fifth left intercostal space, on the midclavicular line. Cardiac diseases might alter the size of the heart or the position of its long axis [3].

The cardiac silhouette reveals the following boundaries:

- Superior: a virtual transverse plane through the sternal angle and the body of T4.
- Inferior: the diaphragm's thoracic surface.
- Anterior: a virtual frontal plane tangent to the anterior surface of the pericardium.
- Posterior: a virtual frontal plane tangent and posterior to the tracheal bifurcation, the pulmonary veins, and the pericardium of the left atrium.

- Lateral: the right and left mediastinal pleura.
- Anatomically, the heart is related:
- Anteriorly: to the sternocostal wall.
- Posteriorly: to posterior mediastinal viscera, including the thoracic esophagus.
- Laterally: to the pleural cavities and their contents.

Weight and Size

The weight and size of the heart vary depending on age, sex, height, epicardial fat, general nutritional status, additional pathology, and body mass index.

The average weight (adult) is $\approx 325 \pm 75$ g in males and $\approx 275 \pm 75$ g in females. Compared by Laennec to the subject's right fist, the heart has an anteroposterior diameter of 14–16 cm, a transverse diameter of 12–15 cm, and a maximum circumference of ~25 cm, with smaller dimensions in females [3].

The size of an empty heart logically differs from that of a blood-filled one, a fact that must be considered by cardiac surgeons when planning the length of vascular conduits used for coronary artery bypass grafting (CABG).

Surface Projections

The area of relative cardiac dullness is located between the third and fifth intercostal spaces, extending from the left sternal border to the midclavicular line while the area of absolute cardiac dullness is more limited, located between the fourth and sixth intercostal spaces, slightly to the left sternal border (between the sternum and the cardiac notch of the left lung).

The projection of the heart on the vertebral column corresponds to the cardiac vertebrae (of Giacomini) T4–T8.

The heart auscultation points are:

- The aortic valve is in the second intercostal space at the right sternal border.
- The pulmonary valve in the second intercostal space at the left sternal border.
- The tricuspid valve in fourth and fifth intercostal spaces at the right sternal border.
- The mitral valve in the fifth intercostal space at the left midclavicular line.
- The Erb point in the third intercostal space along the left sternal border, a key auscultation point for both mitral and aortic valves [4].

Cardiac External Morphology

The heart is pyramid-shaped, presenting either 4 faces (square pyramid) or 3 faces (triangular pyramid), a base, and an apex according to various anatomical schools. More relevant to clinical practice is to describe the heart as triangular pyramid, with a sternocostal or anterior surface (*facies sternocostalis*), a lateral surface

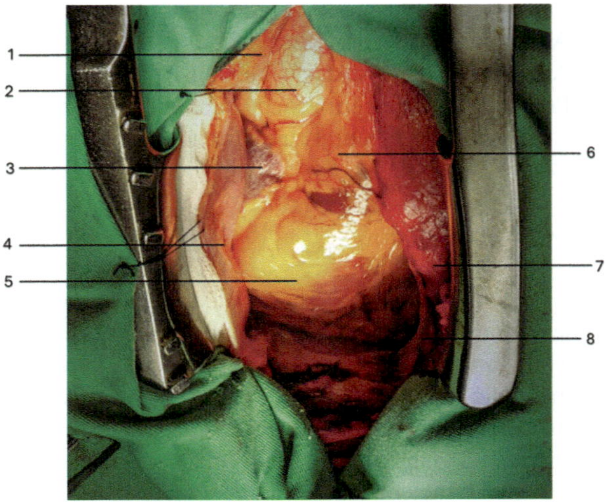

Fig. 2.2 The heart: intraoperative aspect: sternocostal surface: 1—superior vena cava; 2—ascending aorta; 3—right auricle; 4– right lung; 5—right ventricle; 6—pulmonary trunk; 7—left lung; 8—pericardium. (Cardiac surgery image, collection of the Institute of Cardiovascular Diseases, Iasi, Romania)

(pulmonary, left) (*facies pulmonaris*), and a diaphragmatic (inferior) surface (*facies diaphragmatica*), as well as superior, inferior, right, and left borders, and an inferolateral oriented apex [3].

The sternocostal surface is convex, oriented anteriorly, superiorly, and to the right, formed by the RA and right auricle, the right atrioventricular groove, the RV, and the pulmonary outflow tract (*conus arteriosus*) (Fig. 2.2).

Occasionally, a part of the LV may contribute to the anterior surface of the heart (Fig. 2.3).

The lateral or *left surface* presents an atrial or posterior segment with the left auricle wrapping around the left lateral surface of the pulmonary artery, and a ventricular segment, the lateral surface of the LV. The marginal branches of the circumflex artery are accessed for implantation of bypass grafts.

The diaphragmatic or inferior surface is flat and horizontal, related to the tendinous diaphragm. It presents a narrow posterior atrial segment and a broad anterior ventricular segment divided by the posterior interventricular groove into an extensive right ventricular area and a more restricted left ventricular area.

The superior border is primarily represented by the LA.

The right or acute border corresponds to the RA and RV. Near the cardiac apex, the right border is intersected by the anterior interventricular groove, creating the notch of the cardiac apex. The right marginal artery, a collateral branch of the right coronary artery, is visible and surgically accessible along this border.

The left, oblique, obtuse, or *pulmonary border* is mainly formed by the LV, while *the inferior border* of the heart, less pronounced, is formed by both ventricles.

The cardiac apex, the junction of the inferior and left borders at the apex of the LV, corresponds to the fifth intercostal space, situated approximately 6,5 cm from the left parasternal line.

The base is exclusively formed by the atria, separated by the interatrial groove. The opening of the inferior vena cava (IVC) is situated low on the

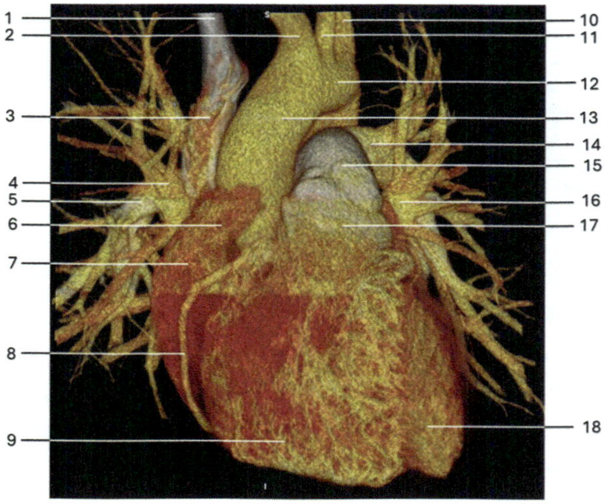

Fig. 2.3 CT VRT reconstruction: the sternocostal surface of the heart: 1—right brachiocephalic vein; 2—brachiocephalic trunk; 3—superior vena cava; 4—right superior pulmonary vein; 5—right pulmonary artery; 6—right auricle; 7—right atrium; 8—right coronary artery; 9—right ventricle; 10—left subclavian artery; 11—left common carotid artery; 12—aortic arch; 13—ascending aorta; 14—Left pulmonary artery; 15—pulmonary trunk and valve; 16—left superior pulmonary vein; 17—conus arteriosus; 18—left ventricle. (Collection of the Institute of Cardiovascular Diseases, Iasi, Romania)

narrow posterior surface of the RA, while more superiorly, lies the opening of the superior vena cava (SVC). These two veins appear to extend into one another, forming a purely vascular right wall (*sinus venosus*) separated from the actual atrial wall by the *sulcus terminalis*. Leftwards, the posterior surface of the LA occupies most of the cardiac base and receives the four pulmonary veins (two left and two right) (Fig. 2.4).

Cardiac Grooves

The coronary (atrioventricular) groove incompletely encircles the heart, being interrupted by the *conus* or infundibulum of the RV.

Anteriorly, the atrioventricular groove separates the RA from the RV, containing the coronary artery and the small cardiac vein.

Posteriorly, the coronary groove separates the LA from the LV and contains the coronary sinus, the great cardiac vein, and the circumflex branch of the left coronary artery.

The interventricular groove marks the position of the underlying interventricular septum between the right and left ventricles. On the anterior surface of the heart, the interventricular groove leaves the coronary groove to the left of the infundibulum and follows a sigmoid curve toward the diaphragmatic surface, on the right flank of the cardiac apex. On the diaphragmatic surface of the heart, the interventricular groove is directed cranially and rejoins the coronary groove, forming the *crux*

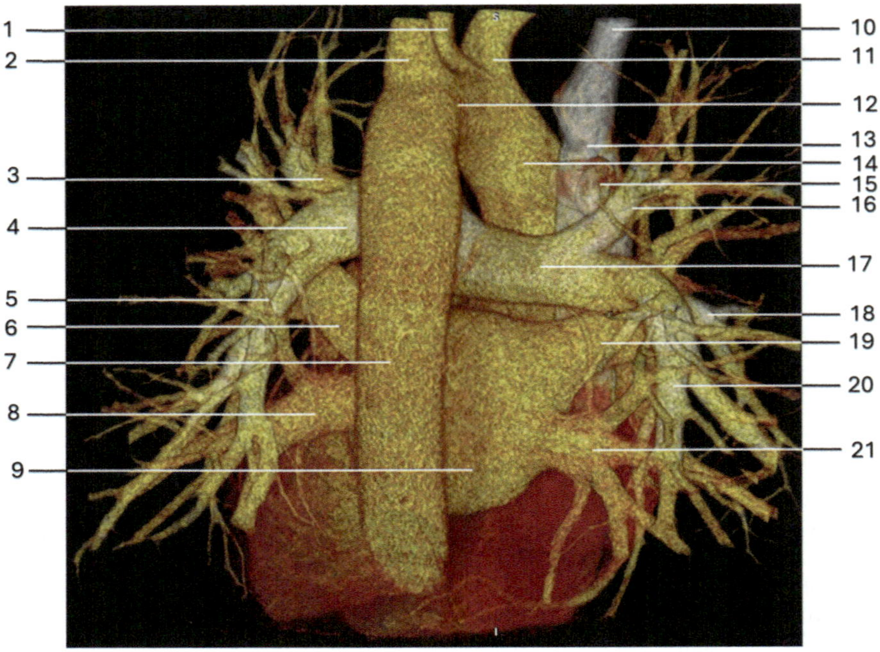

Fig. 2.4 CT VRT reconstruction: the base of the heart: 1—left common carotid artery; 2—left subclavian artery; 3—left upper lobe pulmonary artery; 4—left pulmonary artery; 5—left lower lobe pulmonary artery; 6—left superior pulmonary vein; 7—descending aorta; 8—left inferior pulmonary vein; 9—left atrium; 10—right brachiocephalic vein; 11—brachiocephalic trunk; 12—aortic arch; 13—superior vena cava; 14—ascending aorta; 15—opening of azygos vein; 16—right upper lobe pulmonary artery; 17—right pulmonary artery; 18—right middle lobe pulmonary artery; 19—right superior pulmonary vein; 20—right lower lobe pulmonary artery; 21—right inferior pulmonary vein. (Collection of the Institute of Cardiovascular Diseases, Iasi, Romania)

cordis. The anterior part of the interventricular groove contains the anterior interventricular branch (left anterior descending artery) of the left coronary artery and the great cardiac vein of Galen, while the posterior part contains the posterior interventricular branch (posterior descending artery) of the right coronary artery and the middle cardiac vein.

The interatrial groove, slightly visible in its posterior segment, separates the atria and is covered anteriorly by the pulmonary trunk and aorta.

Cardiac Internal Morphology

The right heart and the left heart are separated by a septum. The atrium is a globular, roughly spherical cavity that opens anteriorly into the ventricle, a pyramidal cavity with two openings at its base: an atrioventricular orifice, which connects the atrium to the ventricle, and an arterial orifice, which allows ventricular emptying.

The right heart receives deoxygenated blood and propels it into the pulmonary circulation, where it becomes oxygenated; operating under low pressures, it maintains an average perfusion pressure of about 15 mmHg in the pulmonary artery. The central venous pressure (right atrial pressure) ranges between 0 and 5 mmHg [5].

The Right Atrium (RA)

The RA, cuboidal in shape, is located between the openings of the SVC and IVC and receives systemic venous blood through the two vena cavae and cardiac venous blood through the coronary sinus.

The RA consists of two morphologically and embryologically distinct segments: the anterior segment, derived from the primitive atrium, and the posterior segment, derived from the right horn of the *sinus venosus*, known as the *sinus venarum*. The junction between the venous component and the true right atrium projects externally at the *sulcus terminalis*, while internally it is marked by the *crista terminalis,* tangent to the right edges of the openings of the two vena cavae [5].

The anterior segment walls reveal muscular ridges formed by parallel bundles of muscle fibers called the pectinate muscles. Representing the sinus portion of the atrium, the smooth posterior segment extends between the openings of the two vena cavae, leftward to the interatrial groove and rightward to the *crista terminalis*.

Externally, the RA presents in craniocaudal direction the following structures: superior cava vein (SVC), right auricle, coronary sulcus (separating the RA from the RV), *sulcus terminalis*, inferior cava vein (IVC).

Anatomically, given the triple obliquity of the heart, the RA is related to the SVC (superiorly); pericardium, right lung, and right mediastinal pleura (anteriorly); right pulmonary veins and LA (posteriorly); pericardium, right phrenic nerve, pericardiophrenic vessels, mediastinal surface of the right lung, and right mediastinal pleura (laterally); ascending aorta and LA (medially); IVC and tendinous part of the diaphragm (inferiorly). Notably, the right lung and right mediastinal pleura are located anterolateral to the right atrium (RA), while the left atrium (LA) is located posteromedially; the interatrial septum is oriented obliquely, positioning the RA anterior and to the right of the LA.

The right auricle (appendage) is a triangular extension with muscular walls and a broad base, anterior to the RA and overlapping the right flank of the ascending aorta.

The RA is cuboidal in shape, presenting the following walls with the corresponding features [3]:

- Superior wall: opening of the SVC (approximately 20 mm in diameter) and ostium of the right auricle.
- Inferior wall: opening of the IVC (approximately 30 mm in diameter) with the Eustachian valve, an endocardial flap situated between the IVC and RA and extending superiorly to the interatrial septum anterior to the *limbus* of the *fossa ovalis*; and the opening of the coronary sinus (approximately 12 mm in diameter) with the Thebesian valve, located anterior and to the left of the IVC opening. Occasionally, the opening of the coronary sinus may be covered by a multi-

perforated tissue named the Chiari network. The inferior wall contains the *sinus band* (a prominence originating at the level of the Eustachian valve and extending toward the septal wall, containing the tendon of Todaro) and *Koch's triangle,* which contains the atrioventricular node (Aschoff-Tawara) and the initial portion of the His bundle. The Koch triangle is delineated by the tendon of Todaro (superior), the tricuspid valve (inferior), and the opening of the coronary sinus (lateral).

- Anterior wall: right atrioventricular orifice with the tricuspid valve.
- Medial (septal) wall: interatrial septum, featuring a central depression called the *fossa ovalis*, which corresponds to the fetal interatrial communication (*foramen ovale*). The *fossa ovalis* is bordered by a prominent ridge, the *limbus of the fossa ovalis* (Vieussens' ring).
- Lateral wall: features the pectinate muscles, horizontal muscular ridges, which arise from the *crista terminalis* and extend into the right auricle. The *crista terminalis* is the terminal part of the smooth atrial wall, originating at the junction between the right auricle and the RA, and running parallel to the openings of the SVC and IVC; at the cranial end of the *crista terminalis* lies the sinoatrial node. The lateral wall of the RA is used for creating pouches for venous cannulation during cardiac surgery involving extracorporeal circulation and represents the usual surgical approach to the RA. Surgical access can be achieved through a vertical, posterior, or arcuate incision.
- Posterior wall: smooth, derived from the *sinus venosus*, contains the intervenous tubercle of lower (formed by the reflection of the pericardium on the right pulmonary veins) and small openings for the small cardiac veins.

Right Ventricle (RV)

The right ventricle (RV), located anteriorly and to the left of the RA, receives blood from the RA and sends it to the lungs via the pulmonary trunk. The RV extends from the right atrioventricular orifice (tricuspid valve) to the cardiac apex and forms most of the anterior surface of the heart. The RV is oriented cranially to the left, extending with the infundibulum (*conus arteriosus*), up to the pulmonary valve. The wall of the RV is one-third the thickness of the LV wall and becomes progressively thinner as it extends toward the apex compared to the base.

The most anterior heart chamber, the RV, is related through the pericardium to the posterior surface of the sternocostal wall, left pleura, and anterior margin of the left lung (it is a vulnerable structure in case of redo sternotomy). The interventricular septum lies behind it, while the right auricle and pulmonary trunk are situated above. Inferiorly, the RV relates to the tendinous part of the diaphragm on which it rests.

The RV presents an inflow component, which supports and surrounds the tricuspid valve, and an outflow component, the infundibulum, which ends with the pulmonary valve. These components form an obtuse angle relative to each other. The aortic root is connected to the infundibulum by a thin band of collagenous tissue named *conus ligamentosum.*

The RV and LV are separated by the interventricular septum, consisting of a proximal membranous part and a distal muscular part.

The RV is triangular pyramidal in shape, described with 3 walls, a base, and an apex:

- Anterior wall: forms ¾ of the heart's sternocostal surface. Separated from the anterior thoracic wall by the pericardium, left pleura, and the anterior border of the left lung, the anterior wall permits a surgical approach through either a horizontal (transverse) incision from the anterior right coronary groove to the anterior interventricular groove or a vertical (longitudinal) incision along the axis of the pulmonary artery. The anterosuperior surface has an oblique, dorsoventral orientation, from right to left, and is bounded by the anterior interventricular groove and the right margin of the heart, forming the anterior wall of the infundibulum. The muscle fibers at this level are oriented in the direction of blood flow.
- Inferior (diaphragmatic) wall: smooth, concave inward, with a reduced thickness of 5 mm related through the pericardium to the diaphragm central tendon and the adjacent muscular portion (left diaphragmatic dome).
- Septal wall: represented by the interventricular septum protruding into the ventricle (convex), is relatively thin in the upper (infundibular) half. A horizontal muscular ridge named the supraventricular crest (Wolff's crest) is located in the middle segment. Muscular and thick (10 mm) in most of its extent, the septal wall becomes membranous and thin near the ventricular base. Its left side faces the left ventricle, while its right side consists of two segments: an anterior interventricular segment, and a posterior atrioventricular segment, slightly larger, separating the RA from the LV. The boundary between these two zones is marked on the right side of the septum by the attachment of the tricuspid valve, thus explaining the existence of abnormal communications (fistula) between the RA and LV.

The infundibulum tendon interconnects the pulmonary annulus and the posterior part of the infundibulum to the root of the aorta, attaching to the wall of the non-coronary sinus. Inferiorly, the tendon connects to the membranous interventricular septum.

The borders of the RV shadow the intersection of its walls, the lateral being the most prominent one (acute border).

The apex of the RV does not correspond to the cardiac apex and describes several trabeculae that intersect and form the cavernous or spongy part of the RV.

The base of the RV is oriented cranially, posteriorly, and to the right, featuring two non-coplanar orifices:

- The right atrioventricular orifice, oriented posterocaudally, is approximately 35–38 mm in diameter.
- The pulmonary artery orifice is positioned anterosuperior, opening at the top of the infundibulum and containing the semilunar valves.

The internal surface of the inflow and outflow tracts differs; the supraventricular crest and the septomarginal trabecula mark the transition.

The supraventricular (Wolff's) crest divides the RV into an *inflow tract* (trabeculated walls, oriented inferiorly) and an *outflow tract* (smooth walls, oriented superiorly). The supraventricular crest is an oblique muscular ridge situated between the right atrioventricular orifice and the pulmonary artery orifice. Concave anteriorly and to the right, it stretches from the interventricular septum to the anterior wall. The anterior leaflet of the tricuspid valve is partially attached to this crest. The septal insertion fuses with the septomarginal trabecula.

The walls of the inflow tract present many trabeculations, especially at the apex, while the outflow tract has smooth walls and is directed toward the pulmonary valve, upward, posteriorly, and to the left. A segment of the *conus arteriosus* forms part of the interventricular septum, called the infundibular (conal) septum, separating the outflow tracts of the RV and LV. The smooth walls of the outflow tract are thought to increase ejection velocity.

Many irregular muscular columns (*trabeculae carneae*) project from the walls of the RV inside the cavity (especially the inflow tract) and can be classified into:

- First-order muscular columns (papillary muscles or pillars): broad-based with a free apex, giving rise to *chordae tendinae* attached to the tricuspid valve leaflets.
- Second-order muscular columns: detached from the ventricular wall at their midpoint and attached to the wall at both ends. The septomarginal trabecula (*Tandler moderator band*) is a second-order muscular column extending from the anterior wall to the septal wall at the level of the anterior part of the supraventricular crest, which it extends, and has a posterior and rightward concavity. The septomarginal trabecula, containing the right bundle branch, is a morphologic marker of the RV used to correctly identify the heart chambers of patients with congenital heart diseases [3].
- Third-order muscular columns: simple muscular projections from the ventricular wall.

Analogous to the pectinate muscles of the RA, *trabeculae carneae* are also found, to a lesser extent, in the left ventricle (LV).

Three papillary muscles, anterior, posterior, and septal, have also been described as part of the RV. The *anterior papillary muscle*, originating close to the RV apex, is the largest and can be single or double-headed. It stretches the *chordae tendinae* attached to the anterior and posterior leaflets of the tricuspid valve. The *posterior papillary muscle* is smaller, gives chordae to the posterior and septal leaflets, and attaches to the free posterior wall. The *septal papillary muscle*, also called the conal papillary muscle, is small but functionally significant. It originates at the level of the interventricular septum, at the base of the outflow tract (the end of the supraventricular crest), corresponding to the junction between the smooth and rough portions of the RV. It gives chordae mostly to the septal leaflet [5].

Right Atrioventricular (Tricuspid) Valve

The atrioventricular valve complex consists of the annulus, valve leaflets, and the supporting tension apparatus formed by the papillary muscles and *chordae tendineae*.

The right atrioventricular orifice is an oval or triangular opening with rounded angles and a long axis of 35–40 mm, traditionally thought to accommodate three of the operator's fingers. The orifice is angled approximately 45° to the sagittal plane, directed obliquely, anterolateral to the left, slightly caudal. Triangular in shape, its borders are described as anterior, posterior, and septal, corresponding to the bases of the three valve leaflets [6].

The tricuspid annulus is an anatomically imprecise term, inconsistently used in medical-surgical practice. While the mitral annulus is anchored through two major collagen structures—the right and left fibrous trigones—only the right fibrous trigone anchors the tricuspid annulus. This thick part of the tricuspid annulus corresponds to the insertion of the septal leaflet and the anteroseptal commissure. However, most of the annular circumference is in direct contact with the myocardium. The anterior and posterior leaflets attach directly to the myocardium. This less reinforced part of the annulus distends during functional valve regurgitation.

The annulus consists of dense connective tissue and is part of the fibrous skeleton of the heart. Medially, it attaches to the membranous part of the interventricular septum. From the right fibrous trigone, a series of paired, curved, endocardial tendons detach (*fila coronaria*), partially limiting the annular circumference.

The tricuspid valve presents three leaflets: anterior, posterior, and septal. Each leaflet consists of a dense connective tissue core continuous with the annulus and two endocardial layers.

The anterior leaflet partially separates the inflow and outflow tracts of the right ventricle and is limited between the anteroseptal and anteroposterior commissures. The anterior leaflet is the largest and attaches to the posterolateral part of the supraventricular crest, extending along the membranous septum and reaching the anteroseptal commissure.

The posterior leaflet, entirely mural, is placed between the anteroposterior and posteroseptal commissures, extending along the free lateral wall and the posterior part of the interventricular septum.

The septal leaflet is placed between the posteroseptal and anteroseptal commissures, attaching mainly to the septal wall and partly to the posterior one. Near the center of the valve, its attachments form an angle marking the transition between the posterior and septal surfaces.

Each leaflet presents three zones:

- The rough zone, opaque, with numerous *chordae tendinae* insertions on the ventricular surface. The atrial surface of the rough zone comes into apposition with the similar surface of the adjacent valve at the closure line.
- The smooth (clear) zone, translucent, is the insertion point of a few *chordae tendinae*, and also contains a thin fibrous center.
- The basal zone, extending 2–3 mm from the annulus, is a thick innervated and well-vascularized structure that contains connective tissue.

The contraction of the papillary muscles stretches the *chordae tendinae* attached to the leaflets, preventing atrial prolapse during ventricular systole. The total leaflet surface is double the valve opening area, allowing overlapping during closure (good coaptation). The leaflets remain in relative apposition during ventricular filling due to blood flow and the tension exerted by the tendinous cords. When ventricular filling decreases, the leaflets approach, without closing. Valve closure is achieved through ventricular contraction, which triggers complete leaflet apposition.

The junction between two leaflets is called the commissure and bears the name of the two adjacent leaflets (anteroseptal, posteroseptal, anteroposterior).

- Anteroseptal commissure: the basal insertion of the tricuspid valve reaches its highest point at the level of the membranous interventricular septum, at the junction of the anterior and septal surfaces of the RV. This region is easily identified and marks the commissure between the anterior and septal leaflets. At this level, there is a fan-shaped chordae, originating from the septal papillary muscle.
- Anteroposterior commissure: corresponds to the right border of the ventricle and attaches to a fan-shaped cord. The anterior papillary muscle is usually directed toward this commissure and also serves as a surgical landmark.
- Posteroseptal commissure: the most difficult to delineate, is usually marked by a muscular column located in the middle of the posterior surface. The posteroseptal commissure extends the most.
- *Chordae tendineae* are composed of multiple layers of elastic fibers, an inner collagen core, and an outer layer of endothelial cells and support the leaflets [7]. Two types of *chordae tendinae* are described:
  - False chordae of variable number and size that connect the papillary muscles to each other or to the ventricular wall.
  - True chordae originating from the apex of the papillary muscles, sometimes from their base or directly from the ventricular wall, attach to valve leaflets.

Depending on the distance from the marginal insertion of the leaflets, Tandler classifies the tendinous cords into first, second, and third-order chordae (free margin, 6–8 mm beyond, and basal insertion). Lam and Silver consider that due to their morphology, there is a higher variability of the *chordae tendinae*, describing fanlike commissural, rough zone, strut, basal, and cleft chordae.

First-order Tandler chordae include commissural chordae, rough zone chordae of the anterior and posterior leaflets that insert into the free margin of the leaflets; second-order Tandler chordae include rough zone chordae of the anterior and posterior leaflets that insert beyond the free margin, strut chordae of the anterior leaflet, and main stem or cleft chordae of the posterior leaflet, while third-order Tandler chordae only include basal chordae of the posterior leaflet.

The tricuspid valve generally presents 25 *chordae tendinae*.

The papillary muscles have been discussed previously.

The Pulmonary Valve

The pulmonary valve, the ejection valve of the RV, is located above the infundibulum with a cranial, left, and slightly posterior orientation. The diameter of the pulmonary valve varies between 20 and 22 mm [5].

The pulmonary valve consists of three semilunar cusps: anterior, right (posterior), and left (posterior). Structurally, each pulmonary cusp consists of an endocardial fold with a dense connective tissue core. The adjacent cusps are interconnected by the valvular commissures and attach to the wall through a U-shaped (semilunar) fibrous valve ring, anchored simultaneously to the right ventricular infundibulum and the pulmonary trunk.

At the center of each free cusp margin lies a nodular condensation called Morgagni's nodule. The three Morgagni nodules ensure complete cusp coaptation during diastole. Opposite the semilunar cusp, the arterial wall presents three dilatations or sinuses (of Valsalva), with thin walls and a crescent-shaped area, the *linea alba,* corresponding to the annulus.

The left heart receives oxygenated blood (99% saturation) from the lungs and propels it into the systemic circulation. High pressures prevail in the left heart, ensuring an average perfusion pressure in the arterial system of about 100 mmHg [3].

Left Atrium (LA)

The left atrium (LA) varies in shape from ovoid to approximately cuboidal, featuring thick walls (approximately 3 mm) and a small blood volume under normal circumstances. The LA is situated along the midline, behind the RA and above the LV. The cavity and walls of the LA originate from the primitive atrium and the proximal segments of the pulmonary veins, which are incorporated into the primitive atrium during embryogenesis.

The obliquely oriented LA is comparably narrower than the RA and contains more trabeculated walls. The two cavities are separated by the interatrial septum.

The left side of the LA is covered by the initial segments of the pulmonary trunk and ascending aorta. Anteroinferior and to the left, the LA connects with the base of the LV through the mitral valve. On the superior left aspect of the LA, opens the left auricle, with a narrow base and of variable shape. This structure is generally described as a "chicken wing".

The posterior wall of the LA has an approximately quadrilateral shape, forms almost the entire base of the heart, and contains the opening of the pulmonary veins. The LA also forms the anterior wall of the oblique pericardial sinus.

The left auricle and the vestibule of the LA are derived from the primitive atrium, while the rest of the LA originates from the primitive pulmonary vein. Disorders in the process of atrial morphogenesis can lead to insufficient incorporation of the pulmonary veins and CHD development (congenital heart disease), such as *cor triatriatum.* The LA side of the interatrial septum is derived from the *septum primum.* Except for the pectinate muscles of the left auricle, the smooth walls of this atrium cause difficulty in differentiating the two parts of the LA.

While traditionally, surgical access to the left atrium for closed-heart mitral commissurotomy was obtained through the left auricle, the new approach is through the right pole, behind the interatrial groove, in front of the right pulmonary veins. To preserve sufficient tissue for closing the left atrium and thus avoid stenosis or obstruction of a pulmonary vein, the newer technique involves dissecting the interatrial groove for about 1 cm and incising the atrial wall as far as possible from the right pulmonary veins.

The defining elements of the LA are the four pulmonary veins: right, left, superior, and inferior.

These veins are enclosed in a serous pericardial sheath along with the IVC and SVC. In certain situations, near the ostium of the left inferior pulmonary vein, the oblique vein of the left atrium may be identified; this structure drains into the coronary sinus and represents the end of the embryonic left common cardinal vein.

Cuboidal in shape, the LS reveals the following six walls [3]:

- Anterior wall: contains the left atrioventricular orifice with the bicuspid or mitral valve.
- Lateral wall: communicates with the left auricle at the boundary with the anterior wall.
- Superior and inferior walls: smooth, without distinctive features.
- Medial (septal) wall: formed by the interatrial septum, which anterosuperiorly has an arcuate or semilunar fold; this structure is upwardly concave, corresponding to the flap valve of the oval foramen.
- Posterior wall: contains the ostia of the four pulmonary veins (2 right and 2 left).

The left auricle, irregular in shape and with a narrow ostium and containing pectinate muscles, is the lateral extension of the left atrium surrounding the pulmonary trunk.

The left atrium is cranially related to the left main bronchus and the right pulmonary artery, from which it is separated by the transverse pericardial sinus.

The LV is inferior and to the left of the LA while the initial segments of the ascending aorta and pulmonary trunk are situated in front. Posteriorly, the LA is separated from the esophagus by the oblique pericardial sinus. Additional posterior rapports are with the descending thoracic aorta, thoracic duct, hemiazygos, and pulmonary veins. Laterally, the LA is related to the left lung and left pulmonary veins.

Left Ventricle (LV)

The LV receives oxygenated blood from the LA and pumps it through the aorta to all tissues of the body. Compared to the RV, the structure of the LV is consistent with its role as a pump that assures a pulsatile blood flow in the high pressures of the systemic arteries. Described as having an ellipsoidal or conical shape, the LV is longer and narrower than the RV and extends from the base corresponding to the coronary groove toward the apex of the heart. The long axis of the LV is oriented ventrally and to the left.

The LV forms the apex, the left surface of the heart, and contributes to the sternocostal and diaphragmatic surfaces, except for the aortic and pulmonary trunk emergence sites. The base of the LV is superficially separated from the LA and left auricle by the left side of the coronary groove. The anterior and inferior interventricular grooves mark the insertion of the interventricular septum on the ventricular wall.

The myocardium of the LV is three times thicker compared to the RV, measuring approximately 8–12 mm, which increases intraventricular pressure by about threefold [4].

The coronary sinus runs along the posterior left portion of the atrioventricular groove beneath the mitral valve annulus. This particularity gives a certain degree of vulnerability to iatrogenic lesions during valve surgery.

The sternocostal surface of the LV is slightly concave to the left, corresponding to the obtuse margin of the heart.

Above and to the left, the LV is related to the left pleura, the left lung (lingula), the left phrenic nerve, and left pericardiophrenic vessels. The LA is also situated above the LV. Medial to the LV is the interventricular septum, while the diaphragm (tendinous part) lies beneath. The anterior and posterior interventricular grooves separate the two ventricles on the surface of the heart. The anterior groove (*sulcus*) contains the left anterior descending artery and the great cardiac vein, while the posterior groove contains the posterior descending artery and the middle cardiac vein. The left (obtuse) margin of the heart is marked by the marginal branch of the circumflex artery. The left coronary groove, containing the circumflex artery and the great cardiac vein, marks the separation between the LV and LA on the surface of the heart.

Described as a conical structure, the LV presents two walls:

- Lateral: free wall facing toward the left lung; extends through the apex slightly forward and downward.
- Medial: corresponds to the interventricular septum.

These walls present a few *trabeculae carneae*, particularly in their anterior half.

Theoretically, to facilitate description, two blunt borders can be distinguished: one anterosuperior and the other posteroinferior, which separate the two surfaces of the left ventricle. In practice, these borders are nearly indistinguishable on the heart.

The apex is rounded, covered with *trabeculae carneae*, which give it a reticular appearance.

The base is occupied by the left atrioventricular orifice at the bottom and to the left, and the aortic orifice at the top and to the right.

The LV cavity is divided by the anterior leaflet of the mitral valve into an inflow tract and an outflow tract. The inflow tract has irregular walls and lies inferiorly and to the left of the anterior leaflet, while the outflow tract is shorter and narrower compared to the pulmonary infundibulum and is directed toward the right and upward.

The smooth part of the outflow tract, adjacent to the aortic valve, represents the aortic vestibule.

The LV presents two papillary muscles: anterolateral and posteromedial. The anterolateral papillary muscle is larger and often multigastric, originating from the sternocostal myocardium.

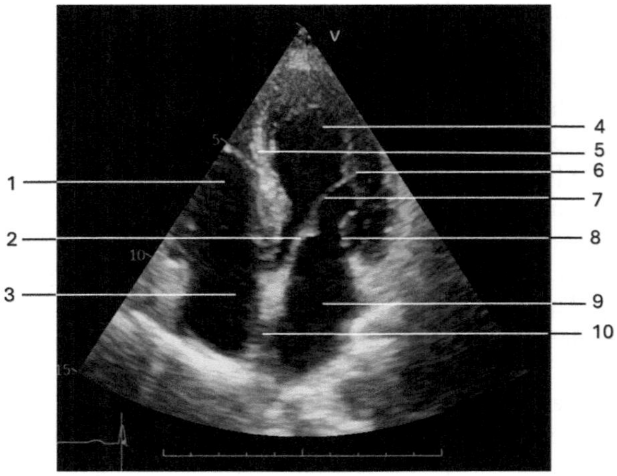

Fig. 2.5 Left ventricle and the mitral valve: 1—right ventricle; 2—anterior mitral leaflet; 3—right atrium; 4—left ventricle; 5—interventricular septum; 6—posteromedial papillary m.; 7—*chordae tendinae*; 8—posterior mitral leaflet; 9—left atrium; 10—interatrial septum. (Ultrasound image, collection of the Institute of Cardiovascular Diseases)

The left ventricle is rarely approached surgically, except in cases of coronary heart disease complications (aneurysm) or the implantation of a left ventricular assist device. An incision is performed at the center of the pathological area in the case of an aneurysm, or near the apex for the implantation of a drainage cannula for ventricular assistance.

The Mitral Valve

Like the tricuspid valve, the mitral valve apparatus consists of the annulus, valve leaflets, papillary muscles, and tendinous chords (Fig. 2.5).

The valve inserts along the entire circumference of the mitral annulus. The free edge of the mitral valve has several indentations, two of which are constant: the anterolateral (or anterior) and posteromedial (or posterior) commissures. These commissures divide the valve into an anterior (septal, large) leaflet and a posterior (mural, small) leaflet. The mitral annulus is a junction zone that provides attachment to the left atrial and ventricular muscle fibers and the mitral valve. It is a flexible structure anchored to the right and left fibrous trigones. The right fibrous trigone is located at the center of the heart and represents the confluence of fibrous tissue from the mitral and tricuspid valves, the membranous septum, and the posterior aspect of the aortic root. The left fibrous trigone is formed by the confluence of fibrous tissue from the left edges of the aortic and mitral valves.

The left atrioventricular orifice is an oval aperture, narrower than the right (allowing the insertion of only two fingers) and measuring 2.7–3.5 cm in diameter.

The mitral orifice is oriented at approximately 45° in the sagittal plane, coplanar but posterosuperior to the tricuspid orifice, posteroinferior, and to the left of the aortic orifice [8].

The ventricular surface is oriented anterolaterally, to the left, and inferiorly toward the left ventricular apex.

The Mitral Annulus

The mitral annulus is a fibrous structure composed of connective tissue, part of the fibrous skeleton of the heart. It is a D-shaped saddle-like structure, with its anterior and posterior points directed toward the LA and the medial and lateral points toward the LV. The anteromedial part of the mitral annulus, forming the straight edge of the "D", shares a common wall (the aortomitral curtain) with the aortic annulus at the attachment of the noncoronary and left coronary cusps. These fibrous attachments make this part more rigid than the posterior annulus, accounting for a greater circumferential length and propensity toward dilation. Annular dilations observed in organic or functional mitral regurgitation develop at the expense of the posterior part of the annulus. The mitral annulus is a dynamic structure throughout the cardiac cycle, influenced by LA and LV contraction and filling [8].

Subendocardial conical fibrous tendons partially surround the atrioventricular junction orifice.

The myocardium is primarily oriented perpendicular to the annulus. However, some LA myocardial fibers are parallel to the mitral annulus and are thought to have intrinsic contractility, thus playing a role in annular movements. Some authors describe the mitral annulus as a fibromuscular ring due to these fibers [8].

Mitral Valve Leaflets

The mitral valve is described as a continuous veil attached circumferentially to the mitral annulus. The free edge has two cleavages, the anterolateral and posteromedial commissures, that divide it into anterior and posterior leaflets. Histologically, mitral leaflets present four layers: peripherally disposed *atrialis* and *ventricularis layers*—thinner, contain elastic fibers; *fibrosa*—contains thick collagen fibers and is responsible for tensile strength; and *spongiosa*—loose connective tissue containing mainly glycosaminoglycans and proteoglycans, responsible for valve flexibility and shock absorbance [8].

The aortic (anterior, anteromedial) leaflet: large, semicircular, or triangular, attaches to approximately two-fifths of the annulus and usually is nonscalloped or presents superficial indentations. The *fibrosa* layer extends toward the aortomitral curtain between the right and left fibrous trigones. The leaflet has a clear and a rough zone separated by a ridge on the atrial surface, while an additional basal zone only exists for the posterior leaflet. *Chordae tendinae* typically split into three cords before inserting on the ventricular aspect of the rough zone. During diastole, the rough zones of the two leaflets are adjacent to one another. From the rough zone to the valvular annulus, a clear zone is described, devoid of tendinous chord insertions. The fibrosa contains extensions of the *chordae tendinae* inserted at the rough zone. Surgeons divide the anterior leaflet into 3 regions, A1, A2, and A3, that oppose the scallops of the posterior leaflet. During passive ventricular filling and atrial systole, the smooth atrial surface continuously directs blood flow toward the apex of the LV. After the onset of ventricular systole and mitral closure, the ventricular part of the clear zone transforms into a smooth surface of the subaortic intervalvular septum, limiting the subvalvular aortic vestibule and defining the boundaries of the terminal part of the LV outflow tract.

The mural (posterior, posterolateral) leaflet attaches to three-fifths of the annulus and is divided by two clefts into 3 scallops numbered from anterolateral to posteromedial: P1, P2, and P3. Like the anterior leaflet, the posterior leaflet presents a rough and a clear zone separated by a ridge, together with an additional basal zone, 2–3 mm thick in the middle scallop (P2), vascularized and receiving a few basal *chordae tendinae* extending from the adjacent ventricular wall. While open, the leaflets are parallel to the ventricular wall. When closed, they protrude into the atrium, but do not prolapse. The apposition line between the leaflets is limited by the previously described ridge between the rough and the clear zone.

A subendocardial nerve plexus was identified on the atrial aspect of the mitral leaflets. Afferent nerve endings are sensitive to local pressure and changes in leaflet tension, suggesting a neural basis for interactions between the mitral valve and the central nervous system [9].

Chordae tendinae

Part of the subvalvular apparatus, *chordae tendinae* are fibrous strings extending from the papillary muscles or ventricular walls to the mitral leaflets or commissures [9].

Morphologically, two types of *chordae tendinae* are described [8]:

- *False chordae tendinae* are fibromuscular bundles that may interconnect the papillary muscles or two points of the ventricular wall without attaching to the mitral valve.
- *True chordae tendinae* can be classified according to their leaflet attachment into commissural, rough, and basal. *Chordae tendinae* attached to the rough zone can be further divided into primary (attached to the free edge) and secondary (attached to the ventricular aspect of the leaflet). Primary chordae are thinner and composed mainly of collagen, while secondary chordae are thicker and more extensible.

Chordae tendinae attaching to commissural regions have a particular morphology: after a common trunk, they branch and spread like a fan to insert on the free edge of the commissural regions. Some fibers of these chordae continue to the base of the posterior mitral leaflet. One commissural chorda is destined to the anterior (anterolateral) commissure, the other to the posterior (posteromedial) commissure. The boundaries of a commissural region are defined by the extent of insertion of the branches arising from the commissural *chordae tendinae*. The branches of the posterior commissural chordae are longer, thicker, and have a wider insertion than their anterior counterpart.

The chordae for the anterior leaflet attach exclusively to the rough zone. Two primary chordae originating from the anterior and posterior papillary muscles stand out due to their thickness and length. These chordae insert on the ventricular surface of the anterior leaflet near the closure line (at 4–5 o'clock position on the posterior side and 7–8 o'clock on the anterior side). They rarely divide before inserting into the leaflet. Primary chords are present in over 90% of cases. Other rough zone chords split shortly after their origin from the papillary muscle into three branches: one branch attaches to the free edge of the leaflet; another branch attaches near the closure line, and an intermediate branch attaches between the previous two.

Ruptures of the anterior leaflet chordae are severe, especially of the primary ones. In cases of elongation, surgical shortening mainly concerns the primary chordae.

Chordae tendinae for the posterior leaflet are of three types:

- *Cleft chordae*, specific to the posterior leaflet, give rise to radial branches that fan out and attach on the sides of a cleft.
- *Basal chordae,* also specific to the posterior leaflet, arise either as a single trunk directly from the left ventricular wall or a trabecula fanning out just before attaching to the basal zone. This type is found in approximately two-thirds of cases.
- *Rough zone chordae* are similar to their anterior leaflet counterparts, though generally shorter and thinner. The posterior leaflet does not receive primary chordae.

Chordae for the anterior commissure and the adjacent halves of the anterior and posterior leaflets arise from the anterior papillary muscle. Chordae for the posterior commissure and the adjacent halves of the anterior and posterior leaflets arise from the posterior papillary muscle. On average, 25 chordae attach to the mitral valve with no significant variation based on sex.

Papillary Muscles

There are two papillary muscles in the left ventricle: the anterolateral (or anterior) and posteromedial (or posterior) papillary muscle. Each muscle provides chordae to the corresponding halves of both leaflets. They originate at the junction of the middle and apical thirds of the left ventricular wall. Often, the anterior papillary muscle consists of a single head while the posterior is formed by two or sometimes even three. The apex of the papillary muscles usually marks the respective commissures.

Morphological studies, both cadaveric and medical imaging-based, have identified up to ten types of papillary muscles. Their forms vary widely, from broad-based muscles scarcely protruding from the ventricular myocardium to free-standing, conical "glove finger" muscles or small projections giving rise to long *chordae tendineae* [10].

Generally, papillary muscles are parallel to the long axis of the LV cavity, this geometry being altered in case of LV dilatation.

The anterior papillary muscle is supplied either by the left anterior descending artery via a diagonal branch or a marginal branch of the circumflex artery.

The posterior papillary muscle is supplied either from the circumflex or the right coronary artery, depending on the coronary dominance, being thus more vulnerable to ischemia in case of coronary artery disease.

The Aortic Valve

The aortic valve is situated at the ventriculo-aortic junction, the convergence of the left ventricle and aorta. Unlike the mitral valve, there is no true annulus, but a virtual annulus marking the junction and joining the nadirs of aortic cusps. This virtual ring is of marked importance for prosthetic valve sizing and positioning (Fig. 2.6).

The aortic valve is part of the aortic root, the "centerpiece" of the heart. This centerpiece comprises 6 different structures: aortic valve cusps (leaflets) and their attachments, the sinuses of Valsalva, the interleaflet trigones, the sinotubular junction, and the virtual annulus [11]. The aortic valve is in the superior wall of the LV, to the right of the mitral valve, and posterior to the pulmonary valve.

The aortic virtual annulus is ovoidal in shape and oriented cranially, to the right, and front. The circumference of the annulus is 6.5–7 cm, the diameter ranges between 2 and 2.3 cm, while the occlusion surface area of the valve is ~3.5 cm^2 [3].

The ventriculo-aortic junction is surrounded by three semicircular collagenous condensations, the attachments of aortic cusps to the aortic wall. These semicircular condensations form a crown-shaped fibrous structure sometimes termed the *annulus*, although this name is rather incorrect, as the word *annulus* describes a circular structure. The crown-like structure divides the aortic root into sub- and supravalvular regions. Beneath each commissure lies an interleaflet trigone, an extension of the LV outflow tract. The trigone between the right and non-coronary cusps continues the membranous part of the interventricular septum (*pars membranaceea septi*) and faces the RV. Part of His bundle is contained by this septum and can be injured during aortic valve surgery. The trigone between the left and con-coronary cusps continues with the aorto-mitral curtain and the anterior mitral leaflet [12].

Like the pulmonary valve, the aortic valve consists of three cusps (leaflets), right, left, and posterior (non-coronary). The right and left cusps face the pulmonary valve. Each cusp consists of endocardial folds with a thickened central fibrous

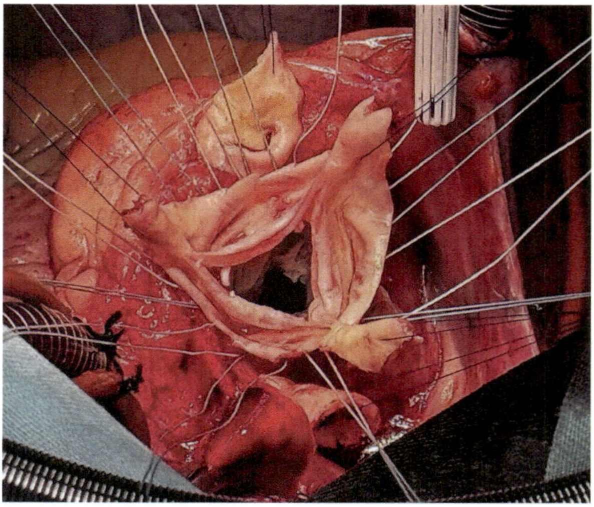

Fig. 2.6 The heart: intraoperative aspect: surgical exposure of the aortic valve for Tirone David intervention. (Cardiac surgery image, collection of the Institute of Cardiovascular Diseases, Iasi, Romania)

lamina. The cusps attach to the wall of the aortic root in a semilunar fashion, with the nadir marking the virtual annulus and the zenith at the level of the sinotubular junction. Each cusp comprises a basal part (the semicircular attachment), a belly, and a thicker free margin presenting the apposition zone termed *lunulae*. Each *lunulae* contains a central nodular thickening, the nodule of Arantius. The surface of the valve facing the ventricle is smoother compared to the surface facing the aorta. The lack of cusp apposition is the substrate of valve regurgitation and can be caused by root enlargement without intrinsic valve alterations. Surgical repair is possible in case of aortic valve regurgitation by correcting the geometry of the aortic root without replacing the valve.

The aortic root wall contains three pear-like dilatations corresponding to the three cusps, named the sinuses of Valsalva. In cross-section, the aortic root appears clover-shaped due to the sinuses. The left and the right sinuses give rise to the coronary arteries and contain at their base an extension of the ventricular myocardium, while the non-coronary sinus wall is completely arterial. In 40% of cases, the right conus artery originates independently from the right coronary sinus.

The non-coronary sinus, facing the fibrous skeleton and mitral annulus, is located cranially to the membranous part of the interventricular septum and the entry site of the left bundle branch.

The three sinuses are not symmetrical, the left coronary sinus being the smallest, while the non-coronary sinus is the tallest and the largest of the three and most prone to aneurysmal dilatation.

The upper limit of each sinus extends beyond the height of the cusps, forming a complete circumferential supravalvular ridge, the sinotubular junction. The asymmetry of the three sinuses tilts the sinotubular junction 5.5-11° relative to the virtual annulus. The understanding of aortic root morphology is crucial for treating ascending aorta aneurysms as recreation of sinus-like spaces ensures a physiologic blood flow and an adequate coronary artery perfusion during diastole [12].

The trileaflet design of the aortic valve is hemodynamically optimal because it minimizes resistance during opening and perfectly seals the orifice during closure. The free edge length equals twice the aortic annulus radius when closed and covers one-third of the circumference (approximately 2 × radius) when open. With 2 cusps, the free edge must stretch from 2 × radius when closed to 3 × radius when open. With 4 cusps, the free edge would be too long relative to the vessel circumference.

Heart Structure

The heart is a primarily muscular organ contained in the pericardial sac and lined internally by the endocardium, which continues with the vascular endothelium. The cardiac surface is covered by the visceral layer of the serous pericardium (epicardium).

The serous pericardium's reflections around the great vessels form the oblique and transverse pericardial sinuses or cul-de-sacs. The oblique sinus is formed by the pericardial reflections surrounding the *venae cavae* and the pulmonary veins behind

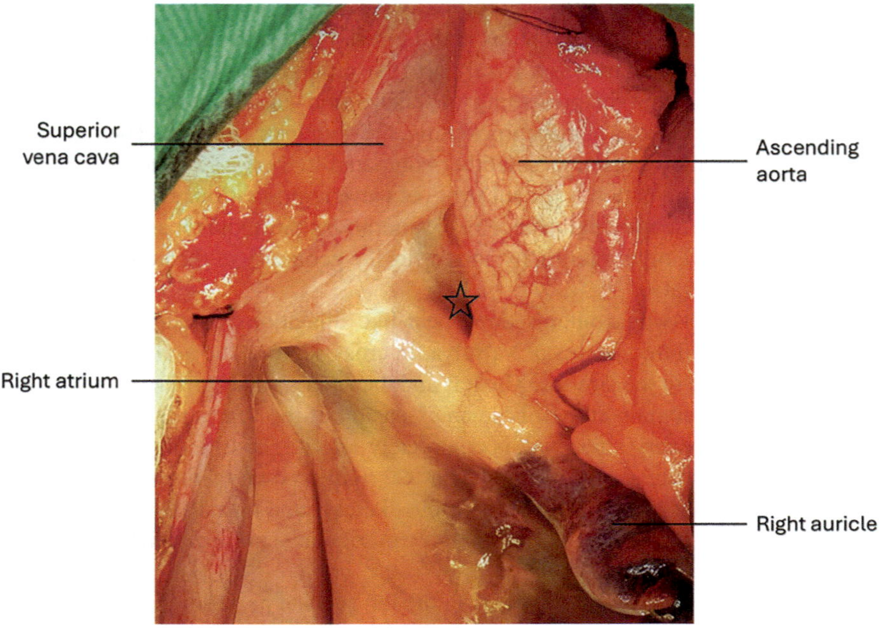

Fig. 2.7 The heart: intraoperative aspect: the right opening of the transverse pericardial sinus. (Cardiac surgery image, collection of the Institute of Cardiovascular Diseases, Iasi, Romania)

the left atrium while the transverse sinus, "L" shaped, separates the serous sheaths of the arterial and venous pedicles of the heart from one another. The floor of the transverse sinus is represented by the angle between the atria and great arteries, the posterior wall by the LA while the roof is formed by the right pulmonary artery. The transverse sinus can be accessed by a right and a left opening, the right opening being limited by the superior vena cava, ascending aorta, and RA while the left opening is limited by the pulmonary trunk, left auricle, and left pulmonary artery (Fig. 2.7). The transverse sinus is used in cardiac surgery for clamping the aorta or pulmonary artery.

This muscular mass, or myocardium, consists of atrial and ventricular fibers that attach to a framework of fibrous tissue.

The Fibrous Skeleton of the Heart

The fibrous tissue of the heart is concentrated at the atrioventricular septum and around the mitral, tricuspid, aortic, and pulmonary valves, forming the fibrous skeleton that anchors the valves. It serves both as the origin and insertion sites for the atrial and ventricular myocardium, provides mechanical stability to the heart, and insulates the atrial from ventricular chambers, thus being essential for normal conduction through the atrioventricular bundle.

The fibrous skeleton of the heart is organized around the centrally located aortic root and comprises of the right and left fibrous trigones, the interleaflet trigones of the aortic root, the interventricular membranous septum, the aorto-mitral curtain, the valvular annuli, the tendon of Todaro, and the conus ligament.

The four valvular orifices are not in the same plane: in an apical-to-basal direction, the tricuspid valve is the most apical, followed by the mitral, aortic, and pulmonary valve. In an anterior-to-posterior direction, the pulmonary valve is the most anterior, and the mitral valve is the most posterior. The aortic and pulmonary valves are angled at 90° to each other, while the mitral and tricuspid valves are saddle-shaped [13].

The right and left fibrous trigones reinforce the aorto-mitral curtain: the right fibrous trigone is the junction point of the aortic, tricuspid, and mitral valve annuli, while the left fibrous trigone lies between the aortic valve and the anterior mitral leaflet. The right fibrous trigone, together with the interventricular membranous septum and the tendon of Todaro represents the central fibrous body. The trigones are used for anchoring sutures during mitral annuloplasty.

The aortic and pulmonary valve annuli are connected by the conus ligament. Fibroelastic tissue from the right and left trigones contributes to forming the mitral and tricuspid annuli. A narrow collagenous band extends anteriorly from the trigones to the aortic and pulmonary annuli.

The membranous interventricular septum represents an inferior extension of the central fibrous body, attaches to the muscular interventricular septum, and provides insertion for the right and posterior aortic semilunar cusps.

The tendon of Todaro, a fibrous extension of the membranous septum, connects to the Eustachian valve of the inferior vena cava.

The atrioventricular (AV) bundle (of His) penetrates the central fibrous body, dividing into left and right bundle branches either at the apex of the muscular septum or near the right and posterior aortic cusps. This non-conductive fibrous tissue separates the atrial and ventricular myocardium. The AV node delays the impulse before it reaches the bundle of His. Accessory pathways (Kent bundle) can bypass the AV node, leading to pre-excitation (Wolff-Parkinson-White syndrome).

Heart Blood Supply

Arterial Blood Supply

The heart is primarily supplied by the left and right coronary arteries, which arise from the ascending aorta just above the respective semilunar valves. Their main trunks run along the coronary (atrioventricular) grooves, forming a crown-like structure around the base of the heart. From this "crown", two arterial loops branch off:

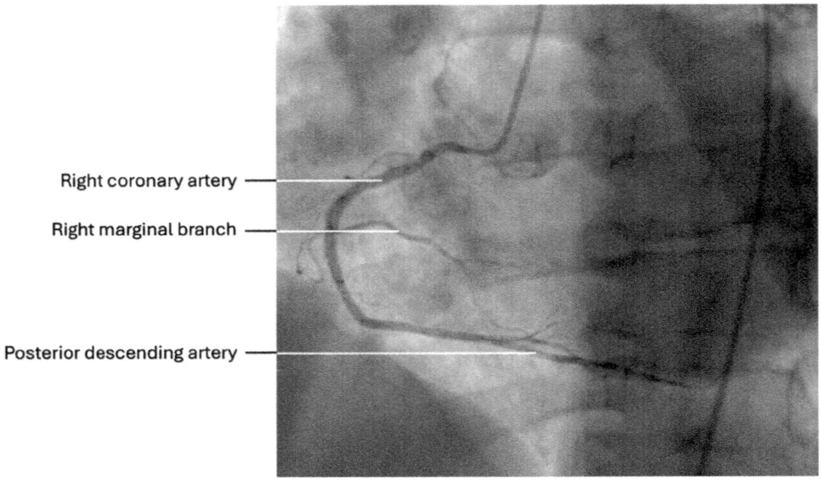

Fig. 2.8 The right coronary artery. (Coronary angiography image, collection of the Institute of Cardiovascular Diseases, Iasi, Romania)

- An anterior-inferior loop following the anterior and inferior interventricular grooves.
- A posterosuperior loop, less prominent and variable, situated in the interatrial grooves.
- Smaller arterial branches emerge from these loops to supply different regions of the heart.

The Right Coronary Artery

The right coronary artery (RCA) arises from the right coronary sinus, 4–5 mm in diameter, C-shaped, courses in the right coronary groove, and is divided into three segments [3]:

- Proximal segment: short (15–25 mm), directed anteriorly and slightly upward, from the aorta to the right coronary groove, between the right atrial appendage and the pulmonary trunk.
- Middle segment: runs vertically in the right coronary groove, curving around the right heart border.
- Distal segment: follows the inferior right coronary groove toward the *crux cordis* (Fig. 2.8).

The branches of the coronary arteries are detailed in Table 2.1.

In case of coronary artery bypass grafting (CABG), the right coronary artery is typically accessed in its third segment and can be directly grafted using arterial or venous grafts.

Table 2.1 Branches of the coronary arteries

Right coronary artery	Left coronary artery
Collateral:	*Terminal:*
Conal branch	Anterior interventricular (descending) artery
Sinuatrial nodal branch	Conal branch
Atrial branches	Short right ventricular branch(es)
Anterior ventricular branches	Diagonal branch(es)
Right marginal (acute) artery (ies)	Septal branch(es)
Retroventricular branch (es)	Circumflex artery
Terminal:	Atrial branches
Posterior interventricular (descending) artery	Left marginal (obtuse) artery (ies)
Atrioventricular node branch	Posterolateral branch (es)
Septal branches	

The Left Coronary Artery

The left coronary artery (LCA) arises from the left coronary sinus and comprises a short left main (LM) trunk (5 mm diameter, up to 25 mm long) that courses behind the pulmonary trunk before dividing into its terminal branches (Fig. 2.9, Table 2.1).

The left anterior descending (LAD) artery courses in the anterior interventricular groove, wrapping around the apex. It is accompanied by the great cardiac vein (GCV) on its left flank; the right tributaries of the GCV may cross over the artery, complicating surgical access. The distal two-thirds of LAD are superficial and easily accessible for CABG beneath the epicardium. The first septal branch (often the largest) may supply the AV bundle and the right bundle branch. The second septal branch travels in the septomarginal trabecula to the anterior papillary muscle. The first diagonal branch is usually the largest and may originate as a third terminal branch of the LCA named ramus intermedius (RI).

The circumflex (Cx) artery mirrors the RCA, courses in the left coronary groove, curving around the left heart border, closely related to the left auricle, great cardiac vein, mitral annulus, and coronary sinus.

The "*triangle of Brocq and Mouchet*" traditionally termed "*avascular*" is limited between the LAD, circumflex artery, and great cardiac vein [5].

Practically no cardiac region receives a uniform, well-defined arterial supply; however, there are preferential zones for each coronary system where the arteries exhibit typical features. The branches supplying the right heart chambers are slender, superficial, and quickly taper off. In contrast, the branches supplying the left ventricle, regardless of their origin, are larger and give off collateral vessels that penetrate deep into the myocardial thickness, branching extensively in a fine, rich arborization that reaches the endocardium. When examining the distribution of arteries on the heart's surface, a balance is observed between the development of the left and right coronary systems.

Three possible vascular patterns can be identified:

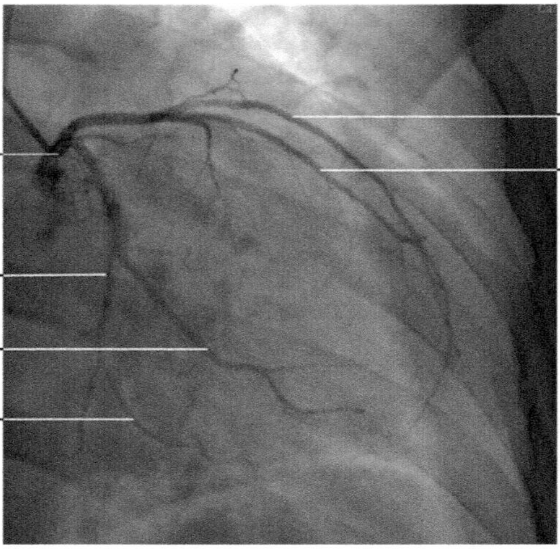

Fig. 2.9 The left coronary artery. (Coronary angiography image, collection of the Institute of Cardiovascular Diseases, Iasi, Romania)

- Right-dominant coronary system (70%): the PDA and posterolateral ventricular branch originate from the RCA that supplies part or all of the heart's inferior surface, in the latter case becoming the exclusive vascular source;
- Left-dominant coronary system (20%): Cx supplies part—or even all—of the inferior surface of the left ventricle, becoming exclusive and potentially providing the PDA;
- Balanced, co-dominant, coronary arteries (10%): both arteries supply the inferior surface of the heart, the PDA emerging from the RCA.

Based on the most common arterial distribution patterns, an average boundary between the two vascular territories can be defined. At the atrial level, this boundary runs to the left of the interatrial septum. Thus, the right coronary artery supplies not only the right atrium but also the interatrial septum and part of the left atrium.

At the ventricular level, on the anterior surface of the heart, the dividing line between the two territories starts at the midpoint of the pulmonary infundibulum, running parallel to the anterior interventricular groove about 1 cm to its right. It then curves around the right border of the heart to reach the inferior surface, where it meets the middle portion of the left inferior coronary groove.

The interventricular septum has a dual blood supply from both the left and right coronary systems. The apical third of the septum is entirely vascularized by the left coronary artery. In the basal two-thirds, LCA supplies the cranial two-thirds (via anterior septal arteries), while RCA supplies the basal third (via inferior septal arteries).

Coronary dominance is thus determined by which artery gives rise to the PDA. The LAD and PDA form the inferior-anterior arterial loop, critical for compensating occlusions. In case of the cardiac conduction system, the SA node artery most often originates from the RCA (67%), sometimes from the LCA (26%), and exceptionally from both (7%). The SA node artery terminates by branching within the sinoatrial node, passing either anterior or posterior to the SVC. The AV node is supplied by the RCA in 85% of cases through an inferior septal artery, which initially runs superiorly and posteriorly, approaching the atrioventricular node from its right side, bends at a right angle beneath the aortic valve, and then extends anteriorly, branching within the AV node. In 15% of cases, the AV node is supplied by the LCA. The AV bundle and its branches usually receive their arterial blood supply from an anterior septal artery. The vascularization of the cardiac conduction system explains the conduction disturbances observed during certain myocardial infarctions [5].

A segmental anatomy of the coronary arteries has been developed by the American Heart Association (AHA) and is widely used to characterize coronary lesions. According to this classification, the coronary arteries can be divided into 15 segments, with an additional 3 segments according to coronary variants [14]:

1. RCA:
   - Proximal segment (1).
   - segments according to coronary Middle segment (2).
   - segments according to coronary Distal segment (3).
   - FPDA (4).
2. LM (5):
   - LAD:
     - Proximal segment (6).
     - Middle segment (7).
     - Apical segment (8).
     - First diagonal branch (D1) (9).
     - Second diagonal branch (D2) (10).
   - Circumflex artery (Cx):
     - Proximal segment (11).
     - Obtuse marginal branch (OM) (12).
     - Distal segment (13).
     - Posterolateral branch (PL) (14).
     - Posterior descending artery (PDA) (15).
   - Additional segments:
     - Posterolateral branch of the RCA (RPL) (16).
     - RI (17).
     - Posterolateral branch (LPL) of the circumflex artery (18).

Based on the coronary vascularization, the Cardiac Imaging Committee of the Council on Clinical Cardiology of the American Heart Association divided the LV into 17 segments that can be used for describing kinetic anomalies: 6 basal, 6 mid, and 5 apical [15].

Venous Blood Supply

Venous blood supply typically consists of three systems: the coronary venous system, the small cardiac veins (veins of Galen), and the smallest cardiac veins (veins of Thebesius).

Coronary Venous System

A system primarily including the coronary sinus, which drains into the RA, it is 3–5.5 cm long (dependent on the site of the drainage of the posterolateral vein) and 5–15 mm wide, with an ampullary shape, located in the right portion of the inferior left coronary groove. It also represents the terminal segment of the left SVC, whose proximal part atrophies during embryological development and becomes the oblique vein of the left atrium (vein of Marshall). At the ostium of the coronary sinus lies a crescent-shaped valve, the Thebesian valve. An additional valve, the valve of Vieussens, usually marks the end of the GCV and the beginning of the coronary sinus.

The coronary sinus drains to the RA nearly all the venous blood from the heart and receives [16]:

- The great cardiac vein (GCV) originating at the apex of the heart; this structure ascends in the anterior interventricular groove (usually to the left of the LAD), makes a right-angle turn to enter the left coronary groove, and then continues as the coronary sinus.
- The middle cardiac vein (MCV) which runs in the inferior interventricular groove, near the PDA.
- The small cardiac vein (SCV) which runs in the inferior right coronary groove, near the RCA.
- One or several lateral and inferior veins.
- The oblique vein of the atrium.

Of particular interest for electrophysiology is the coronary sinus (route for mapping and ablation of left accessory pathways) and the posterolateral vein of the LV (usually draining to the GCV, or directly to the coronary sinus and a potential target for placing a left ventricular lead).

Small cardiac veins (Veins of Galen) are primarily anterior right ventricular veins that drain directly into the right atrium, passing either below or (more commonly) above the RCA. The most important of these is the vein of Galen.

Smallest Cardiac Veins (Veins of Thebesius) are tiny veins in the cardiac walls that drain directly into the heart chambers, predominantly the right-sided cavities but occasionally the left as well [3].

Lymphatic Vasculature

Cardiac lymphatic capillaries are organized into a subendocardial and mid-myocardial network that drains to subepicardial lymphatic vessels and then to collectors accompanying the coronary arteries and coronary sinus toward the base of the heart to reach the tracheobronchial lymph nodes.

Nerve Supply of the Heart

Cardiac activity is regulated by both extrinsic innervation and the intrinsic autoregulated heart conduction system.

Extrinsic innervation originates from the cardiac plexuses, formed by branches of the right and left vagus nerve (parasympathetic) and the sympathetic trunk. From the cervical sympathetic ganglions originate 3 cardiac nerves (superior, middle, and inferior) which contain postganglionic fibers derived from T1-T4 (T5) thoracic ganglions and supply the cardiac plexuses.

The vagus nerve (cranial nerve X) provides preganglionic parasympathetic collateral cardiac branches, divided into three groups [17]:

- Upper cardiac nerves arise just below the inferior ganglion; they follow the vagus in the neck and join the superficial cardiac plexus.
- Middle cardiac nerves originate from the recurrent laryngeal nerves, cross behind the brachiocephalic trunk, and join the deep cardiac plexus.
- Lower cardiac nerves are direct branches that originate from the vagal trunks; they connect to the superficial and deep cardiac plexuses.
- Sympathetic postganglionic and parasympathetic preganglionic fibers converge into two cardiac plexuses:
- The superficial cardiac plexus located between the aortic arch and the division of the pulmonary trunk, is formed by the left superior sympathetic cardiac nerve and the lower cardiac parasympathetic nerve. The Wrisberg parasympathetic ganglion is associated with the superficial cardiac plexus and is located adjacent to *ligamentum arteriosum*.
- Deep cardiac plexus, located anterior to the tracheal bifurcation, is formed by cervical sympathetic cardiac nerves and the cardiac branches of the vagus and recurrent laryngeal nerves.

From the superficial and deep cardiac plexuses detach direct atrial branches and small coronary plexuses (right and left), surrounding the coronary arteries. Anastomoses between these small plexuses form the subepicardial plexus, while finer branches from the coronary plexuses contribute to the subendocardial plexus. The sympathetic nervous system increases cardiac activity (positive chronotropy, inotropy, lusitropy, and dromotropy) while the parasympathetic nervous system decreases it.

The cardiac conduction system is a network of specialized cardiac muscle cells able to initiate and conduct the electrical impulses coordinating cardiac contractions. It is modulated by sympathetic and parasympathetic influences and consists of nodal structures and specialized fiber bundles.

The sinoatrial (SA) node was discovered by Keith & Flack in 1907 located in the right atrium near the superior vena cava ostium, beneath the sulcus terminalis. Its surface projection is in an area limited by 4 points:

- Superior: the SVC 2 mm above the cavoatrial junction.
- Inferior: the RA wall 4 mm below the junction.
- Right: sulcus terminalis 20 mm lateral to the junction.
- Left: sulcus terminalis 5 mm medial to the junction.

Surgeons must pay special attention to this area as the SA node is very superficial (1 mm beneath the surface) and can be easily injured. SA node dysfunction is also linked to ischemia of its nourishing artery.

The atrioventricular (AV) node was discovered by Aschoff & Tawara in 1906. It is located within the interatrial septum beneath the surface of a triangular space named Koch's triangle, and whose limits were previously described. It is adjacent to the left ventricular outflow tract, between the right coronary and non-coronary aortic cusps. Thus, it is vulnerable to infarction, fibrosis, or iatrogenic injury during aortic or mitral valve surgery.

The SA and AV nodes are interconnected by 3 internodal tracts:

- Anterior tract: curves around the SVC and descends the interatrial septum to reach the AV node.
- Middle tract: loops behind the SVC and RA to reach the interatrial septum in its middle part.
- Posterior tract: follows the crista terminalis to reach the posterior aspect of the AV node.

The AV bundle (His bundle) originates from the anteroinferior aspect of the AV node. It passes through the central fibrous body and then runs along the posteroinferior aspect of the interventricular membranous septum. It can be injured during aortic or mitral valve surgery. Within the interventricular septum, it is divided into:

- The right bundle branch (RBB): descends through the septomarginal trabecula to reach the anterior papillary muscle.
- The left bundle branch (LBB): branches like a fan under the left septal endocardium and reaches the anterior and posterior papillary muscles.
- Accessory atrioventricular pathways have been described and are associated with various forms of preexcitation syndromes:
- Kent bundle (associated with Wolff-Parkinson-White syndrome).
- Atrio-Hisian fibers (accelerated AV conduction).
- Mahaim fibers (tachycardia).

References

1. Tachdjian G, Brisset S, Courtot A-M, Schoëvaërt D, Tosca L. Chapitre 3 – Cœur et vaisseaux. In: Embryologie et Histologie Humaines. Paris: Elsevier Masson; 2016. p. 41–65.
2. Houyel L. Embryologie du cœur normal. EMC – Cardiologie. 2009;4(2):1–26. https://doi.org/10.1016/S1166-4568(09)47030-X.
3. Tinica G, Furnica C. Tratat de anatomie. Sistemul cardiovascular. Volumul I. Cordul. Iasi: Editura Universitatii Alexandru Ioan Cuza; 2022.
4. Chillon S, Blaisius D, Pasi N, Ou P, Laissy JP. Radio-anatomie sectionnelle du cœur et des vaisseaux thoraciques. EMC – Radiologie et imagerie médicale-Cardiovasculaire– Thoracique-Cervicale. 2018;36(3):1–17. https://doi.org/10.1016/S1879-8535(18)35258-9.
5. Latrémouille C, Lintz F. Anatomie du cœur. EMC – Cardiologie-Angéiologie. 2005;2(3):231–51. https://doi.org/10.1016/j.emcaa.2005.07.005.
6. Yucel E, Bertrand PB, Churchill JL, Namasivayam M. The tricuspid valve in review: anatomy, pathophysiology and echocardiographic assessment with focus on functional tricuspid regurgitation. J Thorac Dis. 2020;12(5):2945–54. https://doi.org/10.21037/jtd.2020.02.42.
7. Ritchie J, Warnock JN, Yoganathan AP. Structural characterization of the chordae tendineae in native porcine mitral valves. Ann Thorac Surg. 2005;80(1):189–97. https://doi.org/10.1016/j.athoracsur.2005.02.011.
8. Ho S. Anatomy of the mitral valve. Heart. 2002;88(Suppl 4):iv5–iv10. https://doi.org/10.1136/heart.88.suppl_4.iv5.
9. Boudoulas KD, Pitsis AA, Boudoulas H. Floppy Mitral Valve (FMV) – Mitral Valve Prolapse (MVP) – mitral valvular regurgitation and FMV/MVP syndrome. Hell J Cardiol. 2016;57(2):73–85. https://doi.org/10.1016/j.hjc.2016.03.001.
10. Xalxo N, Kaur S, Chauhan M, Sharma E, Sophia L, Agarwal S, Jain P. Papillary muscles: morphological differences and their clinical correlations. Anat Cell Biol. 2025;58(1):44–53. https://doi.org/10.5115/acb.24.210.
11. Paulis RD, Salica A. Surgical anatomy of the aortic valve and root—implications for valve repair. Ann Cardiothorac Surg. 2019;8(3):21–313. https://doi.org/10.21037/acs.2019.04.16.
12. Charitos EI, Sievers H-H. Anatomy of the aortic root: implications for valve-sparing surgery. Ann Cardiothorac Surg. 2013;2(1):53–6. https://doi.org/10.3978/j.issn.2225-319X.2012.11.18.
13. Saremi F, Sánchez-Quintana D, Mori S, Muresian H, Spicer DE, Hassani C, Anderson RH. Fibrous skeleton of the heart: anatomic overview and evaluation of pathologic conditions with CT and MR imaging. Radiographics. 2017;37(5):1330–51. https://doi.org/10.1148/rg.2017170004.
14. Leipsic J, Abbara S, Achenbach S, Cury R, Earls JP, Mancini GJ, Nieman K, Pontone G, Raff GL. SCCT guidelines for the interpretation and reporting of coronary CT angiography: a report of the society of cardiovascular computed tomography guidelines committee. J Cardiovasc Comput Tomogr. 2014;8(5):342–58. https://doi.org/10.1016/j.jcct.2014.07.003.
15. American Heart Association Writing Group on Myocardial Segmentation and Registration for Cardiac Imaging, Cerqueira MD, Weissman NJ, Dilsizian V, Jacobs AK, Kaul S, Laskey WK, Pennell DJ, Rumberger JA, Ryan T, Verani MS. Standardized myocardial segmentation and nomenclature for tomographic imaging of the heart. Circulation. 2002;105(4):539–42. https://doi.org/10.1161/hc0402.102975.
16. Habib A, Lachman N, Christensen KN, Asirvatham SJ. The anatomy of the coronary sinus venous system for the cardiac electrophysiologist. Europace. 2009;11(Supplement 5):v15–21. https://doi.org/10.1093/europace/eup270.
17. Wink J, van Delft R, Notenboom RGE, Wouters PF, DeRuiter MC, Plevier JWM, Jongbloed MRM. Human adult cardiac autonomic innervation: controversies in anatomical knowledge and relevance for cardiac neuromodulation. Auton Neurosci. 2020;227:102674. https://doi.org/10.1016/j.autneu.2020.102674.

3 Evolution of Cardiac Interventions: From Traditional Surgery to Minimally Invasive and Transcatheter Strategies

Magued Zikri

Introduction

The dynamic evolution in the management of cardiovascular pathologies has followed an accelerated path over the last decades.

Offering a less invasive and frequently faster intervention, catheter-based procedures first found their role in cases deemed not amenable to surgery.

The innovations of these techniques, whether hybrid or catheter-based, were linked to the progress of imaging modalities and material engineering, which refined and adopted novel applications at that time.

A complementary and frequently synergistic relation bourgeoned over time to offer customized solutions integrating surgery, interventional cardiology, and imaging.

The classic surgical approach via a full sternotomy and central cannulation for cardiopulmonary bypass is presently one of many other options that can be customized to different clinical scenarios by experienced surgical teams.

Partial upper sternotomy, clamshell transverse sternotomy, and limited anterolateral thoracotomy with peripheral vacuum-assisted cannulation are presently all available.

Intermittent fibrillation was largely replaced by cardioplegia delivered antegrade and/or retrograde, and with different composition and additives, inferring better myocardial preservation for longer duration.

Enhanced thoracoscopic visualization and innovative instrumentation, culminating in robotic surgery, have made limited-access surgery safe and reliable.

The recovery period to full activities following a shorter hospital stay is coupled with a better quality of life and is the main drive in favor of limited access surgery.

M. Zikri (✉)
Cardiothoracic Surgery, Cairo University, Cairo, Egypt

G. Tinică, A. Burlacu (eds.), *Surgical, Hybrid and Minimally Invasive Structural Cardiac Interventions*, https://doi.org/10.1007/978-3-032-16676-0_3

The scope of the following text is to provide a bird's-eye view of such progress as it addresses the management of ischemic heart disease, valvular pathologies, arrhythmia management, and, finally, congenital malformations in a trial to illustrate the benefits of having different modalities customized to individual clinical scenarios.

Some techniques replaced the preceding ones, while others helped to morph the ones that followed.

Some iatrogenic complications that resulted from one were found to be related to the other.

Ischemic Heart Disease

It was the serendipitous selective engagement of the coronary ostium during left heart angiography by Sones at the Cleveland Clinic that could, for the first time, identify the location and severity of stenotic lesions. A pivotal point in time that heralded the birth of precise coronary artery bypass grafting.

The pioneering collaboration of Favaloro and Sones at the same institution, initially using a reversed saphenous vein graft and later that of Green, who performed and refined the direct left internal mammary anastomosis, established surgical revascularization as a new modality for treating ischemic heart disease [1–2].[1]

Although left internal mammary implantation has set the gold standard for the long-term longevity of bypass grafting, it is the use of a reverse saphenous vein graft, an easier conduit to harvest and anastomose, that has allowed this operation to rapidly gain worldwide popularity.

As surgeons and support personnel gained familiarity with coronary surgery, adding multiple arterial conduits was demonstrated to benefit the long-term results of surgery [3].

Beating heart surgery was introduced soon after, allowing exposure through limited incisions and avoiding the systemic inflammatory response triggered by cardiopulmonary bypass.

A wide array of gadgets was subsequently developed to facilitate exposure and stabilization while maintaining distal coronary perfusion during graft anastomosis.

In Zurich, back in the early 1980s, Gruentzig introduced the concept of balloon angioplasty, which was initially tested in peripheral stenotic lesions in larger arteries.

That has rapidly evolved into lower-profile, miniaturized balloons, steerable guide wires, and later, atherectomy devices and Rotablator, to deal with heavy plaque burdens and calcified vessels.

---

[1] "In 1992 when I delivered the honorary lecture at the American Association for Thoracic Surgery meeting, I presented what I believe the principal characteristics of a prospective cardiovascular surgeon should be, and the ten commandments of a master surgeon. The principal thrust was that the person of vital importance is the patient, who should enjoy privileges and our total devotion. We must demonstrate responsibility, energy, intensity and enthusiasm for the work at hand".

The introduction of coronary stents revolutionized interventional cardiology by providing stability to the ballooned area, thereby improving vessel patency.

Initially, bare metal stents were used, followed by a myriad of current drug-eluting stents that claim better control of reparative, lumen-encroaching tissue reaction. Moreover, research on stents made of materials that can be degraded or absorbed offers an interesting concept [4].

With the readiness of cardiology teams for the around-the-clock "stent for life" concept, most emergency surgical interventions in the setting of acute MI are today seldom resorted to, except in salvage situations dealing with ventricular free wall, ventricular septal, or papillary muscle disruption.

The scope of indications for catheter-based interventions has broadened to address chronic total occlusions and acute thrombotic lesions, utilizing, respectively, retrograde coronary artery cannulation and thrombus retrieval devices.

The use of IVUS, an intravascular ultrasound imaging technique, helped better characterize the intraluminal and intramural morphology of the coronary arteries, which further enhanced guided PCI, especially in stent restenosis.

The introduction of mechanical circulation support via IABP and later on veno-venous ECMO further extended the scope of management in acute clinical post-infarction settings and patients with severe left ventricular dysfunction undergoing complex PCI [5].

With the availability of two valid modalities to treat ischemic heart patients, the heart team concept emerged to provide the best clinical practice tailored to the patient's profile, on the one hand, and the location, extent, and nature of the lesions, on the other. Consultation of the heart team is at the center of major societies' recommendations, reflecting its importance for best practice.

Combining the gold standard long-term patency of the left internal mammary artery through a minimal approach to the left anterior descending artery, hybrid procedures were advocated, with PCI offered for the other lesions.

Concluding notes by Bruce Lytle with an insight into where we stand today and where we are heading, I am quoting:

> Randomized studies have not shown an advantage for off-pump surgery. There are data supporting the use of multiple arterial grafts, and they are used in an increasing number of operations but still in a minority. A small number of surgeons practice minimally invasive surgery, but those concepts often clash with those of complete revascularization.
>
> It is important to note that these changes make the bypass operation more difficult, whereas advances in percutaneous transluminal coronary angioplasty have often made those procedures more generic [6].

Structural Heart Disease

Valve Prostheses

(A) Mechanical Prostheses:

The improvement in design and material of mechanical prostheses resulted in smaller gradients for a given annular orifice and reduced thrombogenicity.

Best suited for the younger age group due to its longevity, this category of valve requires lifelong anticoagulation and frequent monitoring of INR levels.

The concept of a ball-and-cage, initially introduced in 1967 and with a longevity of up to 40 years, was largely replaced by the tilting disc valve design, which was subsequently modified into a bi-leaflet central flow configuration.

The use of a biocompatible, highly resistant material, pyrolytic carbon, proved to be the state-of-the-art material first used for the leaflets, then for the entire casing of the valve [7].

(B) Bio prosthetic valves:

Cadaveric homografts are sterilized after retrieval and stored refrigerated at 4 °C in an antibiotic solution without tissue fixation. The limited availability of that valve and technical requirements at the time of its implantation reflected negatively on its wide application, despite its superior hemodynamics and demonstrated longevity.

Xenografts, whether porcine valves or pericardial valves, all require a process of glutaraldehyde tissue fixation to eliminate cellular immunogenicity. This comes with a price, exposing tissue to active calcification, setting the stage for Achilles tendon durability.

Zero-pressure fixation, alternatives to glutaraldehyde use, tissue decellularization, and the use of genetically modified animal valves are all being explored to reduce structural bio-prosthesis deterioration [8].

Aortic Valve Procedures

Aortic valve replacement and repair have a proven track record for addressing various aortic valve and aortic root pathologies and can also address annular reconstruction in cases of extensive calcification and/or infection.

Limited upper sternotomy or high anterior thoracotomy gives direct access to the valve in a suitable aortic root configuration. This was further aided by the use of a "sutureless" aortic valve prosthesis to expedite surgery and hence recovery.

Autologous pericardial tissue has been utilized to augment leaflet tissue to regain valve competency. The mid- to long-term result of the Osaki procedure, which involves refashioning a measured Tri-leaflet configuration, is pending.

Trans-catheter aortic valve implantation(TAVI) was initially introduced back in 2012 for critical aortic stenosis with impaired left ventricular function in advanced age with multiple comorbidities that were judged to be of extremely high surgical risk.

Given the favorable mid-term results and the less-invasive nature compared to surgical AVR, the indications were initially extended to moderate-risk patients and subsequently to low-risk surgical patients in a younger population.

An emerging trend is to offer TAVI to asymptomatic patients with a high gradient before the onset of deleterious left ventricular remodeling.

A new set of clinical scenarios emerged related to the longevity of the crimped biological valve used, and the concept of valve-in-valve came to life, with its annular size limitations and hence high gradients.

It is worth noting that surgical AVR following TAVI is a delicate operation entailing the extraction of the valve and, in some situations, the reconstruction of the aortic annulus [9].

The ongoing development of lower-profile valve delivery systems with improved longevity of leaflet tissue will further enhance their widespread use.

Mitral Valve Procedures

Echocardiography of the mitral apparatus complex enabled the proper identification of the pathology at hand and helped determine the best strategy for both surgical procedures and percutaneous interventions.

Presently, high-resolution TEE imaging and real-time three-dimensional reconstruction are valuable tools available intra-procedurally to guide interventions.

Conservation of the native mitral valve has been a priority to avoid a thrombogenic prosthesis in a frequently enlarged and possibly fibrillating left atrium.

The now near-obsolete closed mitral commissurotomy for pure rheumatic mitral stenosis was gradually replaced by balloon-based valvotomy, first introduced by Inoue in 1981, which proved highly effective in symmetrical non-calcified leaflet fusion.

Regurgitant myxomatous mitral pathologies and ruptured chordae have benefited from ring-supported repairs, as pioneered by Carpentier in Paris, France, and Cosgrove in Cleveland, Ohio.

The edge-to-edge repair advocated at surgery by Alfieri found its application in the catheter-based mitral clip for central mitral regurgitation.

It is applicable for central regurgitation of myxomatous lesions and in a dilated left ventricle with displacement of the papillary muscles.

The concept of ring support for the mitral annulus, with its documented efficacy in mitral valve repair, may be successfully applied to a coronary sinus sling currently under development.

Additionally, dealing with para prosthetic leaks proved to be amenable to precise identification and is controlled by occluders, even in the case of multiple locations [10].

Role of Echocardiography in Percutaneous

Mitral Valve Interventions

The continuum of to-and-fro concepts between the heart team members is well exemplified by the innovations mentioned above.

Cardiac Dysrhythmias

Cardiac Pacemakers

From the basic ventricular pacing-ventricular sensing pacemaker that required epicardial surgical electrode placement, the field of electrophysiology has come a long way.

Smaller pacemakers with extended battery life presently offer safety and convenience, including remote monitoring. Dual-chamber pacemakers with sensors that detect increased activity and adjust the paced rhythm accordingly are presently available.

Cardiac Resynchronization Therapy

It has been resorted to in pacing mode for advanced intraventricular conduction delays in heart failure, resulting in an increase in cardiac output, reverse remodeling, and improved myocardial efficiency [11].

Hemodynamic Effects of Long-Term Cardiac Resynchronization Therapy: Analysis by Pressure-Volume Loops

The original surgically inserted AICD got replaced by smaller versions utilizing endocardial sensing and delivery electrodes that are lifesaving in resistant ventricular dysrhythmias [12].

Accessory Pathways Ablation

This rare congenital anomaly consists of abnormal conductive tissue between the atria and ventricles that perpetuates a reentrant pathway responsible for incapacitating tachycardia.

It was initially ablated surgically using a combination of sharp dissection of the AV groove and cryolesions, after precise identification of the AP location via intraprocedural epicardial mapping. Such surgery was replaced mainly by radiofrequency catheter-based ablation, which has a high success rate.

Newer mapping methods have been recently introduced to improve the localization of the accessory pathway [13].

Atrial Fibrillation

Atrial fibrillation is a common clinical presentation of valvular and ischemic heart disease. AV nodal ablation and ventricular pacing were historically resorted to in patients with incapacitating atrial fibrillation.

The initial curative approach for resistant paroxysmal and permanent atrial fibrillation was advocated by James Cox, who developed an animal model mimicking the multiple reentrant circuits that perpetuate atrial fibrillation and hence designed an intricate set of bi-atrial lesions required to interrupt them.

The complexity of the final product, the Cox maze IV cut and saw operation, limited its permeation in training programs.

It was the introduction of energy delivery devices, first as an adjunct to transmural lesions during left heart surgery and later through percutaneous ablation using steerable catheter tips, that made the myriads of lesion sets, and more specifically pulmonary vein isolation, more readily applicable, aided by real-time three-dimensional cartography [14].

Again, advances in electrophysiology, real-time endocardial recording, and cartographic reconstruction were milestones for the applications of these techniques.

A hybrid approach, involving a thoracoscopically delivered set of epicardial lesions on the left atrial posterior wall, was used in select centers to complement endocardial catheter-based lesions.

Left Atrial Appendage Control

Being the notorious nidus for thrombus formation in atrial fibrillation, obliteration of the mouth of the left atrial appendage has been a routine step in dilated atria during left heart open surgeries.

Both a thoracoscopic left side approach of ligation at the appendage base away from the circumflex coronary artery and use of an endocardial occluder passed trans-septally to the left atrium are available in today's armamentarium, guided by the morphology of the left atrial appendage [15].

Congenital Heart Disease

The evolution of management of congenital heart diseases has demonstrated the complementary roles of catheter-based procedures in conjunction with staged or complete surgical repair.

One of the earliest interventions, back in 1966, is the Raskind Atrial septostomy in TGA, which is offered to heavily cyanotic newborns and is presently widely used globally. Additionally, it has the potential to be performed echo-guided bedside in the Neonatal ICU [16].

Pulmonary valve stenosis is a common congenital anomaly, and its management depends on the patient's age, presenting symptoms, ejection fraction, and gradient across the valve. Pulmonary balloon valvuloplasty is indicated in newborns presenting with cyanosis. The choice between catheter-based and surgical valvuloplasty is guided by the clinical presentation [17].

Additionally, at the level of the right ventricular outflow tract, one interesting application to complement the results of Tetralogy of Fallot with pulmonary valve regurgitation is transcatheter pulmonary valve implantation [18].

Patent ductus arteriosus was traditionally best treated by cutting and suturing of both ends, or by simple ligation in the neonates via a left high thoracotomy.

That being said, today the standard of care is transcatheter ductal closure using a variety of available occluders. Alternatively, in selected cases where ductal flow is vital, ductal stenting can be applied.

Ductal ligation can also be performed during the correction of other congenital anomalies before going on bypass.

Rarely does a patch repair need to be resorted to in the short and wide ductus.

In older patients with calcified ductal tissue, the safest approach is either transcatheter or transpulmonary artery during a brief period of circulatory arrest [19].

Coarctation is a genetically transmitted pathology resulting in different degrees of caliber restriction in the thoracic and/or abdominal aorta, causing resistant differential hypertension and the subsequent acceleration of coronary artery disease.

Management depends on age at presentation, with surgery preferred in the neonates and early childhood for its long-term satisfactory results. Surgical options include resection and end-to-end anastomosis, interposition graft, and reversed subclavian patch. For older individuals, a bypass graft from the left subclavian artery to the descending aorta is helpful.

When non-surgical repair is preferred, balloon dilation and/or stenting can be used, utilizing covered or uncovered stents. This is particularly useful in post-balloon aneurysmal dilation [20].

Closure of atrial and ventricular septal defects:

ASD closure best exemplifies the progress of both surgical closure and transcatheter device occluders.

From the pre-heart-lung machine era, which advocated for inverting the left atrial appendage, to inflow occlusion, to CPB patch repair, to minimally invasive thoracoscopy or robotic-enabled procedures, the entire history of cardiac surgery is recalled.

VSD closure remains primarily in the surgical domain. Neonates can be treated via a hybrid trans-ventricular staged procedure. At sternotomy, while off bypass, a wire is introduced through the RV free wall through the defect, and an occluder is delivered under echo guidance. In adults, muscular and membranous VSDs can be treated both retrogradely and later antegrade in selected cases. The incidence of heart block is significantly higher in membranous VSD. Larger occluders are available for post-infarction VSD and might be lifesaving.

The trial and error of different occlusion devices development is also fascinating.

From stainless steel hooks equipped with initial devices to Nitinol that can be repositioned and retrieved, the precision and safety of such devices have advanced to their current status, making the procedure the leading choice for all sizes and types of ASD situations [21].

Hypertrophic Cardiomyopathy

Hypertrophic cardiomyopathy is a better-understood congenital condition, with tailored management dictated by clinical presentation and utilizing pharmacological, surgical, catheter-based, and arrhythmia control tools.

Definitive treatment by myomectomy has gained worldwide popularity over time, with a steadily increasing number of procedures and relief of symptoms in up to 95% of cases.

Control of the obstructive muscle mass is also tackled by septal artery alcohol injection, with a success rate of 85% in experienced hands, and is currently performed at a steady rate, though reserved for the elderly and those with high surgical risk.

Mavacamten, a new myosin-modulating medication, when used in combination with beta blockers, is beneficial for early, mild cases with few symptoms.

Detection algorithms to identify patients at high risk for sudden cardiac death are utilized for prophylactic AICD implantation.

Onset of atrial fibrillation, a common complication with HCM, is managed by anticoagulants and other previously described interventions when AF is incapacitating.

Refractory non-obstructive systolic dysfunction culminating in heart failure might need, on rare instances, heart transplantation [22].

Concluding Remarks

The general consensus favoring minimally invasive procedures in all medical interventions will eventually lead to the development of a new specialty that encompasses both the diagnostic and therapeutic aspects of cardiovascular disease.

Real-time four-dimensional imaging will guide both catheter-based interventions and minimally invasive surgical procedures with unsurpassed accuracy.

This is already in wide practice in the interventional vascular domain of the thoracoabdominal aorta and of the visceral, peripheral, and neurovascular arterial tree.

Complex situations related to all cardiac pathologies will remain in the realm of the operating room. Forward designing of fellowship training needs to keep such factual realities in perspective.

To conclude, I would like to quote words from the 24th Louis F. Bishop Lecture by Gorlin, delivered 30 years ago. He formulated two words of caution while describing coronary angioplasty that are still valid today and can be rightfully projected on the endless new possibilities of minimally invasive procedures, whether surgical or via percutaneous interventions:

> The first one is the operator's fascination by novel techniques and hardware made available at an ever increasing frequency. That, paired with peer pressure and industry-driven marketing, should not jeopardize clinical safety and best care delivery backed by good judgment and operator training. The second one relates to financial ethics. Two procedures with similar outcomes may have either an immediate or a cumulative significant cost difference. The answer looks straightforward at the level of macroeconomics when a given budget has to be allocated to a certain pathology. It gets much more complicated both at the institution and at the operator level whereby a conflict of interest resides. This is further amplified when self-referral comes into play.

The answer to that problem is complex. Third-party payers looking at actuarial cost do have an input on that. More important is a well-informed patient that is given time to discuss the options at hand and both the immediate and longer time outcomes [23].

References

1. Favaloro RG. Critical analysis of coronary artery bypass grafting: a 30-year journey. J Am Coll Cardiol. 1998;31:1B–63B. https://doi.org/10.1016/s0735-1097(97)00559-7.
2. Green GE, Stertzer SH, Reppert EH. Coronary arterial bypass grafts. Ann Thorac Surg. 1968;5:443–50. https://doi.org/10.1016/s0003-4975(10)66377-1.
3. Lytle BW, Blackstone EH, Loop FD, Houghtaling PL, Arnold JH, Akhrass R, McCarthy PM, Cosgrove DM. Two internal thoracic artery grafts are better than one. J Thorac Cardiovasc Surg. 1999;117(5):855–72. https://doi.org/10.1016/S0022-5223(99)70365-X.
4. King S III. The development of interventional cardiology. JACC. 1998;31(4, suppl B):64B–88B. https://doi.org/10.1016/s0735-1097(97)00558-5.
5. Yang H, Luo L, Song Y, Cao J, Chen J, Zhang F, Tan Y, Zheng Y, Sun Z, Qian J, Huang Z, Ge J. ECMO versus IABP for patients with STEMI complicated by cardiogenic shock undergoing primary PCI: a Chinese National Study and propensity-matched analysis. Hellenic J Cardiol. 2024; https://doi.org/10.1016/j.hjc.2024.09.008. (in press)
6. Lytle B. Evolution of coronary surgery. Circulation. 2024;150(17):1311–2. https://doi.org/10.1161/CIRCULATIONAHA.124.070918.
7. Gott VL, Alejo DE, Cameron DE. Mechanical heart valves: 50 years of evolution. Ann Thorac Surg. 2003;2003(76):S2230–9. https://doi.org/10.1016/j.athoracsur.2003.09.002.
8. Kostyunin AE, Yuzhalin AE, Rezvova MA, Ovcharenko EA, Glushkova TV, Kutikhin AG. Degeneration of bioprosthetic heart valves: update 2020. J Am Heart Assoc. 2020;9(19) https://doi.org/10.1161/JAHA.120.018506
9. Hawkins RB, Deeb GM, Sukul D, Patel HJ, Gualano SK, Chetcuti SJ, Grossman PM, Ailawadi G, Fukuhara S. Redo surgical aortic valve replacement after prior transcatheter versus surgical aortic valve replacement. J Am Coll Cardiol Intv. 2023;16(8):942–53. https://doi.org/10.1016/j.jcin.2023.03.015.
10. Cavalcante JL, Rodriguez LL, Kapadia S, Tuzcu EM, Stewart WJ. Role of echocardiography in percutaneous mitral valve interventions. J Am Coll Cardiol Img. 2012;5(7):733–46. https://doi.org/10.1016/j.jcmg.2012.03.010.
11. Steendijk P, Tulner SA, Bax JJ, Oemrawsingh PV, Bleeker GB, van Erven L, Putter H, Verwey HF, van der Wall EE, Schalij MJ. Hemodynamic effects of long-term cardiac resynchronization therapy: analysis by pressure-volume loops. Circulation. 2006;113(10):1295–304. https://doi.org/10.1161/CIRCULATIONAHA.105.540435.
12. Lange PS, Frommeyer G, Kleemann T, Brachmann J, Lugenbiel P, Reif S, Hochadel M, Senges J, Eckardt L. Pacemaker versus defibrillator therapy in patients eligible for cardiac resynchronisation therapy: evidence from the German device registry. J Climb Med. 2025;14(4):1137. https://doi.org/10.3390/jcm14041137.
13. Sudo K, Kuroki K, Asakawa T, Nakagawa K, Asahina C, Tanaka Y, Hasegawa T, Aonuma K, Sato A. a novel wave-speed mapping method for visualizing accessory pathways in Wolff-Parkinson-white syndrome. J Cardiovasc Electrophysiol. 2025;36(2):401–10. https://doi.org/10.1111/jce.16545. Epub 2024 Dec 17
14. Khasnis A, Veerareddy S, Jongnarangsin K, Ip JH, Abela GS, Thakur RK. Evolution of curative therapies for atrial fibrillation. Indian Pacing Electrophysiol J. 2024;4(1):10–25.
15. Nasr GH, Rushworth PM, Donaldson DM. Left atrial appendage closure: therapy overview and future perspective. Cardiol Clin. 2024;42(Issue 3):389–401. https://doi.org/10.1016/j.ccl.2024.02.018.

16. Matter M, Almarsafawy H, Hafez M, Attia G, Elkhier MMA. Balloon atrial septostomy: the oldest cardiac interventional procedure in Mansoura. Egypt Heart J. 2011;63(Issue 2):125–9. https://doi.org/10.1016/j.ehj.2011.08.043.
17. Jayaram NM, Plummer ST, Makhoul M, Steele J, Reardon LC, Sachdeva R, Windom M, Statile C, Parthiban A. Clinical practice algorithm for the follow-up of repaired and unrepaired atrioventricular septal defects. Expert analysis. Am Coll Cardiol. 2025. https://www.acc.org/latest-in-cardiology/articles/2025/02/03/12/17/clinical-practice-algorithm-for-the-follow-up-of-repaired-and-unrepaired-atrioventricular-septal-defects
18. Arvind B, Ramakrishnan S. Pediatric interventional cardiology: breaking new grounds. Ann Pediatr Cardiol. 2022;15(2):109–13. https://doi.org/10.4103/apc.apc_91_22.
19. Schneider DJ, Moore JW. Patent ductus arteriosus. Circulation. 2006;114(17):1873–82. https://doi.org/10.1161/CIRCULATIONAHA.105.592063.
20. Salciccioli KB, Zachariah JP. Coarctation of the aorta: modern paradigms across the lifespan. Hypertension. 2023;80(10):1970–9. https://doi.org/10.1161/HYPERTENSIONAHA.123.19454.
21. Turner ME, Bouhout I, Petit CJ, Kalfa D. Transcatheter closure of atrial and ventricular septal defects. JACC. 2022;79(22):2247–58. https://doi.org/10.1016/j.jacc.2021.08.082.
22. Maron BJ, Rowin EJ, Maron MS. Advances in the management of hypertrophic cardiomyopathy leading to low disease-related mortality in 2023. Am J Cardiol. 2024;212(Supplement, 1):S77–82. https://doi.org/10.1016/j.amjcard.2023.10.073.
23. Gorlin R. Perspectives on invasive cardiology: the 24th Louis F. Bishop lecture. J Am Coll Cardiol. 1994;23(2):525–32. https://doi.org/10.1016/0735-1097(94)90442-1.

Classical Surgical Techniques in Cardiac Surgery

4

Alberto Bacuşcă, Andrei Ţărus, Silviu Stoleriu, Mihail Enache, and Grigore Tinică

Median Sternotomy

The first median sternotomy was performed in 1957 by Dr. Donald Effler and Dr. Lawrence Groves at the Cleveland Clinic. This approach, which involves a vertical incision along the midline from the jugular notch to the xiphoid process, stands out for its advantages in providing superior access to mediastinal structures compared to the previously used bilateral thoracotomy. As a result, median sternotomy quickly became the standard incision for open-heart surgery [1]. Although the technique was initially proposed by Herbert Milton in 1897, it was not widely adopted until the 1950s with the introduction of cardiopulmonary bypass [2, 3]. Since then, median sternotomy has become the most frequently used surgical approach in cardiac operations due to its relatively simple execution, excellent exposure, and favorable safety profile.

Although minimally invasive approaches such as mini-sternotomy or thoracotomy have become more common in selected cases in the last two decades due to aesthetic benefits and faster recovery, these approaches often do not provide the necessary exposure for complex procedures such as coronary artery bypass grafting (CABG), multiple valve replacements/repairs, and correction of congenital cardiac defects.

When performed correctly, this technique is associated with a low rate of complications, including sternal wound infections and sternal instability, and remains

A. Bacuşcă (✉) · A. Ţărus · S. Stoleriu · M. Enache
Cardiac Surgery Department, University of Medicine and Pharmacy "Grigore T. Popa", Iasi, Romania

Cardiac Surgery Department, Institute of Cardiovascular Diseases, Professor Doctor George I.M. Georgescu, Iasi, Romania

G. Tinică
Cardiovascular Surgery, Cardiovascular Diseases Institute, Iaşi & Grigore T. Popa University of Medicine and Pharmacy, Iaşi, Romania
e-mail: grigore.tinica@umfiasi.ro

G. Tinică, A. Burlacu (eds.), *Surgical, Hybrid and Minimally Invasive Structural Cardiac Interventions*, https://doi.org/10.1007/978-3-032-16676-0_4

the most versatile approach. Compared with alternative incisions such as lateral thoracotomy, median sternotomy is often associated with shorter operative times, reduced blood loss, and more efficient intraoperative access, all contributing to improved surgical outcomes [4, 5]. Moreover, widespread use has led to the development of standardized protocols and globally adopted training programs.

Description of the Sternotomy Technique

The patient is placed in the supine position. Anatomical landmarks are identified—the jugular notch, bilateral clavicle, sternum, and costosternal joints, as well as the xiphoid process. The incision typically measures between 18 and 25 cm depending on patient size and the planned procedure's complexity. After the skin incision, the subcutaneous tissue and fascia are dissected with electrocautery to expose the sternal periosteum, with adequate hemostasis performed at the same time. The interclavicular ligament is identified and incised. The xiphoid process is incised, followed by digital dissection of the retrosternal space to detach adipose tissue, sternopericardial ligaments, and to estimate the distance between the sternum and pericardium. The midline sternotomy line is marked with electrocautery. The sternum is then divided longitudinally with a sternotome, ensuring precise midline cutting and avoiding injury to mediastinal structures. Once the sternum is divided, hemostasis is performed both chemically with bone wax and thermally. A sternal retractor is introduced to gently separate the two halves, providing wide mediastinal exposure, including the heart, great vessels, thymus, and pericardium. Placement of the retractor is preferably done in the sternum segment distal to the manubrium to avoid fractures at this level.

After adequate exposure, the pericardium is typically opened vertically in a T-shaped manner and suspended to expose and gently elevate the heart. Depending on the intervention—e.g., valve repair, CABG, or heart transplant—the surgical team continues with the specific procedure.

The sternum is closed using multiple stainless-steel wires in either simple interrupted or figure of 8 configuration in order to achieve firm approximation along the midline and minimize dehiscence risk. Typically, either four figure-8 wires or eight U-shaped wires are used. Ideally, at least one U-shaped wire is placed for every 10 kg of patient body weight. In high-risk patients (osteoporosis, obesity), rigid plates may be used to improve sternal stability. The subcutaneous tissue and skin are then closed in layers, usually with absorbable sutures.

Postoperatively, patients are monitored in the intensive care unit. Early extubation, pain control, and precautions regarding sternal movement—e.g., avoiding lifting weights—are encouraged to promote healing and prevent complications. Although rare, deep sternal wound infections (mediastinitis) remain among the most serious complications of sternotomy, especially in diabetic, obese patients or those in whom both internal mammary arteries were harvested, requiring prompt diagnosis and management.

Sternal Hemostasis in Median Sternotomy

After sternum division, bone bleeding comes mainly from the vascular channels of the spongy bone. This medullary bleeding is usually diffuse and may be abundant, especially in young patients or those with increased bone vascularity.

Hemostasis is achieved through several methods. Traditionally, bone wax—a sterile mixture of beeswax and softening agents—has been applied to the cut sternal edges to produce immediate hemostasis. However, due to its non-absorbable nature and interference with bone healing, concerns have been raised about routine use [6]. One of the first major critiques came from Prof. Dr. Francis Robicsek, who in a 1976 study demonstrated that eliminating bone wax in median sternotomy procedures did not increase postoperative bleeding but might reduce the risk of deep sternal infections and osteomyelitis [7].

Other, more recent studies also support this position. In a large cohort of 5318 patients, Alhan et al. found that bone wax use was associated with a significantly increased risk of sternal dehiscence (2.5% vs. 1.4%), being an independent risk factor [8]. Consequently, many cardiac surgeons now use bone wax sparingly or avoid it entirely, preferring alternatives such as electrocautery, topical hemostatic agents, and careful mechanical closure with steel wires or rigid plates.

Redo Sternotomy

Median sternotomy is the preferred approach for patients requiring reoperation. Re-sternotomy presents specific technical challenges and increased risks compared to primary sternotomy due to dense adhesions, modified and sometimes difficult-to-identify anatomy, and the proximity of cardiac/vascular structures to the posterior sternal table.

Presence of previous cerclage wires may increase the difficulty of the approach but may also assist the surgeon by serving as landmarks and by upward traction to separate the sternum from the mediastinum.

Preoperative imaging plays a critical role; high-resolution contrast-enhanced CT is considered the gold standard for evaluating the relationship between sternum and heart, presence of adhesions, pericardial status (closed or not during the first surgery), bypass graft location, and other mediastinal structures (Table 4.1) [9]. In high-risk patients—especially those with the right ventricle or patent CABG grafts adherent to the sternum—alternative strategies such as femoral or axillary cannulation before re-entry may be used to decompress the heart and provide circulatory support in case of injury.

Intraoperatively, a cautious approach is recommended: oscillating saw with depth control, a sensitive subxiphoid digital dissection to create a safe plane, and gradual division under direct vision. The approach begins caudally, at the projection of the xiphoid process, with digital dissection followed by insertion of a medium-sized gauze between the sternum and pericardium. Old cerclage wires are grasped

Table 4.1 CT imaging in redo sternotomy: enhanced assessment [10, 11]

Assessment parameter	Clinical significance and key observations
Sternum to right ventricle distance	Measurements under 5 mm indicate substantial risk of RV injury. This risk becomes particularly pronounced in patients with prior pericardial stripping. Established anterior adhesions from previous surgery also represent a marker of risk.
Sternum to Aorta & Bypass Graft Proximity	When the distance between graft and sternum measures less than 10 mm, the likelihood of inadvertent graft injury increases significantly. It is essential to carefully identify the patent grafts, especially the left internal mammary artery grafts. Crossing the midline is essential
Sternal Bone Integrity & Hardware Status	CT scanning effectively identifies complications including sternal non-union, wire displacement or migration, and signs of chronic osteomyelitis that may complicate surgical planning.
Mediastinal Configuration & Alternative Approaches	Thorough evaluation of chest dimensions and adhesion patterns allows surgical teams to consider alternative access routes, such as right thoracotomy or minimally invasive techniques

with Kocher clamps to elevate the sternum. Sternotomy progresses cranially, with depth limited by either the wires or the gauze.

Complications include prolonged operative time, increased transfusion requirements, higher rates of sternal wound infection, postoperative bleeding, and higher mortality compared to primary procedures [10].

Sternal Closure

The conventional method uses stainless-steel wires in various configurations (simple interrupted, figure-8, or X). Choosing the correct wire size is important because large-diameter wires may create unnecessarily large holes that can become sources of bleeding, while very thin wires may cut through the sternum in severe osteoporosis or break in patients with higher body weight.

Classically, the number of wires correlates both with sternal size and with patient weight. Although effective in many cases, the method has limitations in patients with obesity, osteoporosis, or diabetes, which may compromise stability and healing. Complications include dehiscence, infection, and prolonged postoperative pain [12]. In recent years, several innovative techniques have emerged:

Polyethylene Suture Tapes

Recent studies exploring the use of high-strength polyethylene suture tapes as an alternative to steel wires have revealed significant advantages. In a retrospective study involving 300 patients randomized into two groups—150 receiving suture tape closure and 150 traditional wire closure—the suture tape group showed significantly lower rates of sternal wound infections (1% vs. 5%, $p = 0.0363$) and sternal dehiscence (0% vs. 5%, $p = 0.0297$). Closure time was also significantly shorter (11 minutes vs. 19 minutes, $p < 0.0001$) [12].

Rigid Plate Fixation Systems (RPFS)

Rigid plate fixation systems using titanium plates provide enhanced mechanical support compared to wires. In a study published by Miazza et al. on 48 high-risk patients, RPFS resulted in a low incidence of deep sternal wound infections (2.1%) and improved healing as demonstrated on CT scans. Another report described successful use of RPFS in minimally invasive cardiac surgeries, with no sternal complications and lower postoperative pain during 1-year follow-up [13].

Bioresorbable Mesh Plates

In recent years, bioresorbable mesh plates have emerged as a promising technique. A retrospective analysis of 218 patients published by Yokoyama showed that those who received a three-piece mesh plate had lower rates of sternal displacement (4% vs. 20%) and substernal hematoma (16% vs. 38%) compared to bioresorbable pins. The mesh group also had significantly less postoperative bleeding [14].

Nitinol Clip Systems

Nitinol, a shape-memory alloy of nickel and titanium, is used in the Flexigrip sternal closure system. The clip becomes pliable at lower temperatures and regains its original shape at body temperature, ensuring a constant closing force. This is particularly beneficial in obese patients (BMI >35), with improved stability and fewer complications [15].

Classical Cannulation Techniques in Structural Heart Interventions

Aortic Cannulation

The first successful heart–lung machine procedure took place on May 6, 1953, when Dr. John H. Gibbon Jr. repaired an atrial septal defect in an 18-year-old female patient at Thomas Jefferson University Hospital in Philadelphia [16]. This operation, which required 26–27 minutes of circulatory support, is considered the origin of modern open-heart surgery [17]. From that moment on, classical cannulation techniques became the cornerstone of cardiopulmonary bypass, providing reliable access to the aorta for arterial flow delivery and to the right atrium for venous return drainage. These methods have been refined to optimize flow, minimize complications, and ensure efficient perfusion. Despite minimally invasive/percutaneous alternatives, traditional cannulation remains widely used for safety, efficiency, and adaptability.

Aortic cannulation is a critical first step in initiating CPB, allowing the return of oxygenated blood from the circuit into systemic circulation. The ascending aorta is the most common site, typically 2–3 cm above the sinotubular junction along the lesser curvature. Palpation of the aorta is essential to identify areas with atheroma plaques and avoid them. After full systemic heparinization, reinforced purse-string sutures are placed with pledgets. Preferably, two such sutures are placed in a

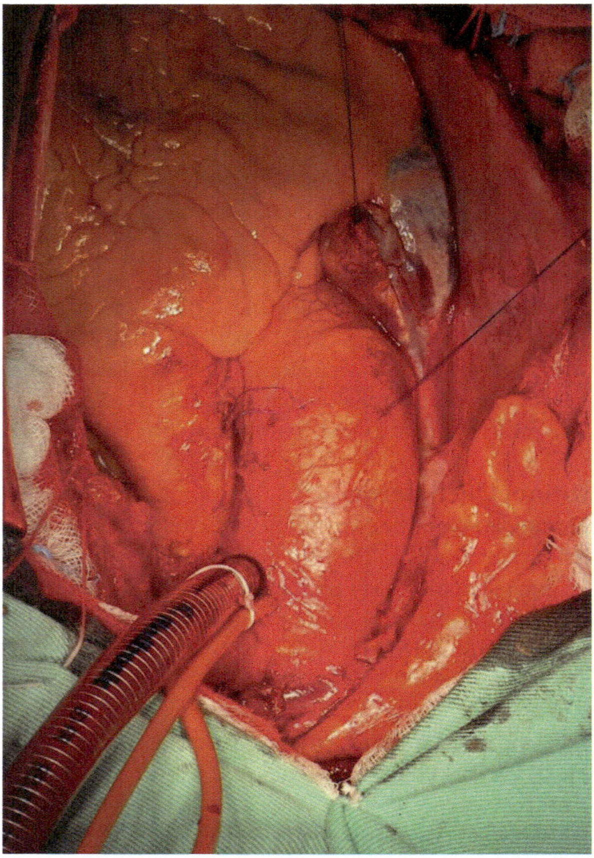

Fig. 4.1 Aortic cannulation—IBCV Iasi collection

contralateral manner that allows them to be tightened simultaneously by both operators. The anesthesiologist is informed of the need to lower the arterial pressure to optimal values below 90–100 mmHg. The 3–0/4–0 Prolene sutures are passed in such a way that they penetrate deeply enough into the aortic wall up to the level of the media, but without producing a transfixing penetration of the wall, in which case a subadventitial hematoma will form in most situations, requiring rapid drainage through adventitial incision.

After circulating and deairing the PVC tubing of the cardiopulmonary bypass circuit, a small incision is made in the center of the purse-strings to remove the adventitia, followed by gentle insertion of the cannula, which is then secured and connected to the arterial limb of the circuit (Fig. 4.1). The procedure becomes more difficult in reoperations, calcified aorta, or aortic pathology (aneurysm, dissection), when alternative strategies or cannulation sites (femoral/axillary artery) are preferred.

Cannula selection depends on anatomy, required flows, and surgical approach. Cannulas vary in design, including straight-tip cannulas (direct axial flow) usually used in routine operations; angled-tip cannulas are preferred in complex procedures to direct the flow away from the aortic wall or cerebral vessels, reducing the risk of jet injury and embolism. Wire-reinforced cannulas are useful in minimally invasive or off-pump procedures to avoid kinking. For cannulation at the level of the aortic arch, special cannulas exist with two side holes to ensure optimal lateral flow to the branches of the aortic arch (brachiocephalic trunk, left common carotid artery, left subclavian artery). Sizes vary from 14 to 24 Fr depending on body surface area and desired pressures.

Potential complications are multiple, with their risk decreasing inversely proportional to the surgeon's experience. The most feared complication is iatrogenic aortic dissection, with an incidence of 0.06–0.23% [18], caused either by direct trauma during cannula insertion or by excessive perfusion pressures, especially in patients with an atherosclerotic or weakened aortic wall. In cases where the purse-strings were not placed adequately (too superficial), there is a risk of hematomas adjacent to the cannulation area, which in extreme cases may progress to dissection. When this occurs, it is necessary to place another purse-string suture sufficiently deep outside the initially placed ones.

Embolic complications are also major, often triggered by manipulation of a calcified aorta or incorrect cannula positioning, which can dislodge atheromatous material, leading to stroke, mesenteric ischemia, or peripheral emboli. Palpation of the ascending aorta before cannulation, or identification of plaques using a sterile intraoperative ultrasound probe, is crucial for direct detection of plaques/calcifications not externally visible. Intraoperative epiaortic ultrasound has significantly improved safety by allowing real-time evaluation of wall integrity and identification of atheroma, reducing the incidence of embolic stroke [19]. Identification of lesions—especially prominent plaques or "porcelain aorta"—helps in choosing an alternative cannulation site, selecting a different cannula, or even reconsidering the entire intervention. The risk of cannulating a severely atherosclerotic aorta outweighs any benefit associated with central cannulation, which is why this action must always be avoided. In patients suspected of having severe atherosclerotic involvement of the ascending aorta (patients known with severe systemic atherosclerosis, multiple severe stenoses or occlusions in the carotid, coronary, renal, mesenteric, or lower-limb territories, etc.), a preoperative CT scan is reasonable to assess the quality of the aortic wall.

Cannula malposition may generate high line pressures, inadequate systemic perfusion, or intimal injury through turbulent flow. Bleeding at the cannulation site remains a risk, though usually controllable with proper suturing technique, especially in patients with fragile aortic tissue or coagulopathy. Rarely, late complications such as pseudoaneurysm at the cannulation site may occur, particularly in reoperations or prolonged procedures [20].

Subclavian Artery Exposure and Cannulation

The choice of auxiliary arterial access—typically the subclavian or femoral artery—depends on anatomy, the nature of the intervention (emergency or elective), and the underlying pathology that needs to be corrected. Both techniques have evolved to provide safe and reliable access with adequate perfusion flows in complex procedures such as aortic dissection repair and minimally invasive cardiac surgery. The use of the right subclavian artery or the brachiocephalic trunk offers important advantages in complex aortic surgery, namely the possibility of antegrade cerebral perfusion (with a lower risk of embolism compared with retrograde methods), the possibility of circulatory arrest for arch procedures with selective cerebral perfusion, though with the disadvantage of potential limb ischemia. Dissection of the subclavian artery requires special attention to avoid injury to the phrenic nerve, brachial plexus, or pleura, as it may lie at considerable depth, especially in obese patients.

Indications for Subclavian Artery Cannulation

- Aortic arch surgery requiring antegrade cerebral perfusion
- Ascending aortic pathology (dissection, atheroma) where direct cannulation is risky

Exposure Approaches

Supraclavicular Approach

A transverse incision is made approximately 1 cm above the clavicle. After division or retraction of the platysma and the omohyoid muscle, the adipose tissue between the scalene muscles is exposed. At this stage, protection of the phrenic nerve is essential. This approach offers good exposure of the proximal structures.

Infraclavicular Approach

This is the most commonly used in practice because it provides exposure of at least 4–5 cm of the subclavian artery. A parallel incision is made immediately below the clavicle, with deeper access through the pectoralis major muscle and the clavipectoral fascia. For optimal exposure, the pectoralis minor may be divided and gently retracted, and the branches of the brachial plexus lifted on tapes or loops. This method is preferred when more distal arterial access is required.

Intrathoracic Approach Via Median Sternotomy

This type of access allows direct visualization of the brachiocephalic trunk and its dissection up to its bifurcation into the right subclavian artery and right common carotid artery. It is particularly useful when precise and controlled intrathoracic cannulation is required, but has the disadvantage of providing only partial cerebral perfusion through the right common carotid artery when circulatory arrest is needed.

Cannulation Techniques

Direct Cannulation

After heparinization, a purse-string suture is placed and followed by a transverse arteriotomy with direct insertion of the cannula. An alternative is advancing the cannula using the Seldinger technique—puncturing the artery with an 18G needle, followed by advancement of a guidewire into the aorta and insertion of the cannula over the guidewire. This method is fast, but carries a higher risk of local trauma or flow restriction by entering in the false lumen in the case of an extended aortic dissection.

Side-Arm Graft

An end-to-side anastomosis of an 8 mm Dacron graft is created on the subclavian artery, followed by insertion of the cannula through the free end of the graft. This minimizes manipulation of the native artery, clears the operative field, and allows repositioning without interrupting the procedure [21]. The disadvantage is the possibility of bleeding from the anastomotic site, especially in cases of excessive cannula manipulation.

Femoral Artery Exposure and Cannulation

Femoral cannulation is widely used for its accessibility and efficiency. It is valuable in emergencies (e.g., type A aortic dissection), when rapid initiation of CPB is critical, or in reoperations to decompress the heart and increase its distance from the sternum. It plays a key role in minimally invasive procedures (valvular and coronary), when central access is limited or undesirable, and in patients with sternal malformations [22].

The common femoral artery is located in the femoral triangle, immediately below the inguinal ligament, lateral to the vein and medial to the nerve—an anatomically predictable relationship that facilitates safe vascular access. Its superficial position and relatively large diameter make it suitable for both open and percutaneous cannulation.

Surgical exposure may be performed either through a longitudinal incision over the femoral pulse or a transverse incision in the inguinal crease. Dissection of the anatomical layers continues until the artery is isolated, which is then controlled proximally and distally with vascular loops. The femoral vein and nerve are protected to avoid iatrogenic injury.

Cannulation Methods

Open (Direct) Cannulation

After heparinization and placement of a purse-string suture, a small arteriotomy is made followed by insertion of the cannula. Reliable in stable elective procedures.

Percutaneous Technique Using the Seldinger Method

This is frequently chosen in emergencies or in high-risk patients. A needle is inserted into the vessel, a guidewire is passed through the needle, then the tract is gradually dilated (sequential dilatation), and the cannula is placed. The entire procedure may be performed completely percutaneously or "open-guided," meaning that after surgical exposure of the artery, the guidewire is inserted under direct vision. In this way, the safety of controlled access is combined with the speed of the percutaneous technique, reducing the risk of injury or malpositioning—especially when anatomy is difficult or the patient is hemodynamically unstable. Percutaneous arterial suture devices may be used to minimize the risk of hemorrhagic complications after removal.

Advantages and Risks

The main advantage is rapid initiation of cardiopulmonary bypass (CPB). In addition, retrograde perfusion obtained through this route may be useful in certain aortic procedures. On the other hand, there are risks: limb ischemia (due to blockage of distal flow), retrograde embolization of atheromatous material to the brain or abdominal organs, as well as propagation of a dissection and malperfusion in patients with a severely atherosclerotic or fragile aorta. For these reasons, good preoperative imaging and intraoperative vigilance are essential [23].

Inferior Vena Cava and Bi-Caval Cannulation

Venous cannulation allows drainage of deoxygenated blood to the heart–lung machine. Two main techniques are used: single IVC (inferior vena cava) cannulation and bi-caval cannulation (SVC + IVC).

Single IVC (Double-Stage Cannula through the Right Atrial Appendage—Fig. 4.2)

It is used when complete isolation of the right atrium is not required (CABG or some valvular procedures without opening the interatrial septum, ascending aorta surgery). A double-stage cannula is used, which allows blood drainage directly from the inferior vena cava and from the right atrium, where blood from the SVC drains. The advantages are fewer cannulation sites, shorter operative time, and lower risk of postoperative bleeding.

Bi-Caval

Essential when exposing/opening the right atrium and the interatrial septum—tricuspid repair/replacement, ASD closure, heart transplantation, intra-atrial tumors. Some surgeons also use this technique for mitral valve procedures through the posterior approach at the interatrial groove because of the risk of opening the right atrium. This technique allows complete occlusion of venous return, keeping the

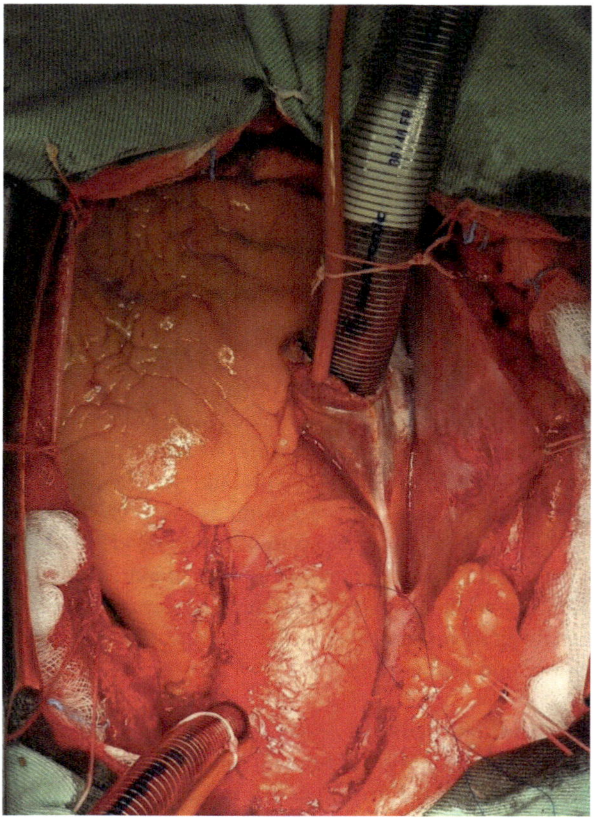

Fig. 4.2 IVC cannulation with dual-stage single cannula—IBCV Iasi collection

operative field completely dry. Snaring both venae cavae prevents backflow and improves exposure.

Cannulas are usually single-stage, straight or curved, and sized according to body surface area (18–30 Fr). The SVC cannula is placed through the superior wall of the right atrium or directly into the superior vena cava, preferably more than 1 cm distal to the cavo-atrial junction where the sinus node is located. The IVC cannula is placed through the inferior wall of the right atrium or directly into the inferior vena cava at the pericardial reflection on the diaphragm. Vacuum-assisted drainage (VAVD) can improve flow in bi-caval settings, especially in minimally invasive procedures.

Although the bi-caval technique provides superior exposure and hemodynamic control in complex right-heart surgery, it is technically more demanding and carries higher risks (air embolism, arrhythmias, injury to the venae cavae) [24]. Single IVC cannulation, though simpler, may result in insufficient drainage and venous distension when complete right atrial isolation is required.

Cardioplegia Solutions: Composition, Delivery, and Clinical Applications

Crystalloid vs. Blood Cardioplegia

Cardioplegia represents the controlled induction of cardiac arrest in diastole for myocardial protection during cardiac surgery. The primary objective is to reduce oxygen consumption, prevent ischemic injury, and preserve function during the period of aortic cross-clamping. Classifications include: composition (crystalloid vs blood), temperature (cold vs warm), route of administration (antegrade vs retrograde), and timing (intermittent vs continuous).

Crystalloid Cardioplegia

These are the most common electrolyte solutions that mimic plasma composition, containing potassium (for cardiac arrest), sodium, calcium, magnesium, and buffering agents. Classic examples include St. Thomas'—with extracellular action and a duration of effect of 20–30 minutes—and Bretschneider, with intracellular action and a duration of action up to 120 minutes [25]. Among the advantages are lower cost and the fact that they are easy to prepare and administer, but their main limitation lies in their low oxygen-carrying capacity due to the absence of hemoglobin, resulting in weaker myocardial protection and a higher risk of myocardial ischemic injury and edema [25, 26].

Blood Cardioplegia

It uses the patient's oxygenated blood mixed with a crystalloid solution in a typical ratio of 4:1 or 8:1, to which electrolytes and other additives are added. Through its hematic content, it offers superior oxygen delivery, better buffering capacity, and an osmolarity close to physiological, providing superior myocardial protection—particularly in high-risk patients such as those with left ventricular hypertrophy, diabetes, or prolonged cross-clamp time [27–29]. Modern protocols, such as the Buckberg regimen, usually include an induction phase, maintenance infusions, and a terminal warm "hot shot" intended to optimize myocardial functional recovery at declamping [30].

Cold vs. Warm Cardioplegia

Cold cardioplegia acts through hypothermia, suppressing myocardial metabolism and reducing oxygen demand, which prolongs tolerance to ischemia. It is generally administered as high-potassium solutions, either blood-based or crystalloid, infused antegrade through the aortic root or retrograde through the coronary sinus. Cold blood cardioplegia is preferred over crystalloid due to its superior oxygen-carrying and buffering capacity. Braathen et al. reported lower postoperative CK-MB and troponin T levels in patients undergoing AVR, compared with cold crystalloid [31]. However, low temperatures can impair mitochondrial respiration and may delay recovery.

Warm (normothermic) cardioplegia aims to maintain enzymatic function and metabolism, limiting ischemia–reperfusion injury. It is typically blood-based, administered intermittently or continuously, often with a terminal "hot shot" before declamping. Intermittent tepid-warm administration has demonstrated lower CK-MB levels and better left ventricular function compared with cold cardioplegia in elective CABG, and has also been associated with reduced inotropic requirements, earlier extubation, and shorter intensive care stays in some studies [32, 33].

Moderate-temperature cardioplegia (28–32 °C) represents a hybrid strategy combining metabolic suppression induced by lower temperatures with avoidance of the biochemical disturbances associated with deep hypothermia. Fiore et al. demonstrated comparable or superior protection compared with cold blood cardioplegia, with lower enzymatic release and reduced inotropic requirements [34].

Route of Delivery: Antegrade vs. Retrograde

Administration of cardioplegia may be antegrade through the aortic root or directly into the coronary ostia, or retrograde through the coronary sinus. The antegrade route is preferred in patients with a competent aortic valve and patent coronary arteries, as it mimics physiological flow (Tables 4.2 and 4.3).

In patients with aortic insufficiency, severe coronary artery disease with significant proximal stenoses where antegrade flow does not adequately perfuse all territories, the retrograde route becomes essential (Table 4.4). The combined approach can improve protection and distribution [35] (Fig 4.3).

Comparative Evidence Across Cardioplegia Strategies

Meta-analyses of RCTs comparing warm blood cardioplegia with cold cardioplegia generally indicate no significant differences in mortality, myocardial infarction, or stroke, but they do show modestly improved postoperative cardiac function for warm techniques in low-risk elective cases [36, 37], as well as reduced levels of necrosis markers (CK-MB, troponin) [38]. Among cold solutions, cold blood cardioplegia has been associated with a reduction in perioperative infarction compared with cold crystalloid cardioplegia [37].

A recent meta-analysis including 15 studies and 2282 patients found no relevant differences in in-hospital mortality between del Nido, Custodiol, blood cardioplegia, and St. Thomas solution. However, del Nido cardioplegia was associated with shorter bypass time, whereas Custodiol was associated with reduced hospital stay, although with limited clinical relevance [39]. Large multicenter analyses suggest

Table 4.2 Types of cardioplegia and their characteristics

Cardioplegia type	Composition	Temperature	Delivery route	Advantages	Limitations	Typical uses
Crystalloid (e.g., St. Thomas')	Electrolyte solution with K+, Mg2+, buffers	Cold (4–10 °C)	Antegrade	Simple, inexpensive, easy to prepare	No oxygen delivery, potential for myocardial edema	Routine CABG, short procedures
Blood Cardioplegia	Patient blood + additives	Cold or Warm	Antegrade or retrograde	Provides oxygen, buffering, physiological properties	More complex setup, blood handling needed	High-risk patients, long procedures, LV hypertrophy
Del Nido	Crystalloid with lidocaine, mannitol	Cold (4–8 °C), single dose	Antegrade	Long single-dose protection, reduces interruptions	Mostly validated in pediatrics; some adult use only	Pediatric, adult CABG, minimally invasive surgery
Custodiol (HTK)	Intracellular-type crystalloid	Cold (~4 °C)	Antegrade	Long single-dose protection (2–3 hours)	Risk of hemodilution, weaker buffering	Complex, prolonged procedures (transplant, aortic)
Antegrade delivery	Any cardioplegia solution	Cold or Warm	Aortic root	Direct coronary perfusion, simple in normal anatomy	Ineffective if aortic insufficiency or coronary disease	Most surgeries with intact aortic valve
Retrograde delivery	Blood or crystalloid	Cold or Warm	Coronary sinus	Useful in aortic regurgitation, grafted coronaries	Possible inadequate perfusion of right ventricle	Reoperations, aortic valve insufficiency

Table 4.3 Characteristics of antegrade cardioplegia

Characteristic	Details
Solutions used	Any type (crystalloid, blood, Del Nido, Custodiol)
Temperature	Cold or warm
Route	Through the aortic root or directly into the coronary ostia
Advantages	Direct coronary perfusion, simple technique
Limitations	Ineffective in severe aortic insufficiency or advanced coronary stenosis
Typical uses	Most procedures when the aortic valve is competent

Table 4.4 Characteristics of retrograde cardioplegia

Characteristic	Details
Solutions used	Blood or crystalloid
Temperature	Cold or warm
Route	Through the coronary sinus (balloon catheter)
Advantages	Useful in aortic insufficiency, coronary grafts, reoperations
Limitations	Inadequate perfusion of the right ventricle or superficial epicardial branches
Typical uses	Reoperations, severe aortic insufficiency, situations with insufficient antegrade perfusion, CABG with severe proximal stenoses

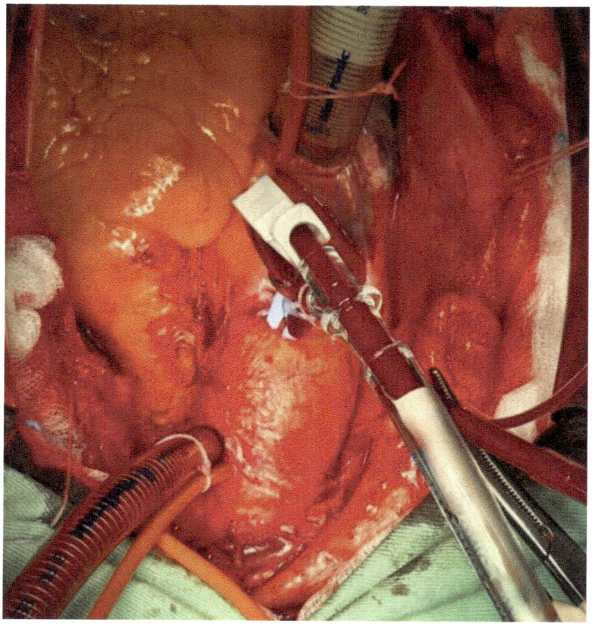

Fig. 4.3 Antegrade cardioplegia delivery—IBCV Iasi collection

potential advantages of del Nido cardioplegia in reducing perioperative mortality compared with the other solutions, while the Custodiol solution may present a lower risk of postoperative atrial fibrillation [39, 40].

In adult RCTs comparing del Nido with cold blood cardioplegia (10 trials, ~1800 patients), del Nido was associated with lower volumes of administered cardioplegia, more frequent spontaneous rhythm recovery, and lower postoperative troponin T and CK-MB levels, while major clinical outcomes (ICU duration, stroke, atrial fibrillation, mortality) remained similar [38].

Cardioplegia cannulas are critical for myocardial protection, facilitating precise delivery of solutions antegrade into the aortic root or retrograde through the coronary sinus. Advances over the past decade have focused on safety, ease of insertion, and monitoring to minimize complications (aortic injury, coronary sinus trauma, inadequate perfusion).

Modern antegrade cannulas often have balloon tips for sealing within the aortic root/coronary ostia, preventing reflux and concentrating delivery. Balloon materials are biocompatible and low-pressure to minimize the risk of intimal injury (dissection). Many cannulas integrate pressure-monitoring ports in the aortic root—essential for avoiding over-pressurization [41, 42].

For retrograde delivery, cannulas have ergonomic curvatures and softer tips to navigate the variable anatomy of the coronary sinus, reducing perforations; pressure monitoring is standard to promptly detect elevated pressures and adjust flow accordingly [43].

Heart Venting in Cardiac Surgery

Venting and deairing techniques are essential in CPB. Their purpose is the decompression of the cardiac chambers—mainly the left ventricle—to prevent distension, reduce wall stress, and optimize exposure. They also facilitate the removal of air accumulated in the cardiac cavities during surgery, reducing the risk of ischemia and air embolism [44, 45]. The sites of introduction of venting cannulas and the techniques used are varied. There are cannulas introduced through the right superior pulmonary vein (RSPV) or directly into the left atrium via the transmitral route, which are particularly effective in mitral/aortic surgery. Alternatively, the aortic root vent is used during aortic clamping to evacuate blood accumulated proximally, especially in patients with an incompetent aortic valve.

There are also left ventricular (LV) apical venting techniques, frequently used in the past in patients with severe ventricular dysfunction or prolonged CPB, reducing wall stress. All these strategies prevent LV overload, preserve myocardial function, and support improved postoperative outcomes in high-risk cardiac surgery [45, 46]. Minimally invasive and robotic procedures have introduced new techniques, including percutaneous and catheter-based methods, for effective decompression with reduced surgical trauma [47].

Proper placement and management of the vent are essential for effective myocardial protection. Insufficient venting may lead to ventricular distension, increased oxygen consumption, and reduced cardioplegia efficacy, whereas excessive or incorrect venting may cause arrhythmias, bleeding, or even structural injury. The most commonly used technique, insertion through the right superior pulmonary vein, involves placing a purse-string suture with 4–0 Prolene from the lateral wall of the left atrium to the pulmonary vein, approximately 1 cm from its orifice into the left atrium. An incision is made in the center of this purse-string with a scalpel, and the transmitral vent cannula is advanced until retrograde flow is observed in the high-pressure pulsatile cannula. The ECG is checked. Contact of the cannula tip with the ventricular wall is identified on the ECG by the presence of extrasystoles. The cannula is withdrawn until these disappear.

Effective deairing is essential for preventing gas embolism, which can produce neurological deficits, myocardial dysfunction, and other embolic phenomena. Combinations of mechanical maneuvers, CO_2 insufflation, and imaging guidance are used. Mechanical maneuvers play a central role in effective intraoperative deairing. Trendelenburg positioning helps divert air away from the cerebral circulation, while lung inflation during weaning from bypass promotes evacuation of bubbles from the pulmonary veins and left atrium. Manual venting, through gentle compression or "tapping" of the heart, facilitates mobilization of residual air from between the muscular trabeculae, while the vent placed in the aortic root allows continuous suction during closure and rewarming, being located at the most superior point of the aorta. Together, these maneuvers form the foundation of modern deairing protocols [48].

Carbon Dioxide (CO_2) Insufflation

CO_2 is denser than air and highly soluble, displacing air from the operative field and reducing the risk of embolism during CPB. It is typically insufflated into the pericardial cavity at 2–5 L/min, creating a CO_2-rich environment that minimizes air retention. Special diffusers promote laminar flow and reduce turbulence. Clinical studies have shown reductions in intraoperative microemboli, supporting the routine use of CO_2 in deairing protocols [49, 50].

Transesophageal Echocardiography (TEE) Guidance

TEE has become indispensable, offering real-time visualization of intracardiac air and precise guidance of maneuvers. It allows detection of small bubbles and evaluation of deairing adequacy, increasing safety through immediate feedback and confirmation of complete evacuation [48].

In Refractory Situations, Direct Aspiration Is Effective

LV venting (catheter via apex or pulmonary vein) for targeted evacuation of air from the LV; aortic root aspiration during closure and rewarming for continuous removal of air from the ascending aorta—especially valuable in complex procedures or difficult anatomy.

References

1. Reser D, Caliskan E, Tolboom H, Guidotti A, Maisano F. Median sternotomy. Multimed Man Cardiothorac Surg. 2015;2015:mmv017.
2. Dalton ML, Connally SR, Sealy WC. Julian's reintroduction of Milton's operation. Ann Thorac Surg. 1992;53(3):532–3.
3. Gerbode F, Braimbridge MV, Melrose DG. Median sternotomy for open cardiac surgery during total heart-lung by-pass. Ann Surg. 1958;76(5):821–4.
4. Daemen JHT, Heuts S, Olsthoorn JR, Maessen JG, Sardari NP. Right minithoracotomy versus median sternotomy for reoperative mitral valve surgery: a systematic review and meta-analysis of observational studies. Eur J Cardiothorac Surg. 2018;54(5):817–25.
5. Burdett CL, Lage IB, Goodwin AT, White RW, Khan KJ, Owens WA, et al. Manubrium-limited sternotomy decreases blood loss after aortic valve replacement surgery. Interact Cardiovasc Thorac Surg. 2014;19(4):605–10.
6. Schonauer C, Tessitore E, Moraci A, Barbagallo G, Albanese V. The use of local agents: bone wax, gelatin, collagen, oxidized cellulose. Hemostasis. 2005:89–96. https://pubmed.ncbi.nlm.nih.gov/15221572/.
7. Robicsek F, Daugherty HK, Cook JW. The prevention and treatment of sternum separation following open-heart surgery. J Thorac Cardiovasc Surg. 1977;73(2):267–8.
8. Alhan C, Arıtürk C, Senay S, Okten M, Güllü AU, Kilic L, et al. Use of bone wax is related to increased postoperative sternal dehiscence. Kardiochir Torakochir Pol. 2014;11(4):385–90.
9. Khan NU, Yonan N. Does preoperative computed tomography reduce the risks associated with re-do cardiac surgery? Interact Cardiovasc Thorac Surg. 2009;9(1):119–23.
10. Roselli EE, Pettersson GB, Blackstone EH, Brizzio ME, Houghtaling PL, Hauck R, et al. Adverse events during reoperative cardiac surgery: frequency, characterization, and rescue. J Thorac Cardiovasc Surg. 2008;135(2):316–23.
11. Akhtar NJ, Markowitz AH, Gilkeson RC. Multidetector computed tomography in the preoperative assessment of cardiac surgery patients. Radiol Clin North Am. 2010;48(1):117–39.
12. Khalpey Z, Kumar UA, Aslam U, Phillips T, Khalpey Z, Cooper A, et al. Improving sternal closure outcomes in cardiac surgery: polyethylene suture tapes vs. steel wires. J Clin Med. 2025;14(1):277.
13. Miazza J, Reuthebuch B, Bruehlmeier F, Camponovo U, Maguire R, Koechlin L, et al. First report on rigid plate fixation for enhanced sternal closure in minimally invasive cardiac surgery: safety and outcomes. Bioengineering (Basel). 2024;11(12):1280.
14. Yokoyama Y, Yamamoto T, Oyama T, Lee J, Machida Y, Endo D, et al. Sternal closure with sandwiched three-piece bioresorbable mesh reduces postoperative hemorrhage: a retrospective study. J Cardiothorac Surg. 2023;18(1):345.
15. Robu M, Rădulescu B, Margarint I, Ştiru O, Antoniac I, Gheorghiţă D, et al. Surgical strategy for sternal closure in patients with surgical myocardial revascularization using mammary arteries. J Cardiovasc Dev Dis. 2023;10(11):457.
16. Hill JD, John H, Gibbon J, Part I. The development of the first successful heart-lung machine. Ann Thorac Surg. 1982;34(3):337–41.

17. Romaine-Davis A. John Gibbon and his heart-lung machine. Philadelphia: University of Pennsylvania Press; 2016.
18. Ram H, Dwarakanath S, Green AE, Steyn J, Hessel EA. Iatrogenic aortic dissection associated with cardiac surgery: a narrative review. J Cardiothorac Vasc Anesth. 2021;35(10):3050–66.
19. Biancari F, Santini F, Tauriainen T, Bancone C, Ruggieri VG, Perrotti A, et al. Epiaortic ultrasound to prevent stroke in coronary artery bypass grafting. Ann Thorac Surg. 2020;109(1):294–301.
20. Niklewski T, Zembala M, Puszczewicz D, Nadziakiewicz P, Karolak W, Zembala M. The use of intraoperative epiaortic ultrasonography in monitoring patients over 75 years old treated with aortic valve replacement. Kardiochir Torakochir Pol. 2017;14(1):10–5.
21. Cavozza C, Campanella A, Pasquale P, Audo A. Percutaneous or side-arm graft right subclavian artery cannulation via median sternotomy. Aorta (Stamford). 2019;7(5):150–3.
22. Tsiouris A, Elkinany S, Ziganshin BA, Elefteriades JA. Open Seldinger-guided femoral artery cannulation technique for thoracic aortic surgery. Ann Thorac Surg. 2016;101(6):2231–5.
23. Werner P, Winter M, Coti I, Kahrovic A, Andreas M, Haberl T, et al. Advantages and disadvantages of femoral versus central cannulation. Innovations (Phila). 2025;20(2):148–57.
24. Puthettu M, Vandenberghe S, Demertzis S. Effect of cannulation site on emboli travel during cardiac surgery. J Cardiothorac Surg. 2021;16(1):181.
25. Ledingham SJM, Braimbridge MV, Hearse DJ. The St. Thomas' Hospital cardioplegic solution: a comparison of the efficacy of two formulations. J Thorac Cardiovasc Surg. 1987;93(2):240–6.
26. Matte GS, del Nido PJ. History and use of del Nido cardioplegia solution at Boston Children's Hospital. J Extra Corpor Technol. 2012;44(3):98–103.
27. Guru V, Omura J, Alghamdi AA, Weisel R, Fremes SE. Is blood superior to crystalloid cardioplegia? A meta-analysis of randomized clinical trials. Circulation. 2006;114(1 Suppl):I331–8.
28. Jacob S, Kallikourdis A, Sellke F, Dunning J. Is blood cardioplegia superior to crystalloid cardioplegia? Interact Cardiovasc Thorac Surg. 2008;7(3):491–8.
29. Sá MP, Rueda FG, Ferraz PE, Chalegre ST, Vasconcelos FP, Lima RC. Blood vs crystalloid cardioplegia in cardiac surgery: a meta-analysis. Perfusion. 2012;27(6):535–46.
30. Boening A, Assling-Simon L, Heep M, Boengler K, Niemann B, Grieshaber P. Buckberg's blood cardioplegia in a rat model of acute myocardial infarction. Exp Gerontol. 2018;104:98–104.
31. Braathen B, Tønnessen T. Cold blood cardioplegia reduces cardiac enzyme levels vs cold crystalloid in AVR. J Thorac Cardiovasc Surg. 2010;139(4):874–80.
32. Dar MI. Cold crystalloid vs warm blood cardioplegia for CABG. Ann Thorac Cardiovasc Surg. 2005;11(6):382–5.
33. James TM, Nores M, Rousou JA, Lin N, Stamou SC. Warm blood cardioplegia: concepts and controversies. Tex Heart Inst J. 2020;47(2):108–16.
34. Fiore AC, Swartz MT, Nevett R, Vieth PJ, Magrath RA, Sherrick A, et al. Intermittent tepid vs cold blood cardioplegia in elective CABG. Ann Thorac Surg. 1998;65(6):1559–64.
35. Jegaden O, Eker A, Montagna P, Ossette J, Vial C, Guidollet J, et al. Antegrade/retrograde cardioplegia in bypass grafting: metabolic RCT. Ann Thorac Surg. 1995;59(2):456–61.
36. Kot TKM, Chan JSK, Froghi S, Lau DHH, Morgan K, Magni F, et al. Warm vs cold cardioplegia in cardiac surgery: meta-analysis. JTCVS Open. 2021;6:161–90.
37. Tan J, Bi S, Li J, Gu J, Wang Y, Xiong J, et al. Different cardioplegia types in cardiac surgery: network meta-analysis. Front Cardiovasc Med. 2022;9:996744.
38. Li C, Xiang H, Yang H, Liu W, Lan W, Luo C, et al. Del Nido vs cold blood cardioplegia in adult cardiac surgery: meta-analysis. J Cardiothorac Surg. 2024;19(1):356.
39. Al-Hasan-Al-Saegh S, Takemoto S, Benenati S, Shafiei S, Yavuz S, Galli M, et al. Myocardial protection in minimally invasive surgery: Del Nido, HTK, and blood cardioplegia. J Clin Med. 2024;13(22):6977.
40. Ler A, Sazzad F, Ong GS, Kofidis T. Del Nido vs St. Thomas cardioplegia in adult and pediatric cardiac surgery: meta-analysis. Perfusion. 2020;35(8):724–35.

41. Lopes JB, Santos CJ. Coronary perfusion pressure during antegrade cardioplegia in CABG. Braz J Cardiovasc Surg. 2017;32(3):171–6.
42. Onorati F, Renzulli A, De Feo M, Santarpino G, Gregorio R, Biondi A, et al. Antegrade blood cardioplegia in LMS disease. J Thorac Cardiovasc Surg. 2003;126(5):1345–51.
43. Orihashi K, Miyashita K, Tashiro M, Kihara K, Kondo N, Yamamoto M, et al. Avoidance of coronary sinus injury during retrograde cardioplegia. Ann Thorac Surg. 2016;102(6):e583–6.
44. Lüsebrink E, Binzenhöfer L, Kellnar A, Müller C, Scherer C, Schrage B, et al. Venting during VA-ECMO. Clin Res Cardiol. 2023;112(4):464–505.
45. Cevasco M, Takayama H, Ando M, Garan AR, Naka Y, Takeda K. LV distension and venting strategies in VA-ECMO. J Thorac Dis. 2019;11(4):1676–83.
46. Breyer RH, Lavender S, Cordell AR. Delayed LV rupture from transatrial vent. Ann Thorac Surg. 1982;33(2):189–91.
47. Mandal K, Alwair H, Nifong WL, Chitwood WR Jr. Robotic mitral valve surgery. J Thorac Dis. 2013:S694–703. https://pubmed.ncbi.nlm.nih.gov/24251030/.
48. Orihashi K, Ueda T. De-airing in open heart surgery: survey and literature review. Gen Thorac Cardiovasc Surg. 2019;67(10):823–34.
49. Nyman J, Svenarud P, van der Linden J. CO_2 de-airing in minimally invasive surgery: a new device. J Cardiothorac Surg. 2019;14(1):12.
50. Persson M, Van Der Linden J. CO_2 de-airing of wound cavity: theory and diffuser comparison. J Cardiothorac Vasc Anesth. 2003;17(3):329–35.

Concept of Minimally Invasive Cardiac Surgery

5

Ghenadie Bostan and Gheorghe Manolache

Introduction

The first minimally invasive cardiac surgeries were performed at the end of the twentieth century, and later began to be widely adopted starting around 2018–2019, when some cardiac surgery clinics began extensively implementing the terminology MICS (minimally invasive cardiac surgery) into their surgical programs. These procedures have become the successors of the remarkable international progress seen with thoracoscopic and laparoscopic surgeries. A significant innovation came from the "Stanford group," which demonstrated that cardiopulmonary bypass with a closed chest and cardioplegic arrest was feasible and safe for mitral valve replacement [1].

A major contribution to the advancement of minithoracotomy techniques came from cardiac procedures performed via mini-sternotomy, which challenged surgeons to step outside their comfort zones.

Minimally invasive cardiac surgery yields more favorable postoperative clinical outcomes compared to sternotomy, specifically regarding postoperative pain,

G. Bostan (✉)
Department of Cardiovascular and Thoracic Surgery, Republican Clinical Hospital "Timofei Mosneaga", Chisinau, Republic of Moldova

Division Cardiovascular Surgery, Institute of Cardiovascular Disease "Prof. Dr George IM Georgescu", Iasi, Romania; https://www.scr.md

G. Manolache
Department of Cardiovascular and Thoracic Surgery, Republican Clinical Hospital "Timofei Mosneaga", Chisinau, Republic of Moldova; https://www.scr.md

G. Tinică, A. Burlacu (eds.), *Surgical, Hybrid and Minimally Invasive Structural Cardiac Interventions*, https://doi.org/10.1007/978-3-032-16676-0_5

a considerable reduction in wound-related complications (infection, dehiscence), better respiratory function, and a significant decrease in the need for blood transfusions.

Patient Selection and Assessment

A thorough patient assessment involves ruling out any history of right or left hemithorax pathology (such as mastectomy, radiotherapy, thoracic trauma, or pleural effusions with possible adhesions). A chest X-ray in three projections and a transthoracic echocardiogram (as a primary investigation) should be performed, as well as arterial and venous Doppler ultrasound of the inguinal region. If necessary, an angio-CT scan can be performed. It's also essential to evaluate the position of the right atrium and ascending aorta relative to the intercostal spaces on imaging. In the case of minimally invasive mitral valve surgery, the aortic valve must be competent.

Atrial fibrillation is not a contraindication for MICS. Usually, patients with a large anteroposterior or lateral thoracic diameter may be excluded from MICS, as exposure of the target valve can be difficult, and any possible intraoperative complication might only be resolved by converting to sternotomy. Likewise, patients with grade III obesity may also be excluded.

There is the following classification to evaluate the ascending aorta position in relation to the sternum (see Fig. 5.1):

This classification offers the possibility to exclude patients who can later present in surgery complications, but also helps choose the right access (anterolateral or axillar).

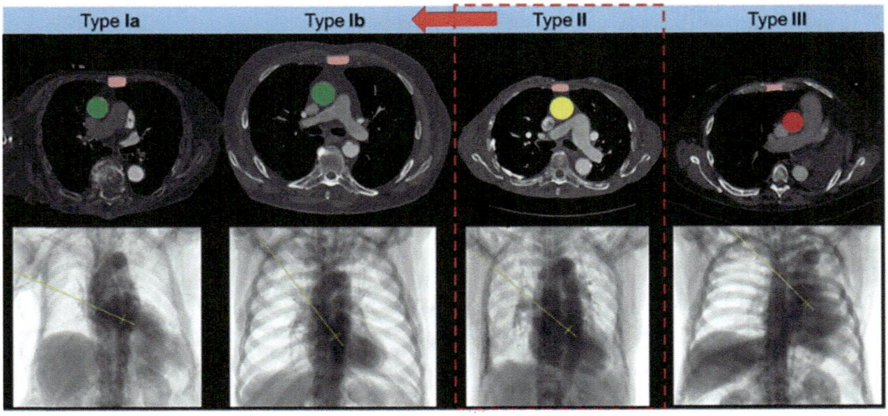

Fig. 5.1 CT planning for RALT access: preoperative ascending aorta-sternal relationship

Cannulation

The development of extracorporeal circulation using peripheral cannulation has had a major impact on the advancement of minimally invasive, endoscopic, and Da Vinci® robotic cardiac interventions. For arterial and venous cannulation, the right common femoral artery and the right common femoral vein are typically used. Preoperatively, a computed tomography angiography (CTA) is performed—especially in patients with atherosclerotic disease. Regional vascular Doppler ultrasound is mandatory for all patients. Often, a *CT protocol for minimally invasive cardiac surgery* is drafted, which describes the thoracic cavity's parameters in relation to the surgical pathology and assesses the patency of the femoral artery and femoral vein.

If the right femoral artery is compromised, the left femoral artery may be accessed, or, in cases of aortoiliac disease, the right axillary artery may be used [3]. When the minimally invasive intervention begins with double-lumen intubation and the right lung is deflated during minithoracotomy, the ascending aorta may be accessed for arterial cannulation—the cannula can be passed either through the working port or via a separate dedicated port. Cannulating the ascending aorta is less traumatic compared to axillary cannulation.

Femoral venous cannulation is guided transesophageally by echocardiography (TEE) at the bicaval junction, confirming that the guidewire enters the superior vena cava and maintains a straight, unbent position (Fig. 5.2). Arterial cannulation is performed after echocardiographic confirmation of the guidewire's position in the descending aorta (see Fig. 5.2). Cardiopulmonary bypass (CPB) is initiated slowly, checking for the absence of arterial resistance, and subsequently, vacuum-assisted venous drainage (VAVD) is gradually installed. Respiratory support can then be paused for the minithoracotomy. In experienced surgical teams, the thoracic and femoral approaches can be performed simultaneously. One can start the cardiopulmonary bypass even in cases of pleural adhesions (which may occur in approximately 2–4% of primary patients).

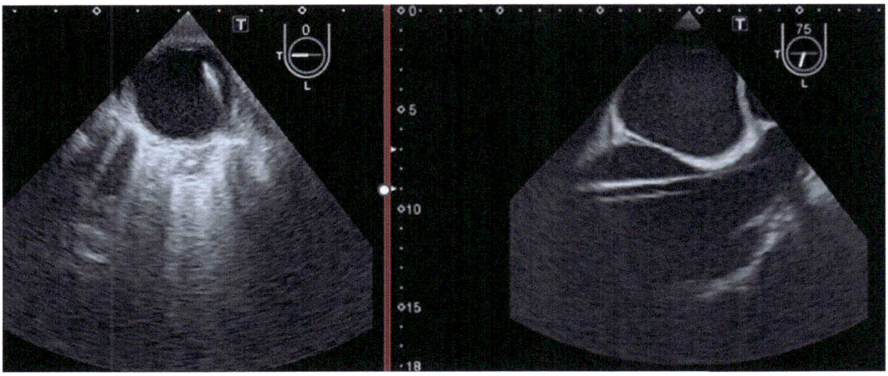

Fig. 5.2 Left: Insertion of the Seldinger in the descending aorta. Right: Insertion of the cannula in the superior vena cava

Venous cannulation in minimally invasive interventions has its own evolution. Initially, surgeries were performed using femoro-jugular cannulation. Later, with the advancement of double-stage cannulas, most interventions can now be performed using only femoral cannulation. Additionally, for multivalvular surgeries or atrial/ventricular septal defects, it's necessary to gain experience in caval clamping (SVC and IVC). For beginner surgeons, it's advisable to perform femoro-jugular cannulation (e.g., for atrial septal defect repair).

Thus, peripheral venous cannulation allows resolving for the following:

1. *MICS for structural left heart pathology* (Mitral valve surgery, Aortic valve surgery, Aortic membrane excision, Left atrial myxoma with a small pedicle, MIDCAB (Minimally Invasive Direct Coronary Artery Bypass)).
2. *MICS for structural right heart pathology* (Tricuspid valve surgery, Atrial Septal Defect, Right atrial myxoma, Ebstein's anomaly repair, MIDCAB).
3. *Fast-Track MICS for combined left and right heart pathology* (Mitral and Tricuspid valve surgery, Aortic, Mitral, and Tricuspid valve surgery, Atrial septal defect, Left atrial myxoma with a large pedicle).

Cardioplegia

Myocardial protection is typically performed antegradely in the aortic root, with a purse-string suture placed on the right side of the ascending aorta. The preferred solutions are Del Nido or Custodiol. TEE control of the aortic root is mandatory during cardioplegia administration, as well as verification of left ventricular filling. In most patients without aortic pathology, cardioplegia can be safely delivered via the aortic root. In patients with aortic regurgitation, it is feasible to administer it through the minithoracotomy using a Long-Debakey cannula inserted directly into the coronary ostia.

In reoperative cardiac interventions or in the absence of aorto-iliac disease, it is preferable to use an endoaortic balloon occlusion (EABO), which provides an arterial line, antegrade cardioplegia, and aortic root suction capability.

The aortic clamp has also evolved in minimally invasive procedures. The Chitwood® DeBakey (see Fig. 5.3) clamp with a rigid body is used when placing

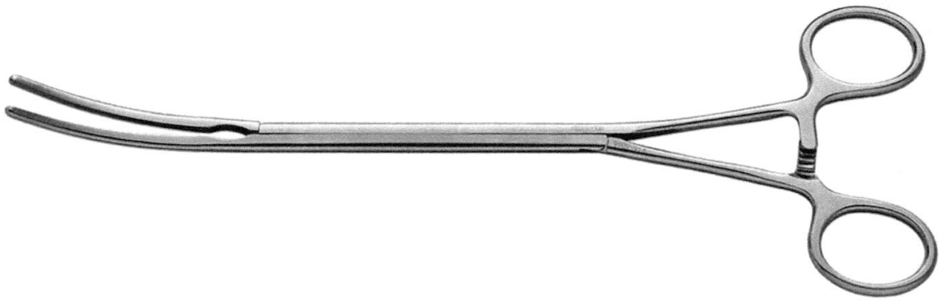

Fig. 5.3 Chitwood® transthoracic aortic clamp

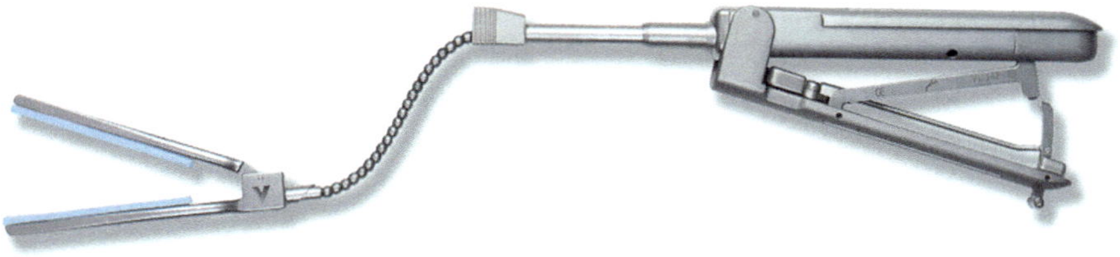

Fig. 5.4 Cygnet® Aortic flexible clamp

the clamp through a dedicated port, though it can also be placed via the minithoracotomy port (albeit somewhat inconveniently). This clamp is also widely used in endoscopic and Da Vinci® robotic procedures [2].

The flexible aortic clamps, Cygnet® or Cosgrove®, are quite commonly used in minimally invasive (see Fig. 5.4) and endoscopic surgeries. They have a fast-track purpose, allowing greater mobility of the ascending aorta and enabling atraumatic displacement of the clamped aorta towards and away from the chest wall. They are very suitable for multivalvular surgeries (mitral and aortic valve surgery or 3-valve procedures) and are very convenient for placement through the minithoracotomy working port.

Surgical Approach

Upper ministernotomy is performed for aortic valve surgery, as well as for replacement of the ascending aorta, and later became possible for aortic root surgery as well. Lower ministernotomy is feasible in some patients for mitral valve surgery and for atrial septal defect repair. It is preferable to first use long surgical instruments in these ministernotomy approaches to gain experience with the new tools—afterward, it is more appropriate to transition to minithoracotomy. The first minithoracotomies (in aortic valve surgery) were performed on the anterior chest wall, in the second or third intercostal space (with or without rib disinsertion) using peripheral cannulation. Later, with the development of valve ligation systems (Knot-pusher or Cor-Knot®) and improvements in valve exposure techniques, the minithoracotomy incision could be moved toward the anterior axillary line.

Similarly, for mitral valve surgery, the initial minithoracotomy is typically performed in the fourth intercostal space, submammary, on the anterolateral side. Subsequently, better exposure can be achieved in the third or fourth intercostal space at the anterior axillary line, although this position is slightly farther from the mitral complex.

Minimally invasive cardiac surgery is also feasible for multivalvular pathology in patients with acceptable thoracic cavity parameters [4–6].

Once these techniques have been refined, it became possible to use a 5 mm or 10 mm endoscope (the 10 mm version providing a broader video recording of the operative field). With the entire team able to visualize the progress of the

Table 5.1 Surgical invasiveness from Carpantier-Loulmet classification

		Incision length	Vision
Level I	Mini-incision	10–12 cm	Direct-vision
Level II	Micro-incision	4–6 cm	Video-assisted
Level III	Micro- or port incision	1–2 cm	Video-directed
Level IV	Port incision with robotic instruments	1–2 cm	Video-directed

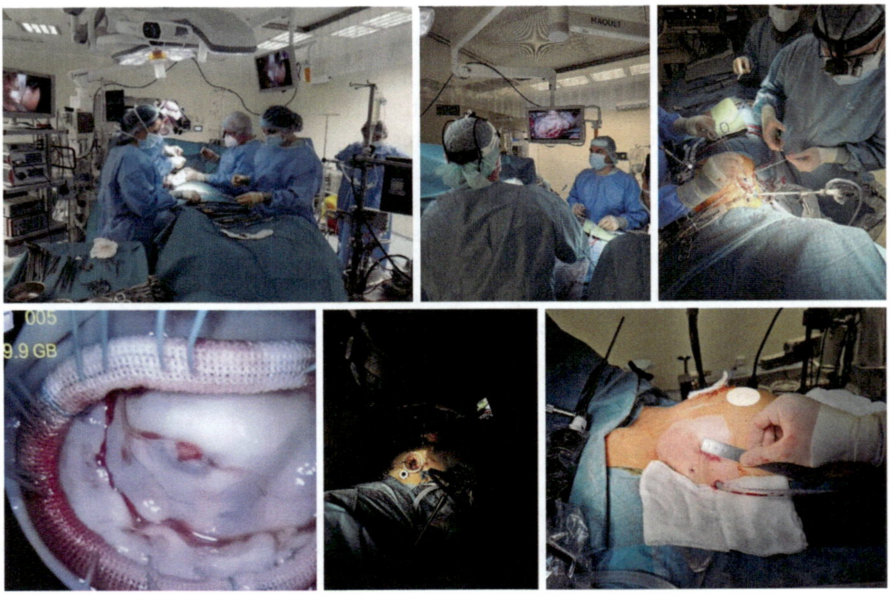

Fig. 5.5 Direct-vision transaxillary Mitral valve plasty

intervention, the thoracoscopic approach can be made even smaller—approximately 2–3 cm—without the need for a metal intercostal retractor, thereby avoiding this source of surgical trauma (see Table 5.1). It is possible to use only an Alexis® wound protector.

In 1996, Carpentier performed the first video-assisted mitral valve repair, through a minithoracotomy using cold fibrillatory arrest, followed soon enough by a surgical team from East Carolina University.

Minimally Invasive Mitral Valve Surgery

After the development of techniques and technologies, it became faster to perform Direct-vision procedures through a 3–4 cm incision (see Fig. 5.5), and Video-assisted procedures through a 2–3 cm incision (see Fig. 5.6). The working port needs to be at least 2–3 cm to allow for the protected insertion of the valve ring or valve prosthesis.

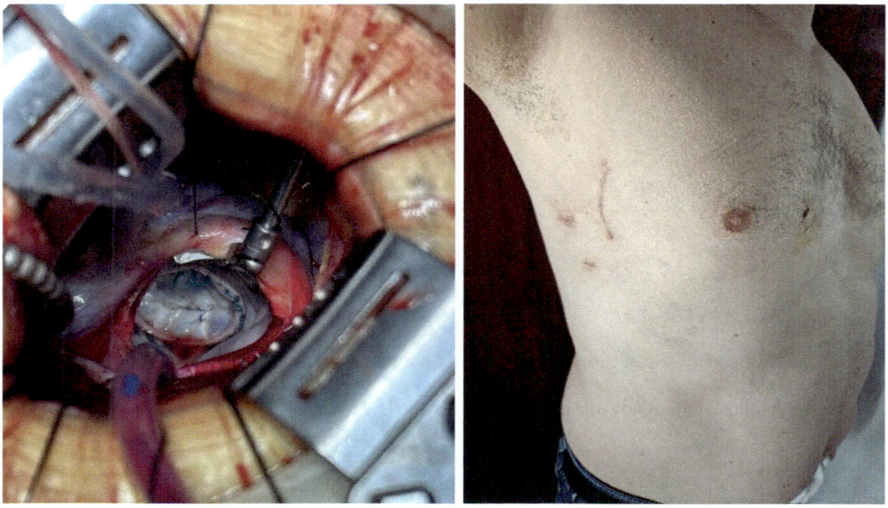

Fig. 5.6 Endoscopic video-assisted mitral valve plasty with 2 monitors

Minimally Invasive Aortic Valve Surgery and Ascending Aorta

Aortic valve surgery is feasible for most pathologies, including both acquired and congenital malformations. Bicuspid aortic valve disease with stenosis in children and adults (weighing over 35 kg, to allow protected femoral access) can be managed this way. Degenerative aortic valve disease in elderly patients is widely treated through minimally invasive valve replacement—it is also considered an alternative to TAVI (transcatheter aortic valve implantation). The advantage of minimally invasive surgery over TAVI is the option to implant either a biological or a mechanical prosthesis.Aortic valve insufficiency can likewise be corrected through minimally invasive valve reconstruction.The ascending aorta can be replaced via a minimally invasive approach as well, especially with the use of a flexible aortic clamp, as it allows for mobility and non-rigid manipulation of the proximal and distal anastomosis sites.

Thus, minimally invasive aortic valve surgery offers two primary techniques:

1. "Miami Method"—an anterior minithoracotomy in the 2nd intercostal space, with or without disinsertion of the 3rd rib (see Fig. 5.7).
2. Trans-axillary Method—using the 3rd intercostal space at the anterior axillary line (see Figs. 5.8 and 5.9).

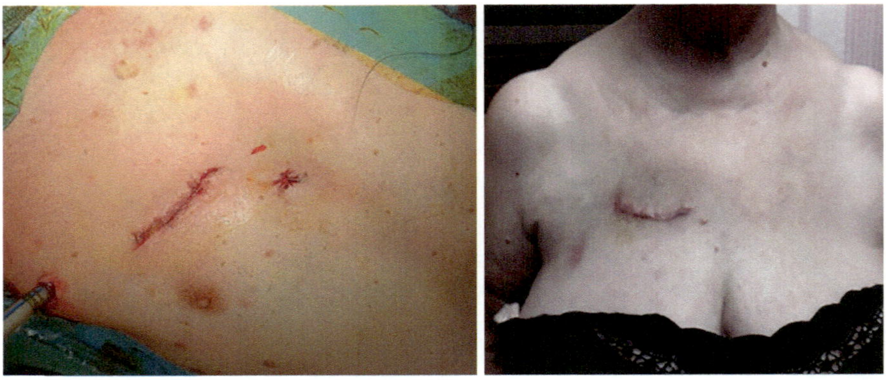

Fig. 5.7 "Miami method" of minimally invasive aortic surgery

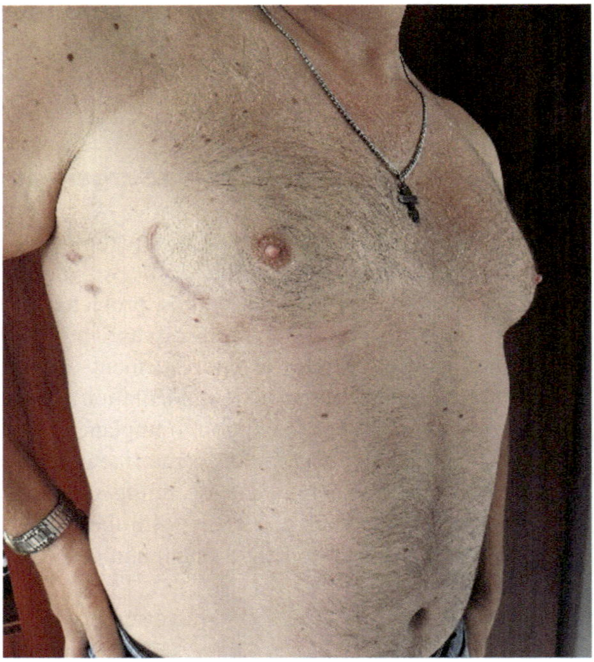

Fig. 5.8 Trans-axillary access for minimally invasive aortic surgery

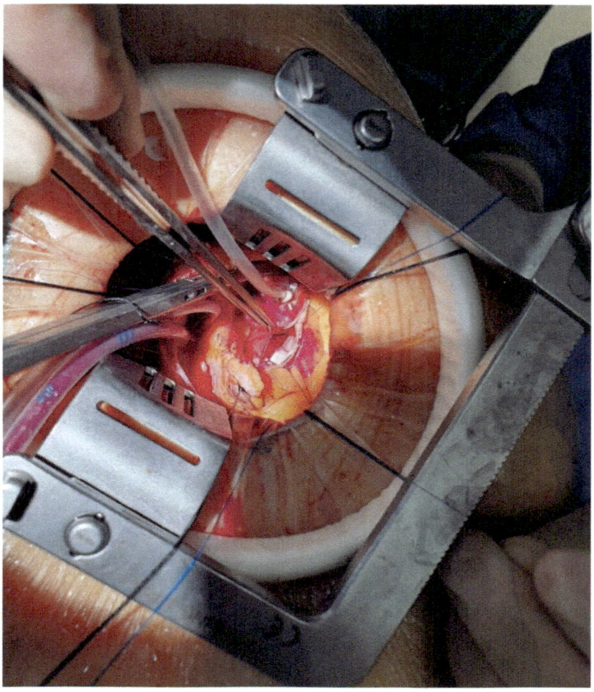

Fig. 5.9 Trans-axillary aortic valve replacement with biological prosthesis and aortic root enlargement, Manouguian technique

Minimally Invasive Direct Coronary Artery Bypass (MIDCAB)

MIDCAB operation is possible to perform for one and all affected coronary arteries via left mini-thoracotomy in the fourth or fifth intercostal space. It is performed with or without cardiopulmonary bypass. The intervention has 2 stages:

1. Mammary artery harvesting with specific retractor (see Fig. 5.10).
2. Performing grafts with simple intercostal retractor (see Fig. 5.11).

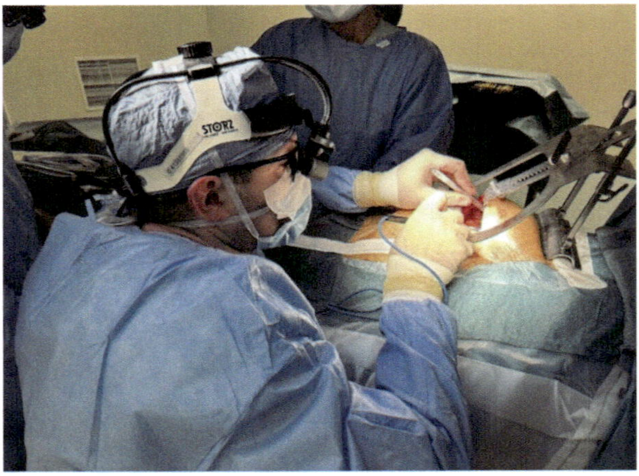

Fig. 5.10 Mammary artery (LIMA) harvesting via fifth intercostal with MIDCAB IMA Retractor

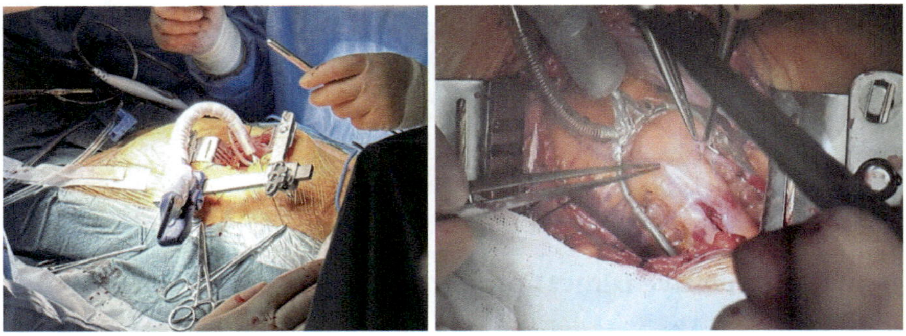

Fig. 5.11 Performing the LIMA-LAD anastomosis with the Octopus tissue stabilizer, OFF-PUMP

Minimally Invasive Complex Surgery (*Mital Valve Plasty: Ring Insertion and 1-Neochord, Tricuspid Valve Plasty and 1 CABG—Saphenous Vein to RCA2*)

With gained experience in all types of minithoracotomies (anterior, anterolateral, and axillary), it is possible to address ischemic lesions of the right coronary artery (RCA) in association with valvular pathology (see Fig. 5.12).

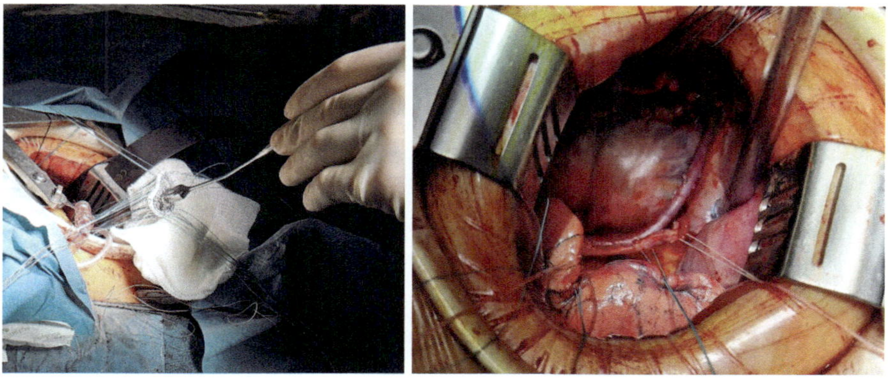

Fig. 5.12 Insertion of the mitral ring. 1 CABG graft (Saphenous vein to right coronary artery)

Minimally Invasive Left Atrial Myxoma Excision

Minimally invasive surgical techniques have gained significant traction and are now standard in mitral, tricuspid, aortic, and coronary surgeries. Left atrial myxoma resection via median sternotomy is established as a safe procedure with low mortality and recurrence rates, still the antero-lateral minithoracotomy approach also provides excellent access to the right atrium, left atrium, aortic root, and interatrial cavity. This approach offers a clear surgical field, enhancing precision during operations. Sondergaard's groove incision and the superior transseptal approach can be effectively performed via minithoracotomy. The superior transseptal approach is reserved for patients with smaller atriums.

Minimally invasive interventions for cardiac myxoma can be addressed through two types of approaches:

- Myxomas with a pedicle insertion smaller than 1 cm^2 can be directly excised through the left atrium.
- Myxomas with a pedicle insertion larger than 1 cm^2 (see Fig. 5.13) require an approach through the right atrium. This access necessitates femoro-jugular cannulation, which also allows for addressing the interatrial septum. With gained experience, it is possible to perform only femoral cannulation using a bicaval (double-stage) cannula (see Fig. 5.14). This cannulation reduces the operative time by approximately 30 minutes.

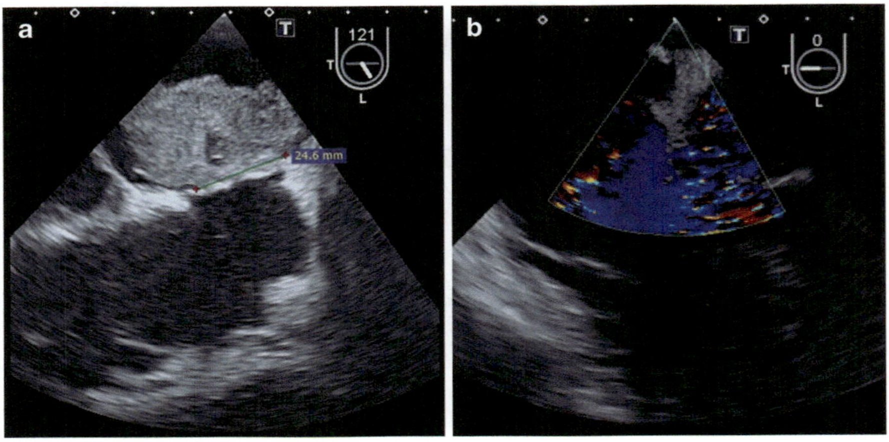

Fig. 5.13 Position of the pedicle insert of the myxoma preoperative(A), and postoperative: septum with autopericardum patch

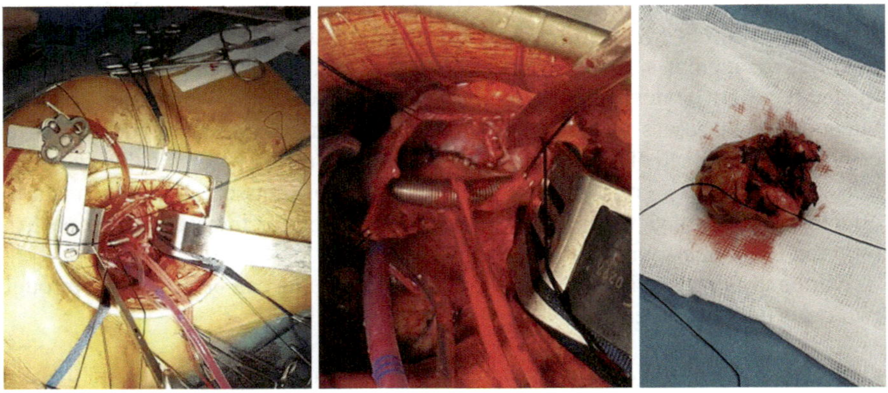

Fig. 5.14 Excision of the myxoma via right anterolateral mini-thoracotomy, only femoral cannulation (intraoperative images)

Minimally Invasive for Pediatric Congenital Heart Defect

The right axillary antero-lateral mini-thoracotomy (see Fig. 5.15) is currently the preferred approach for repairing various moderate congenital heart defects (CHD) in both adults and children as small as 10 kg. This approach offers a direct line of sight to the atrial septum, atrioventricular (AV) valves, and the membranous ventricular septum, facilitating precise repairs. However, it is not recommended for conal septal defects or pulmonary valve procedures, as the right ventricular outflow tract is difficult to access and may result in suboptimal outcomes or residual defects.

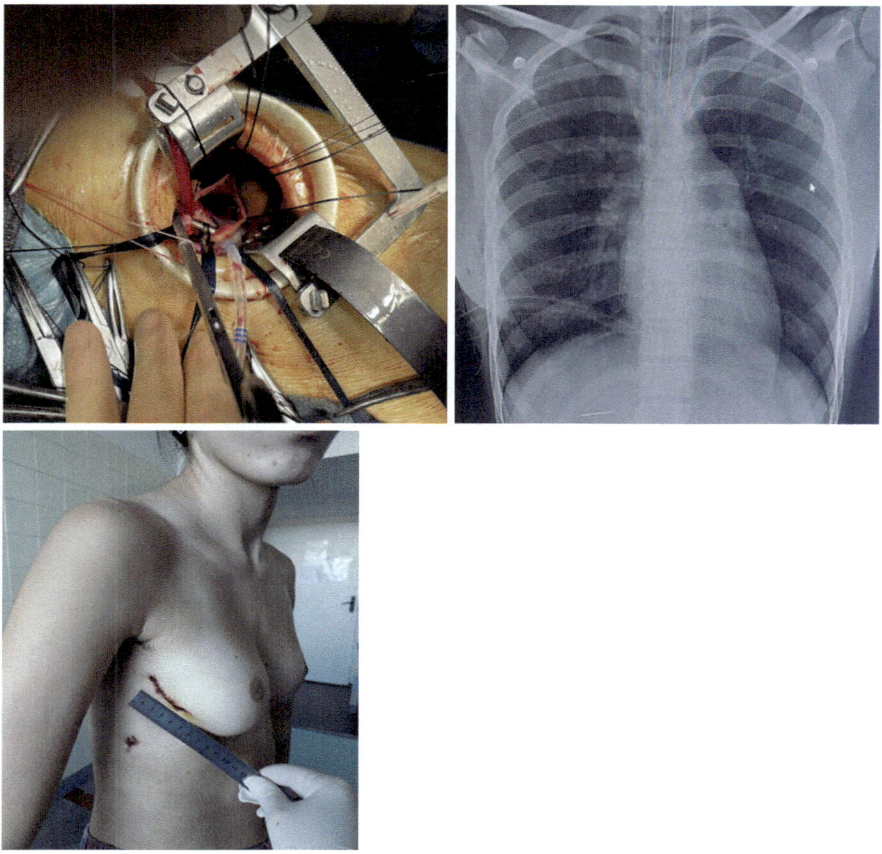

Fig. 5.15 17-year-old girl. Atrial septal defect. Plasty with autologous pericardial patch and tricuspid valve annuloplasty

The axillary region is one of the least muscularly covered parts of the thoracic cage, allowing for less invasive transthoracic access. Additionally, the subaxillary scar is far from the breast and naturally covered by the resting arm, providing excellent cosmetic results regardless of gender.

Initially, this approach was primarily used for closing ostium secundum atrial septal defects (ASD). With increasing experience, its application has expanded to treat other CHDs, such as right-sided pulmonary vein anomalies like PAPVC, including performing the Warden procedure for SVC reinsertion into the right atrial appendage. It has also been used for scimitar vein syndrome, involving off-pump relocation of the anomalous vein to the left atrium, as well as for partial atrioventricular septal defects, subaortic stenosis (SAS), and restrictive peri-membranous ventricular septal defects (VSD).

Overall, this approach combines safety, efficacy, and cosmetic advantages, making it a versatile choice for a broad range of moderate CHD repairs.

Conclusions

- Minimally invasive interventions can be utilized for various heart pathologies, including valvular diseases, tumors, myocardial revascularization, and congenital anomalies. Early clinical results indicated significant advantages, such as reduced surgical trauma, minimal discomfort, quicker recovery times, and a lower risk of infections among all patients.
- In this article, transition from minimally invasive to fully endoscopic heart structural surgery has proved beneficial for patients. The approach featured several advantages, such as smaller incisions, no need for undermining the wound, and the elimination of rib spreading to facilitate better access. The findings indicated enhanced patient outcomes, including less postoperative bleeding and pain, shorter hospital stays, and improved cosmetic results.
- The performed technique for myxoma excision complies with the main oncological criteria of removing the tumor en complex with the interatrial septum. Avoidance of jugular cannulation in minimally invasive cardiac operations reduces trauma.

References

1. Schwartz DS, Ribakove GH, Grossi EA, et al. Minimally invasive cardiopulmonary bypass with cardioplegic arrest: a closed chest technique with equivalent myocardial protection. J Thorac Cardiovasc Surg. 1996;111:556–66.
2. Bates MJ, Randolph Chitwood W Jr. Minimally invasive and robotic approaches to mitral valve surgery: transthoracic aortic crossclamping is optimal. JTCVS Tech. 2021;10:84–8. https://doi.org/10.1016/j.xjtc.2021.09.034.
3. Ramchandani M, Al Jabbari O, Abu Saleh WK, Ramlawi B. Cannulation strategies and pitfalls in minimally invasive cardiac surgery. Methodist Debakey Cardiovasc J. 2016;12(1):10–3.
4. Pfannmuller B, Davierwala P, Hirnle G, et al. Concomitant tricuspid valve repair in patients with minimally invasive mitral valve surgery. Ann Cardiothorac Surg. 2013;2:758–64.
5. Mihos CG, Pineda AM, Davila H, Larrauri-Reyes MC, Santana O. Combined mitral and tricuspid valve surgery performed via a right minithoracotomy approach. Innovations (Phila). 2015;10:304–8.
6. Lamelas J. Minimally invasive concomitant aortic and mitral valve surgery: the “Miami Method”. Ann Cardiothorac Surg. 2015;4:33–7.

6 Minimally Invasive Aortic Valve Surgery

Kerem Oral, Mehmet Ezelsoy, and Belhhan Akpinar

Introduction

Minimally invasive aortic valve surgery is an alternative technique to conventional aortic valve surgery. This technique is characterized by smaller chest incisions compared to those made in sternotomy.

The first minimally invasive AVR (MIAVR) was performed via thoracotomy in 1993 [1]. In 1996, Cosgrove reported the use of mini sternotomy [2]. With the increasing popularity of the transcatheter aortic valve replacement (TAVI) procedure conducted by interventional cardiologists for managing aortic valve disorders, it has prompted cardiac surgery to advance and enhance its practices in this area. Besides having improved cosmetic results MIAVR is associated with less pain, less blood transfusions, less respiratory and wound complications as well as reduced hospital stay. However, most of the studies comparing these techniques are retrospective or propensity score-matched studies which should preclude us from drawing definitive conclusions [3].

One benefit of MIAVR is the avoidance of unnecessary dissections, as it targets only the essential area of the heart. By not fully opening the pericardium, there will be fewer adhesions if a subsequent procedure is needed in the future [4].

The most common approach of minimally invasive aortic valve surgery is widely accepted upper J-sternotomy extending into the right third or fourth intercostal space. Other techniques include right anterior mini thoracotomy (RAT) (with or without endoscopic assistance), right parasternal approach, and transverse sternotomy. The other two techniques will be briefly discussed as they are not widely adopted.

K. Oral · M. Ezelsoy · B. Akpinar (✉)
Cardiovascular Surgery Department, Koc University Hopsital, Istanbul, Turkey

G. Tinică, A. Burlacu (eds.), *Surgical, Hybrid and Minimally Invasive Structural Cardiac Interventions*, https://doi.org/10.1007/978-3-032-16676-0_6

Preoperative Workup

For a successful minimally invasive aortic valve surgery (MIAVS), the patient must be thoroughly evaluated preoperatively, and the surgical plan should be made in advance. The patient's peripheral and cerebrovascular disease, chronic obstructive pulmonary disease (COPD), chest deformity, and history of previous cardiac surgery are all important for the operations as well as coronary artery disease.

To evaluate these conditions, carotid and vertebral color Doppler ultrasonography is routinely performed in all patients with a history of stroke or transient ischemic attack. Chest X-ray imaging does not provide sufficient information about the lungs and thorax. Therefore, contrast-enhanced thoracic computed tomography (CT) should be routinely performed in patients undergoing MIAVS. The lungs should be evaluated in detail for sequelae of previous pneumonia, pneumothorax, pleural adhesions, and the condition of the parenchyma.

In addition, thoracic CT can be used to evaluate the sternum, chest deformities, and retrosternal structures, and is particularly important in the right anterior thoracotomy (RAT) approach.

In patients undergoing MIAVS, peripheral arterial cannulation may be required. To prevent systemic embolisms and dissections that may occur during retrograde arterial perfusion, CT angiography of the lower extremities, pelvis, abdomen, and thorax should be performed. The presence of soft and irregular plaques, and the diameter and tortuosity of the iliofemoral vessels are crucial for selecting the appropriate cannulation site. The size, calcification, and deviation of the ascending aorta, aortic root, and thoracic aorta are also evaluated through the same imaging.

Coronary angiography should be performed in all patients, and the presence of coronary lesions should not preclude MIAVS. Patients eligible for percutaneous coronary intervention before or after surgery should be carefully evaluated, and it should be remembered that minimally invasive procedures can be part of hybrid procedures.

Intraoperative Consideration

A coordinated surgical team is essential to safely perform MIAVS. The collaboration of an experienced anesthesiologist, perfusionist, nurse, and echocardiologist will directly affect the success of the operation. Transesophageal echocardiography (TEE) must be routinely performed intraoperatively.

A single-lumen endotracheal tube may be used although not a must. Even if a thoracotomy is performed, lung retraction can be achieved with mechanical retractors.

Carbon dioxide field flooding can help remove trapped air after the procedure when venting options are restricted. Consequently, passive and some active de-airing can be enhanced by displacing air in the cardiac chambers with CO2, which is highly soluble.

Cannulation Techniques

To operate through small incisions and narrow surgical fields, small and flexible cannulas and instruments may be required. During cardiopulmonary bypass (CPB), proper functioning of the cannula and cross-clamp is critical for a safe MIAVS. This is vital for the procedure, also increases the surgeon's comfort during the operation.

It is very important to decide whether cannulation will be peripheral or central. If peripheral cannulation is chosen, the decision of whether it is performed percutaneously or via surgical incision depends on the appropriateness of the cannula and the surgeon's preference.

Peripheral arterial cannulation can be performed via the femoral or axillary artery. Depending on the MIAVS method used, aortic cannulation can also be done directly on the ascending aorta. Peripheral venous cannulation can be achieved through the right internal jugular vein and femoral vein. Recently, dual-stage cannulas, which are inserted through a single vein, have become increasingly common as an alternative for venous drainage. Regardless of the method, the position of the cannulas must be confirmed with TEE.

This system is routinely used in our hospital and rarely causes drainage issues. One of the most common venous drainage methods is percutaneous femoral vein and direct cannulation of the superior vena cava. Aortic cross-clamping is another step that must be decided during the operation. Although direct cross-clamping of the aorta is the first choice, alternatives such as endoaortic balloon catheters and transaxillary clamping techniques may be used.

Surgical Techniques

Regardless of the surgical technique used, ensuring safe cannulation and cross-clamp placement, and protecting the myocardium are among the most important objectives. After the surgical technique is applied, there must be easy access to the aortic valve, ascending aorta, and aortic arch without compromising surgical comfort. Additionally, in case of a complication, it should be easy to convert to a standard incision. Although many MIAVS techniques have been described, for the sake of simplicity, we can categorize them into four groups (Fig. 6.1):

1. Upper Hemisternotomy (J-Sternotomy)
2. Right Anterior Thoracotomy
3. Transverse Thoracotomy
4. Right Parasternal Approach

Upper Ministernotomy Approach (J-Sternotomy)

The upper ministernotomy approach has been commonly used in MIAVS procedures. The short and safe learning curve has increased the interest in this method. The aortic valve, ascending aorta, and aortic arch are reached through a narrow but deep field, allowing for the surgery to be completed with good exposure.

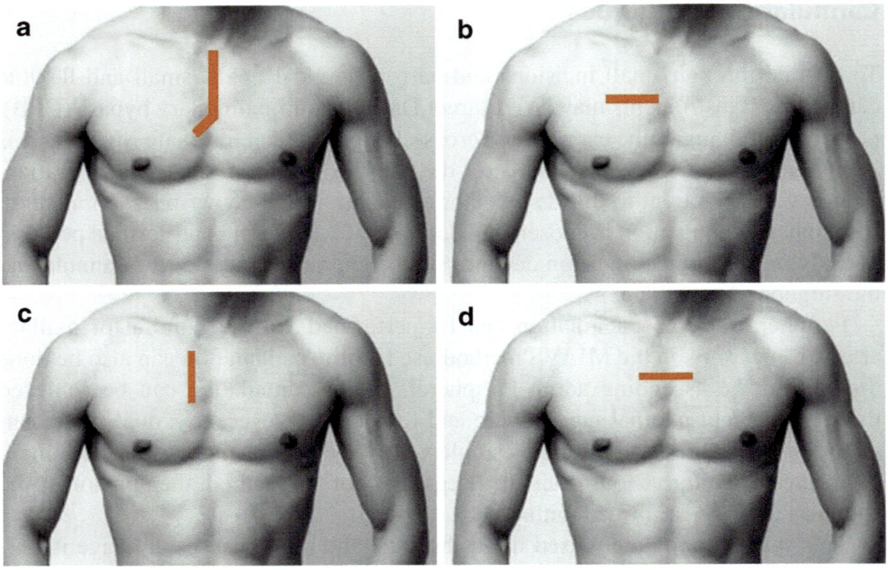

Fig. 6.1 Minimally invasive approaches for aortic valve. (**a**) J-Sternotomy; (**b**) right anterior minithoracotomy; (**c**) right parasternal approach; (**d**) transverse sternotomy. The minimally invasive incision is marked by line. (Image courtesy Ela Ezelsoy)

In this approach, a partial median sternotomy is performed to form a "J" shape toward the right third or fourth intercostal space. Depending on the surgical preference, an "L" or inverted "T" shape can also be used. In this method, venous and arterial cannulation is generally performed directly on the heart and ascending aorta. Sometimes the access to the right atrium can be difficult, especially in cases of long aortas. In these patients, percutaneous femoral venous canulation can be a good option.

After administering general anesthesia, a transthoracic echocardiogram is performed, and the third/fourth intercostal space is distinctly indicated. A saline bag is positioned beneath the shoulder blades to lift the sternum, and external defibrillator pads are applied. Subsequently, a mini sternotomy (upper J type) is carried out in the identified intercostal space. A specially designed sternal retractor (Estech, USA) is utilized to delicately widen the sternum. The patient receives heparin, and the pericardium is opened and secured to the surrounding skin. Cannulation of the ascending aorta and femoral vein is completed, and cardiopulmonary bypass (CPB) is sustained at a temperature of 32 °C with vacuum assistance for venous drainage (Fig. 6.2). In each case, a vent for the right upper pulmonary vein is inserted.

Following the cross-clamping of the aorta, a tepid blood cardioplegic solution is administered, and an oblique aortotomy is performed. The aortic valve and coronary ostia are assessed, and transaortic venting is intermittently carried out after the resection of the valve. The prosthetic aortic valve is positioned using separate pledget sutures in every case. Subsequently, the aortotomy is closed, and de-airing is

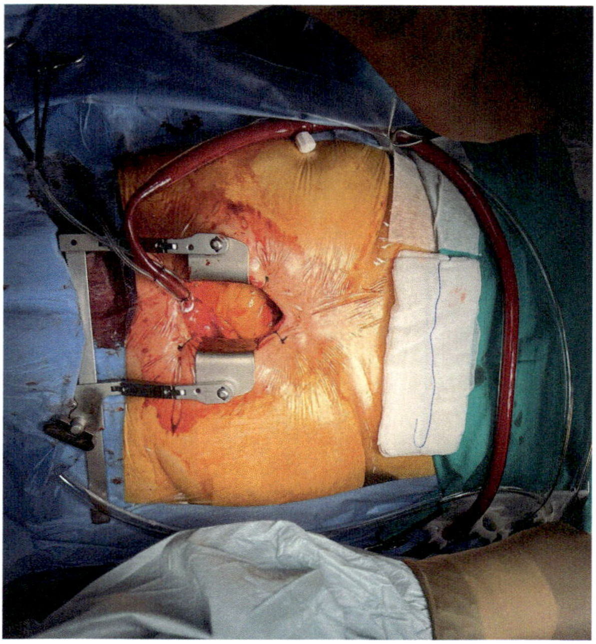

Fig. 6.2 Cannulation sites (ascending aorta and right femoral vein). (Image courtesy CORCYM)

done with the assistance of TOE. Two epicardial pacing wires are inserted, and the patient is gradually weaned off cardiopulmonary bypass (CPB).

One drain is placed in the pericardial space and another in the mediastinum under the sternum (Fig. 6.3). The sternum is closed with three/four wires, and TOE is utilized to check for any pericardial fluid accumulation until the patient leaves the operating room.

Right Anterior Thoracotomy (RAT)

The right anterior thoracotomy approach is one of the most frequently used methods for minimally invasive aortic valve surgery. In this technique, a 4-5 cm incision is made along the anterior axillary line, through the second intercostal space. The pectoralis major muscle is dissected, and the intercostal muscles are incised. After entering the thoracic cavity, a soft tissue retractor and rib retractor are placed. If necessary, one rib can be resected to increase the surgical field.

All patients must undergo a CT scan to clarify the spatial relationship between the intercostal spaces, the ascending aorta, and the aortic valve. Patients can only be considered for this incision if they meet the following conditions: (1) at the level of the main pulmonary artery, more than half of the ascending aorta is positioned to the right of the right sternal border; (2) the distance from the ascending aorta to the sternum does not exceed 10 cm; (3) the angle (the angle formed between the midline and the incline of the ascending aorta) must be greater than 45 degrees (Fig. 6.4).

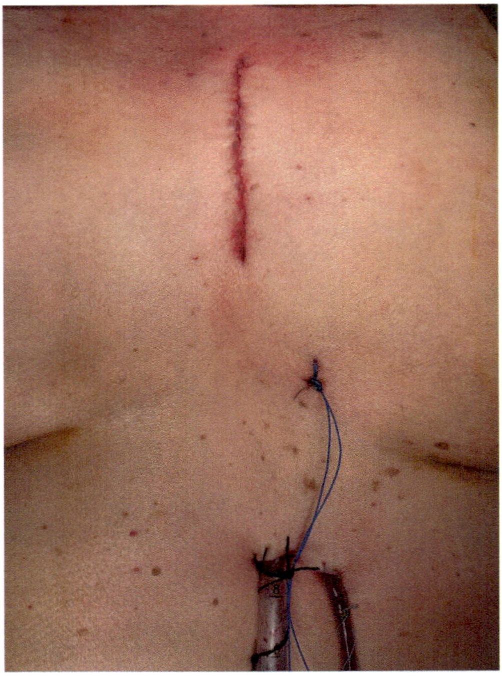

Fig. 6.3 Postoperative scar after aortic valve replacement through a J-sternotomy. (Image courtesy Edwards Intuity)

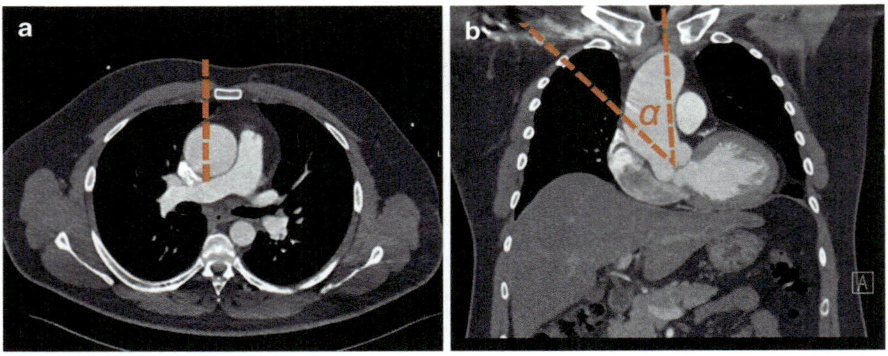

Fig. 6.4 Chest CT-scan preoperative evaluation. (**a**) In the axial view of thorax CT-scans, the ideal exposure of the ascending aorta is more than half of its circumference right sided with respect to parasternal line (scatted line), (**b**) in the coronal view of thorax CT-scans the ideal angle between midline (vertical scatted line) and ascending aorta (obliquus scatted line) is 45° (α angle)

The criteria for excluding the right thoracotomy method include previous cardiac surgery and a history of right-sided radiotherapy. Both parasternal and transverse sternotomy incisions have been discontinued because of complications.

A right anterior thoracotomy is performed through a skin incision 4–5 cm, positioned at the level of the second intercostal space. A soft tissue retractor is placed into the thoracotomy, and a flexible cannula is used for direct aortic cannulation. Next, a percutaneous cannula is advanced via the femoral vein into the right atrium to facilitate venous drainage under transesophageal echocardiography guidance and using the Seldinger technique. Once vacuum-assisted cardiopulmonary bypass (CPB) is established, a left ventricular vent is introduced through the right superior pulmonary vein. Subsequently, the ascending aorta is clamped, and antegrade tepid blood cardioplegic solution is administered either into the aortic root or selectively directed to the coronary ostia.

Since the aortic valve is accessed from a distance and at an angle, special instruments and flexible shaft devices are required. In this technique, the aortic valve is reached through a narrow and shallow surgical field. Compared to the sternotomy approach, it has a more advantageous cosmetic appearance and less postoperative pain [5].

Transverse Thoracotomy

In this technique, a transverse incision is made along the third or fourth intercostal space. A rib retractor is used to expand the surgical area. This approach is particularly preferred in reoperations. The most significant advantage of this method is its cosmetic appearance, as the incision can be made submammary or under the breast in women.However, this approach is rarely used today due to limited exposure and the risk of bleeding from the internal thoracic artery.

Right Parasternal Approach

In this technique, the incision is made just lateral to the sternum, and part of the costal cartilages is resected. It was one of the first described minimally invasive approaches for aortic valve surgery. However, it has fallen out of favor because the limited field of vision complicates the surgery and may lead to more bleeding.

A significant drawback of the parasternal approach was the high rate of lung herniation, which frequently necessitated a subsequent procedure to fix the defect.

Totally Endoscopic Aortic Valve Replacement (TEAVR)

Based on the technique described by Dr. Alaaddin Yilmaz.

Surgical Technique Summary

The totally endoscopic aortic valve replacement (TEAVR) technique, developed by Dr. Alaaddin Yilmaz and his team, aims to provide complete aortic valve replacement without sternotomy using a full endoscopic approach [7]. The operation is performed through five trocars placed in the right hemithorax, allowing for optimal access and visualization.

Peripheral cardiopulmonary bypass is established via the femoral artery and vein. A transthoracic aortic clamp is used, followed by antegrade cardioplegia administration. A transverse aortotomy is performed to expose the aortic valve. After excision of the calcified native valve and annular decalcification, a conventional sutured bioprosthetic valve is implanted.

Step-by-Step Approach

1. Patient is positioned in lateral decubitus. Five trocars are inserted in the right hemithorax.
2. Femoral cannulation is performed and cardiopulmonary bypass is initiated.
3. The aorta is clamped transthoracically and antegrade cardioplegia is administered.
4. Transverse aortotomy is made. The native valve is excised and annulus is decalcified.
5. The bioprosthetic valve is implanted using conventional sutures.
6. The aortotomy is closed and CPB is weaned off.

Advantages

- No sternotomy required—fully endoscopic approach
- Reduced postoperative pain and shorter hospital stay
- Superior cosmetic outcomes
- Ideal for low-risk or younger patients

Challenges and Learning Curve

TEAVR requires advanced experience in minimally invasive cardiac surgery [8]. Mastery of endoscopic visualization, precise port placement, and management of peripheral CPB are critical to the success of the procedure.

Postoperative Period

In patients undergoing minimally invasive aortic valve surgery, postoperative management is similar to that of patients undergoing conventional surgery. However, due to the minimally invasive nature of the procedure, extubation, mobilization, and hospital discharge typically occur earlier [5].

The most common complications are related to peripheral cannulation sites and vascular injuries: hematoma, bleeding, pseudoaneurysm, limb ischemia, seroma, and prolonged lymph leak following dissection of the groin vessels may be encountered [6]. If there is suspicion of any of these, the patient should be evaluated promptly with Doppler ultrasonography or contrast-enhanced imaging. If endoaortic balloon occlusion is used, potential aortic dissection should also be considered.

In addition, all patients should be evaluated postoperatively with echocardiography to assess the prosthetic valve and ventricular function and to detect any pericardial effusion.

Sutureless Aortic Valves

The first sutureless aortic valve was used by Hufnagel in 1952. Over the past two decades, it has re-emerged as a rapidly evolving technology. The "Perceval" valve, developed by Sorin, is a stentless valve made from bovine pericardium mounted on a nitinol frame (Fig. 6.5). The pericardial tissue used in this valve has a

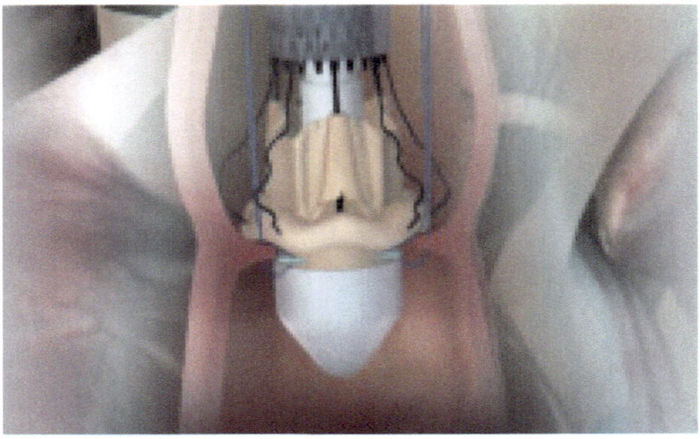

Fig. 6.5 Perceval valve implantation

long-standing history of application in other bioprostheses with proven long-term outcomes, whereas the Perceval valve itself currently has mid-term follow-up data available [9].

The Sorin Perceval valve is particularly favored in minimally invasive cases due to the limited surgical field [10]. Its ease of implantation deep into the aortic root, lack of need for suture tying, and the ability to reposition the valve intraoperatively make it highly suitable for such cases. In contrast to conventional valves, this prosthesis can be seated into the aortic root more quickly and easily using a dedicated holder system after resection of the native valve via a higher transverse aortotomy.

Given the height of the Perceval valve and its pre-mounted state on the holder, the aortotomy incision should be made approximately 2 cm above the sinotubular junction (STJ). Upon deployment, the valve self-expands into the Valsalva sinuses. If a standard aortotomy is performed too close to the STJ, the struts of the valve may protrude outside the incision, complicating closure of the aortotomy.

For implantation, the valve is sized after native valve excision. Three guiding sutures are placed at the midpoint of each leaflet and passed through the corresponding loops on the valve. The prosthesis is then seated at the annular level. After deployment, the guide sutures are removed. As the valve is seated in a nitinol frame, thermal expansion is achieved by applying warm saline, allowing the nitinol to fully expand. Once correct positioning is confirmed, a brief balloon dilation (~30 seconds, 4 atm) can be performed to ensure optimal sealing. During aortotomy closure, sutures must not be passed through the nitinol frame.

Rapid Deployment Bioprostheses

Although not completely sutureless, another rapidly implantable valve system is the "Intuity" valve developed by Edwards. Unlike the Perceval valve, Intuity features a balloon-expandable stented design. It consists of the company's "Magna Ease" bioprosthesis mounted onto a balloon-expandable subannular frame. Its durability is considered equivalent to that of conventional bioprosthetic valves [11].

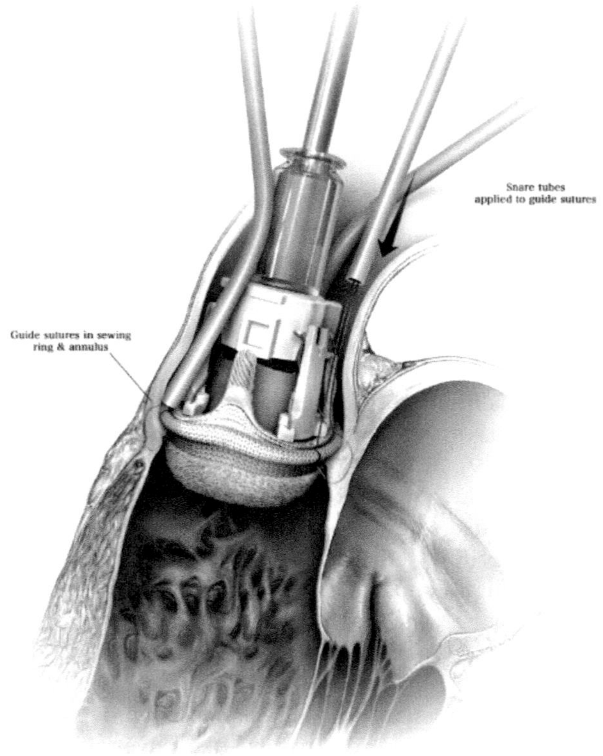

Fig. 6.6 Deployment of Edwards Intuity Elite valve

The Edwards Intuity Elite represents the second-generation design. Due to the thicker stent of the initial model, the Elite version was introduced with improvements. During implantation, three guiding sutures are placed through the center of each cusp and are tied after valve deployment (Fig. 6.6). Initially, a transverse aortotomy above the STJ was recommended. However, anatomical challenges in some patients—especially difficulties in seating the valve and tying guiding sutures—led to a return to the traditional oblique aortotomy approach.

Both the Perceval and Intuity valves can be implanted more quickly than conventional prostheses, offering a significant reduction in aortic cross-clamp and cardiopulmonary bypass (CPB) times, particularly advantageous during minimally invasive AVR procedures [12]. While suitable for calcific aortic stenosis, these valves are not recommended in pure aortic regurgitation, as they rely on annular calcification for anchoring.

Transcatheter Aortic Valve Implantation (TAVI)

Introduction

Transcatheter aortic valve implantation (TAVI), also known as transcatheter aortic valve replacement (TAVR), has revolutionized the treatment of severe aortic stenosis, particularly in patients at high or prohibitive surgical risk. Since its first successful human use in 2002, TAVI has undergone substantial refinement and has become a less invasive alternative to surgical aortic valve replacement (SAVR). The procedure typically involves transfemoral access and eliminates the need for sternotomy and cardiopulmonary bypass.

Indications

TAVI is primarily indicated in patients with symptomatic severe aortic stenosis who are inoperable or at high surgical risk. Severe stenosis is defined by an aortic valve area $<1.0\ cm^2$, a mean gradient >40 mmHg, or a peak velocity >4 m/s. Patient evaluation is conducted by a multidisciplinary Heart Team that considers anatomy, comorbidities, and life expectancy. Recently, TAVI indications have expanded to include intermediate and low-risk patients, reflecting the growing body of evidence for its safety and efficacy [13].

Technical Considerations

The transfemoral approach is the preferred access route due to its minimally invasive nature and superior outcomes [14]. Comprehensive pre-procedural imaging, particularly multidetector CT (MDCT), is essential for evaluating annular size, vascular access, and calcification. The valve is delivered retrogradely through the femoral artery and deployed under fluoroscopic and echocardiographic guidance. Valve choice—balloon-expandable vs. self-expanding—depends on patient-specific factors.

The transapical approach is reserved for patients with unsuitable femoral anatomy. This involves a left anterolateral thoracotomy, with antegrade delivery through the left ventricular apex into the aortic valve and descending aorta. Transapical or transaortic access is considered in patients with narrow iliofemoral vessels.

Outcomes and Complications

Clinical trials have shown that TAVI provides outcomes comparable to SAVR in selected patients, with faster recovery and improved quality of life [15]. Nevertheless, complications such as vascular injury, paravalvular regurgitation, conduction disturbances requiring permanent pacemaker placement, and stroke must be considered.

In the PARTNER 1A trial involving high-risk operable patients with symptomatic severe aortic stenosis, all-cause 30-day mortality was 3.4% in the TAVI group versus 6.5% in the SAVR group ($P = 0.07$), and 1-year mortality was 24.2% vs. 26.8%, respectively ($P = 0.44$). Functional capacity and quality of life improvements in elderly patients were comparable to those in younger patients [16].

In the PARTNER 1B trial comparing TAVI to medical therapy (including balloon valvuloplasty) in inoperable patients, early and late mortality was significantly higher in the medically treated group (50% at 1 year and 90% at 5 years). At 1 year, NYHA class III–IV symptoms were significantly lower in the TAVI group (25.2% vs. 58.0%, $P < 0.001$) [17].

Ongoing innovations in valve design and procedural techniques continue to improve outcomes and reduce complication rates [18].

Discussion

New incisions foreign to traditional cardiac surgeons are now being touted as a new answer to approach cardiac structures.

Aortic valve disease is one of the most common structural heart diseases. Since the first AVR through median sternotomy in 1964, surgeons have been operating conveniently using this method. However, destroying the integrity of the sternum can lead to poor healing especially in elderly and osteoporotic patients and this is a shortcoming affecting postoperative recovery.

Evidence so far demonstrates that MIAVR is associated with a similar mortality and stroke rates as conventional AVR and minimally invasive cardiac surgery is becoming increasingly common [5]. However, as per the Society of Thoracic Surgeons only 22% of cardiac surgical operations are minimally invasive which suggests a reluctance in utilizing these techniques [19].

The major benefit of minimal access aortic valve surgery lies in reducing the trauma associated with gaining exposure without compromising surgical results. Some of the theoretical advantages of these approaches such as decreased postoperative pain, rapid convalescence and early return to work have been confirmed in several clinical studies. However, it must be kept in mind that most of these are retrospective, or propensity score-matched studies. Other suggested benefits such as decreased postoperative complications and other advantages over conventional sternotomy remain to be proven. In addition, quality of life issues including satisfaction with the procedure discomfort and performance of daily activities are difficult to evaluate retrospectively [20].

Minimally invasive techniques should allow the surgeon to continue utilizing tools and approaches familiar to cardiac operations. Mini-sternotomy employs standard retractors, cannulation, and myocardial protection techniques. Should the surgeon need to have access to the entire heart, simple completion of sternal division provides full cardiac exposure. Our clinical experience with over 200 aortic valve operations suggests that mini sternotomy in combination with standard cannulation techniques allows smaller pericardial drainage devices resulting in early extubation, decreased length of stay, and improved patient comfort and outcome.

Limited data comparing different MIAVR techniques are available. A small right anterolateral thoracotomy may be regarded as less invasive and satisfying for the patient. However, from a technical point of view this technique is more challenging with higher risk of perioperative complications due to peripheral cannulation and difficulty in conversion to sternotomy. Totally endoscopic approaches remain the prerogative of high-volume centers who are specialized in implementing this technique. The prolonged CPB and ischemic times represent a drawback for minimally invasive techniques. However, the utilization of rapid deployment aortic valves and automated fastener devices such as Cor-knot has facilitated the adoption of these minimally invasive techniques.

Results of patients undergoing MIAVR with conventional valves have shown favorable results in terms of decreased length of stay in hospital and lower postoperative complications [21]. However, most of these studies are retrospective. Results of SURE and SURD registry have shown that MIAVR using sutureless valve is a safe and reproducible method [21]. Borger et al. have reported a higher incidence of paravalvular leak in the MIAVR group with sutureless valves [21, 22].

Totally endoscopic aortic valve surgery uses certain ports via a small right lateral thoracotomy. No direct visualization and need for special surgical instruments and peripheric cannulation are the disadvantages of the technique. Although Yilmaz et al. have reported excellent results the reported results are limited, and it remains unknown whether this platform may be adopted safely [7, 8].

Several studies comparing MIAVR with TAVI are available. A study comparing two techniques found a lower incidence of pacemaker implants and paravalvular leaks in the MIAVR group. Moreover, stroke rates and vascular complications were also higher in the TAVİ group. However, survival remained similar between the two groups [17].

The therapy decision-making with aortic valve pathologies is open to debate. Although there are guideline recommendations for conventional AVR and TAVI, there are no clear guideline recommendations for MIAVR. Prospective randomized studies comparing MIAVR with TAVI are needed to address this issue.

Conventional aortic valve surgery will continue to be the approach in patients requiring concomitant surgery. The MIAVR techniques represent a valuable alternative for those patients considered to undergo an isolated AVR. The MIAVR combines the advantage of a surgical AVR coupled with the increasing patient demand for minimally invasive procedures. MIAVR procedures should be available in the armamentariums of every cardiac surgeon. Each surgeon should choose the technique that suits him most in terms of patient safety and optimal results.

References

1. Rao PN, Kumar AS. Aortic valve replacement through right thoracotomy. Texas Heart Inst J. 1993;20:307–8.

2. Cosgrove DL, Sabik JF. Minimally invasive approach for aortic valve operations. Ann Thorac Surg. 1996;62:596–7.
3. Jahangiri M, Hussain A, Akowuah E. Minimally invasive surgical aortic valve replacement. Heart. 2019;105(Suppl 2):s10–5. https://doi.org/10.1136/heartjnl-2018-313512. PMID: 30846519
4. Ogami T, Yokoyama Y, Takagi H, Serna-Gallegos D, Ferdinand FD, Sultan I, Kuno T. Minimally invasive versus conventional aortic valve replacement: the network meta-analysis. J Card Surg 2022;37(12):4868–4874. https://doi.org/10.1111/jocs.17126. Epub 2022 Nov 15. PMID: 36378939.
5. Glauber M, Miceli A, Gilmanov D, Ferrarini M, Bevilacqua S, Farneti PA, Solinas M. Right anterior minithoracotomy versus conventional aortic valve replacement: a propensity score matched study. J Thorac Cardiovasc Surg 2013;145(5):1222–1226. https://doi.org/10.1016/j.jtcvs.2012.03.064. Epub 2012 Apr 18. PMID: 22516391.
6. Ortiz D, Jahangir A, Singh M, Allaqaband S, Bajwa TK, Mewissen MW. Access site complications after peripheral vascular interventions: incidence, predictors, and outcomes Circ Cardiovasc Interv 2014;7(6):821–828. https://doi.org/10.1161/CIRCINTERVENTIONS.114.001306. Epub 2014 Nov 11. PMID: 25389345; PMCID: PMC4529288.
7. Yilmaz A, Van Genechten S, Claessens J, Packlé L, Maessen J, Kaya A. A totally endoscopic approach for aortic valve surgery. Eur J Cardiothorac Surg 2022;62(6):ezac467. https://doi.org/10.1093/ejcts/ezac467. PMID: 36165709.
8. Hosoba S, Ito T, Mori M, Kato R, Kajiyama K, Maeda S, Nakai Y, Morishita Y. Endoscopic aortic valve replacement: initial outcomes of isolated and concomitant surgery Ann Thorac Surg 2023;116(4):744–749. https://doi.org/10.1016/j.athoracsur.2023.04.045. Epub 2023 Jun 3. PMID: 37276923.
9. Szecel D, Eurlings R, Rega F, Verbrugghe P, Meuris B. Perceval Sutureless aortic valve implantation: midterm outcomes. Ann Thorac Surg. 2021;111(4):1331–7. https://doi.org/10.1016/j.athoracsur.2020.06.064.
10. D'Onofrio A, Tessari C, Lorenzoni G, Cibin G, Martinelli G, Alamanni F, et al. Minimally invasive vs conventional aortic valve replacement with rapid-deployment bioprostheses. Ann Thorac Surg. 2021;111(6):1916–22. https://doi.org/10.1016/j.athoracsur.2020.06.150.
11. Davies RA, Bandara TD, Perera NK, Orr Y. Do rapid deployment aortic valves improve outcomes compared with surgical aortic valve replacement? Interact Cardiovasc Thorac Surg. 2016;23:814.
12. Sundt TM, Jneid H. Guideline update on indications for Transcatheter aortic valve replacement. JAMA Cardiol. 2021;6(9):1088–9.
13. Ruparelia N, Prendergast BD. Technical aspects of transcatheter aortic valve implantation (TAVI). E-Journal Cardiol Pract Vol. 14, N° 5 2016.
14. Barbanti M, Webb JG, Gilard M, Capodanno D, Tamburino C. Transcatheter aortic valve implantation in 2017: state of the art. EuroIntervention. 2017;13(AA):AA11–21. https://doi.org/10.4244/EIJ-D-17-00567.
15. Smith CR, Leon MB, Mack MJ, Miller DC, Moses JW, Svensson LG, Tuzcu EM, et al..; PARTNER trial investigators. Transcatheter versus surgical aortic-valve replacement in high-risk patients. N Engl J Med 2011;36423:2187–2198. https://doi.org/10.1056/NEJMoa1103510.
16. Leon MB, Smith CR, Mack M, Miller DC, Moses JW, Svensson LG, Tuzcu EM, et al. PARTNER Trial Investigators. Transcatheter aortic-valve implantation for aortic stenosis in patients who cannot undergo surgery. N Engl J Med. 2010;363(17):1597–607. https://doi.org/10.1056/NEJMoa1008232.
17. Glauber M, Bacco L, Cuenca J, et al. Minimally invasive aortic valve replacement with sutureless valves: results from an international prospective registry. Innovations. 2020;15:120–30.
18. Zaid S, Atkins MD, Kleiman NS, Reardon MJ, Tang GHL. What's new with TAVR? An update on device technology. Methodist Debakey Cardiovasc J. 2023;19(3):4–14. https://doi.org/10.14797/mdcvj.1230. PMID: 37213874; PMCID: PMC10198244.

19. Gundry SR, Shattuck OH, Razzouk AJ, Del Rio MJ, Sardari FF, Bailey LL. Facile minimally invasive cardiac surgery via ministernotomy. Ann Thorac Surg. 1998;65(4):1100–4. https://doi.org/10.1016/s0003-4975(98)00064-2. PMID: 9564935
20. Doll N, Borger MA, Hain J, Bucerius J, Walther T, Gummert JF, Mohr FW. Minimal access aortic valve replacement: effects on morbidity and resource utilization. Ann Thorac Surg. 2002;74(4):S1318–22. https://doi.org/10.1016/s0003-4975(02)03911-5. PMID: 12400808
21. Di Bacco L, Miceli A, Glauber M. Minimally invasive aortic valve surgery. J Thorac Dis 2021;13(3):1945–1959. https://doi.org/10.21037/jtd-20-1968. PMID: 33841981; PMCID: PMC8024826
22. Borger MA, Dohmen PM, Knosalla C, Hammerschmidt R, Merk DR, Richter M, Doenst T, Conradi L, Treede H, Moustafine V, Holzhey DM, Duhay F, Strauch J. Haemodynamic benefits of rapid deployment aortic valve replacement via a minimally invasive approach: 1-year results of a prospective multicentre randomized controlled trial. Eur J Cardiothorac Surg 2016;50(4):713–720. https://doi.org/10.1093/ejcts/ezw042. Epub 2016 Mar 2. PMID: 26935407.

Emerging Role of Hybrid Cardiac Procedures

7

Vladimir Kornovski, Petar Uzov, Yordan Krasnaliev, and Tsvetomir Loukanov

Introduction

Nowadays, cardiac surgery faces the challenge of asserting its effectiveness, competing with interventional cardiologists who are expanding their area of intervention on heart disease. Interventional cardiology is becoming more aggressive, and cardiac surgery is introducing increasingly minimally invasive surgical techniques. At first glance, we can think of a struggle between institutions, but in reality it is a matter of cooperation between them, aiming to provide the best of both specialties in the treatment of heart disease and achieving a long-term result. This cooperation called a hybrid strategy in the treatment of heart disease is defined as a combination of catheter-based treatment methods and minimally invasive surgical intervention. This concept combines the treatment options available only in the catheterization room with the options available only to the surgeon in order to reduce surgical morbidity [1]. The first implementation of a hybrid cardiac procedure is done in 1990 by Angelini et al. and the first results are reported in 1996 [2]. With the progressive

Supplementary Information The online version contains supplementary material available at https://doi.org/10.1007/978-3-032-16676-0_7.

V. Kornovski (✉)
Cardiac Surgery at University Hospital, "Sveta Marina", Varna, Bulgaria
e-mail: v.kornovski@svetamarina.com

P. Uzov
Cardiac Surgery, Heart and Brain Hospital, Burgas, Bulgaria

Y. Krasnaliev
Cardiac Surgery, Heart and Brain Hospital, Pleven, Bulgaria

T. Loukanov
Cardiac Surgery, University Hospital Heidelberg, Heidelberg, Germany
e-mail: tsvetomir.loukanov@med.uni-heidelberg.de

G. Tinică, A. Burlacu (eds.), *Surgical, Hybrid and Minimally Invasive Structural Cardiac Interventions*, https://doi.org/10.1007/978-3-032-16676-0_7

evolution of stent technology along with the adoption of minimally invasive surgical approaches, the hybrid strategy became an alternative to standard surgical or interventional techniques for the treatment of different cardiac pathologies [3]. Thus, hybrid procedures can be discussed in coronary diseased patients with the planning of minimally invasive direct coronary artery bypass (MIDCAB) procedure using LIMA to LAD and PCI of non-LAD coronary arteries. The progress in coronary hybrid procedures go further to totally endoscopic coronary artery bypass (TECAB) as a surgical part of the procedure, using only ports and allows for both single and multivessel revascularization and using single or both mammary arteries for conduits [4]. The next and highest level of hybrid revascularization is the introduction of robotic surgical access to coronary revascularization. The first reported case of robotically assisted hybrid revascularization procedure was by Kiaii et al. in 2005 [5]. In high-risk patients with valvular heart disease and concomitant coronary pathology, evolution of the treatment is PCI procedure followed by minimally invasive valve intervention, on direct vision, endoscopically assisted or totally endoscopic valve intervention. The pathology involving the aortic arch and descending aorta is extremely suitable for a hybrid approach with surgical correction of the aortic arch and simultaneously or at a second stage performing an endovascular procedure for the descending aorta.

Summing up, the hybrid strategy in the treatment of heart disease is finding more and more continuity given the increasing complexity of the pathology and the associated increase in operative risk. The hybrid technique makes it possible to use the advantages of surgical correction, with proven long-term results, but through minimal surgical access, combined with the advantages of interventional cardiology. In order to be beneficiaries of the advantages of the hybrid approach to heart disease, it is extremely important to create a working heart team at the institutional level, to establish a program for the development of minimally invasive and hybrid cardiac surgery, in which all members of that heart team and the patient are fully empathetic.

Current Application of Hybrid Procedures

Coronary Artery Disease

The goal of any treatment for coronary artery disease, medical therapy, coronary artery bypass surgery, or percutaneous coronary intervention (PCI) is withdrawal of the symptoms, prolonging the asymptomatic period, and decreasing the incidence of major cardiovascular and neurological events. Coronary artery bypass grafting (CABG) remains the "gold standard" in the treatment of multivessel coronary artery disease and left main disease and has been proven to be a revascularization method with good long-term results. Trials like ASCERT, FREEDOM, and SYNTAX have reported in terms of survival rates superiority of CABG over PCI [6, 7]. Probable reason for this is 95% of patency at 10 years of the left internal mammary artery (LIMA), accorded to its resistance to atherosclerosis and the release of nitric oxide in the coronary circulation, anastomosed to LAD, and no other method of revascularization is known to surpass this result [7–10]. Despite the level of recommendation by the ESC/EACTS 2018 guidelines to use more than one arterial graft, class I for the use of radial artery in high-grade coronary stenosis and class IIa for bilateral internal mammary artery (BIMA) use, this practice is not largely adopted [11]. CABG surgery is unique because of its good results reported from randomized trials and large observational studies in terms of increasing life expectancy in eligible patients compared to any other surgical intervention [8]. In patients with multiple coronary artery involvement, the other main option of revascularization is PCI. Contemporary drug-eluting stents (DES) with their important improvement in patency rates—target lesion revascularization rates are reported to be 3–3.5% at 1 year—are fully competitive with saphenous vein grafts for revascularization of non-LAD coronary artery in CABG [11, 12]. Additionally, PCI is related to fewer periprocedural complications. Accordingly, the hybrid coronary revascularization (HCR) is an emerging method, combining the benefits and eliminating the disadvantages of surgery and stenting, with promising effect on resolution of significant coronary artery disease [13]. The HCR consists in a planned procedure. A combination of minimally invasive direct coronary artery bypass (MIDCAB) and PCI to treat multivessel coronary artery disease.

Patient Selection

All patients diagnosed with coronary artery disease and considered for HCR treatment should be discussed by the institutional "heart-team", reviewing all anatomical, clinical, and procedural factors that may have an impact over the outcomes. The latest 2018 ESC/EACTS guidelines on myocardial revascularization give class IIa for the revascularization of LAD through minimal invasive surgical access in the context of hybrid revascularization if expertise exists [14].

Indications for HCR are [9, 11, 15, 16]:

- Multivessel CAD with complex LAD or left main (LM) lesion with optimal distal anatomy, suitable for CABG and concomitant focal disease of circumflex artery, right coronary artery, or both, suitable for PCI (Fig. 7.1)
- Low to intermediate SYNTAX scores
- No contraindication for dual antiplatelet therapy for 3–12 months
- Patient choice. Patients who refuse median sternotomy
- High probability of complete revascularization as a result of HCR

Other factors to consider HCR indicated for coronary artery diseased patient include overall health status and comorbidities. Thus, an exception for HCR can be discussed in patients ideally considered for standard CABG based on the SYNTAX score [16]. Using the risk stratification provided by Euroscore II and STS score calculators helps the heart-team to evaluate high-risk patients who may profit from the minimally invasive surgical part of the HCR procedure. Frail patients, the presence of severe physiological disorders, obese diabetic patients with high risk of wound infections, chronic kidney disease, severe carotid and neurological diseases, severe aortic calcification, poor quality of venous conduits, previous sternotomy—these are all conditions that pose the patient in high risk for standard open cardiopulmonary bypass surgery and midline sternotomy [17, 18].

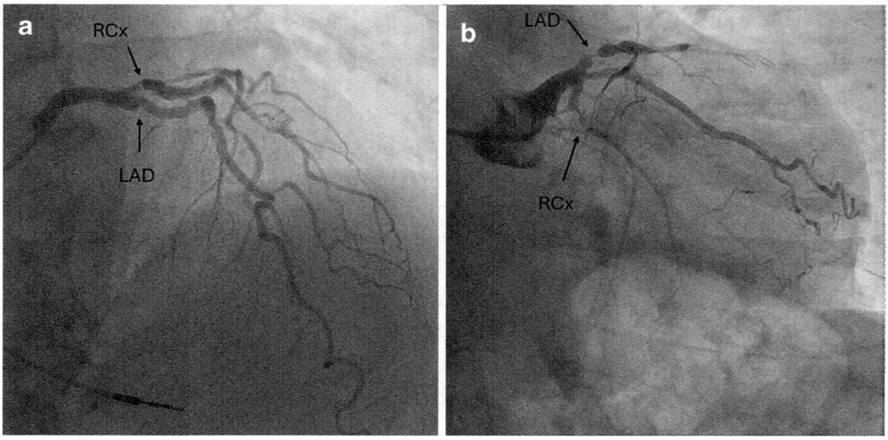

Fig. 7.1 Ideal cases for hybrid coronary revascularization. (**a**) focal stenosis at proximal LAD and proximal RCx coronary arteries. (**b**) proximal LAD stenosis and subtotal occlusion of RCx coronary artery

Contraindications for HCR are [15, 19]:

- Hemodynamic instability or cardiogenic shock. However, if the culprit lesion is non-LAD artery, it may be possible to perform PCI first part of HCR and at the second stage to perform the second part of HCR—MIDCAB
- Stenosis of left subclavian artery or LIMA stenosis
- Calcified or intramyocardial LAD target—considered a relative contraindication
- Left side intrapleural adhesions—considered a relative contraindication
- Pulmonary disease with high risk of intolerance to single-lung ventilation

HCR: The Surgical Procedure

In our institution, the most common surgical approach is performed for the surgical part of HCR—left mini-thoracotomy in the fourth or fifth intercostal space. The patient is positioned on supine position with slightly elevated left part of the chest (Fig. 7.2). General anesthesia is induced and intubation is performed with double-lumen endotracheal tube. Monitoring of arterial blood pressure, central venous pressure, and diuresis is performed on a standard fashion. The operative field is prepared on a manner if conversion to full sternotomy is required to be easily performed. Incision is made in fourth or fifth intercostal space sub-mammary, 6–8 cm of length. After soft tissues and muscles are divided and penetration of left pleural space is performed, the left lung is excluded from the ventilation process. A specific rib retractor is placed, and the harvesting of LIMA is started on direct vision with standard instruments, skeletonized or pedicled (Fig. 7.3). Usually, the full length of LIMA is possible to be reached (Fig. 7.4) (See Video 7.1). After heparinization of the patient and activated clotting time (ACT) of 380–400 seconds is

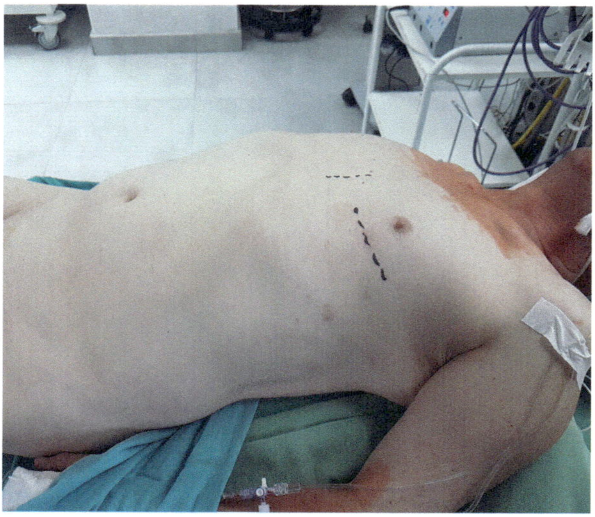

Fig. 7.2 Patient's position for MIDCAB procedure

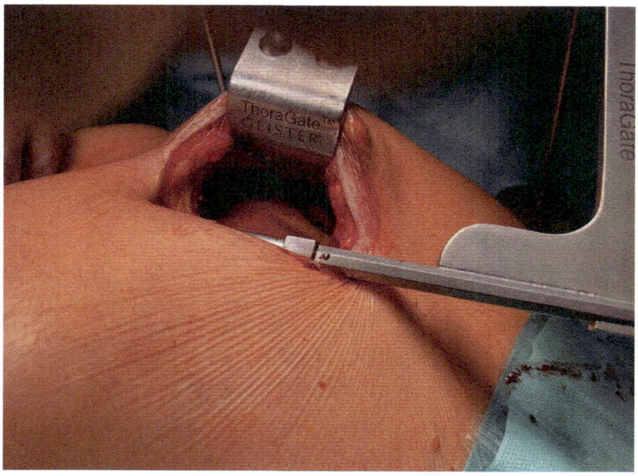

Fig. 7.3 After left pleura entering, specific retractor provides the operative field for LIMA harvesting under direct vision with standard instruments

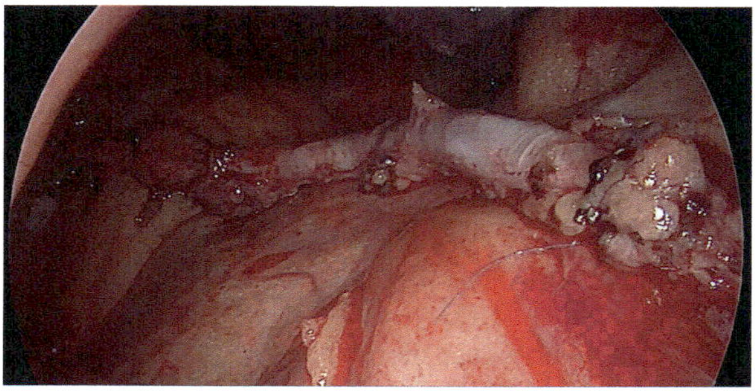

Fig. 7.4 Full length of LIMA is achieved with this surgical access

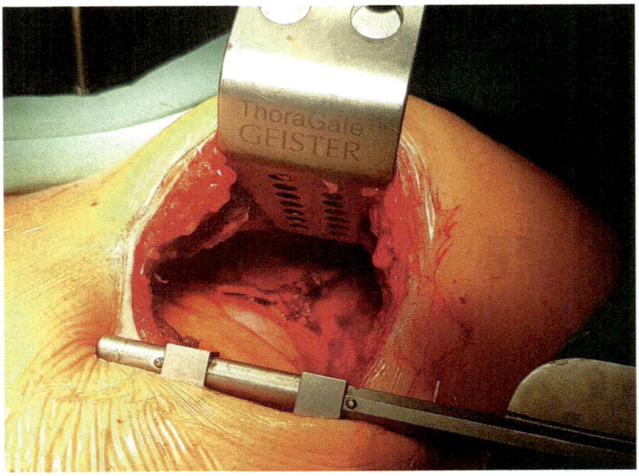

Fig. 7.5 Harvested LIMA just before transection

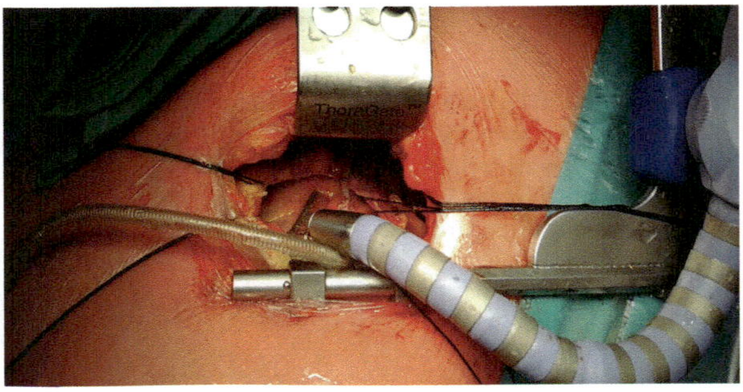

Fig. 7.6 LIMA-LAD anastomosis performed with the aid of Octopus Medtronic Stabilizer

achieved, the pericardium is opened and suspended. The target point of anastomosis on LAD is located and LIMA is transected distally (Fig. 7.5). The LIMA-LAD anastomosis is performed with 8/0 monofilament suture on beating heart, using Octopus Medtronic stabilizer and intracoronary shunt depending on coronary artery diameter (Fig. 7.6). The LIMA-LAD flow is assessed with flow probe based on transit time flow measurements (TTFM) (Fig. 7.7). After neutralization of heparin with protamine sulfate and exact hemostasis is done, left pleural space is drained and the chest incision is closed, placing an intercostal catheter for prolonged analgesia (Fig. 7.8). The MIDCAB procedure can be combined with thoracoscopy or robot assistance in the setting of endoscopically assisted minimally invasive direct coronary artery bypass (EAMIDCAB) and robot assisted minimally invasive direct coronary artery bypass (RAMIDCAB) for minimizing the surgical approach and to have more precision in LIMA harvesting and anastomotic performance [15]. In robotically assisted or endoscopically assisted hybrid procedures, the harvesting of LIMA is performed through three ports, in third, fifth, and seventh intercostal space between mid and anterior axillary lines [17]. After the

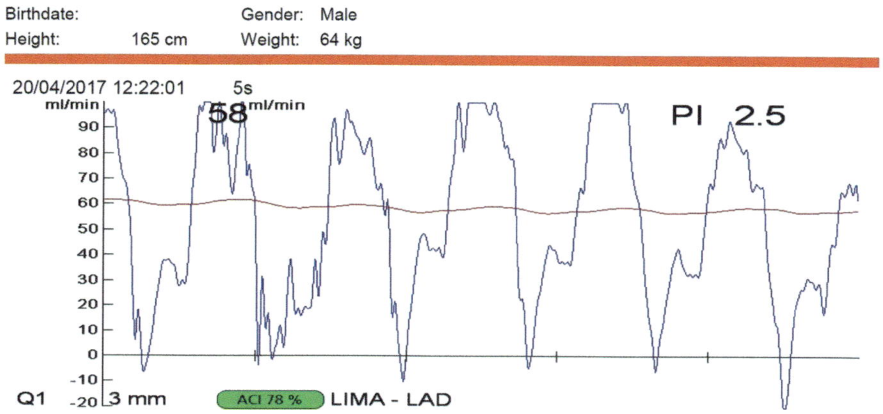

Fig. 7.7 Flowmetric assessment of the graft using TTFM, showing good parameters of the flow (ml/min. and graphic curve showing predominantly diastolic flow) and low pulsatility index

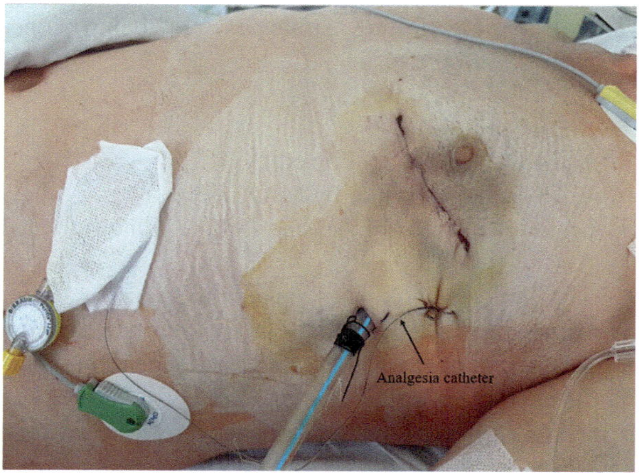

Fig. 7.8 Final stage of MIDCAB procedure with closed skin incision, drainage to left pleura, and catheter for continued analgesia

arterial graft is harvested and the location of the target vessel—LAD is cleared, microthoracotomy of 3 cm is performed. The use of special retractor helps that anastomosis between LIMA and LAD is performed on beating heart on direct vision [11, 17]. The patient is transferred to intensive care unit and extubated as soon as physiological and hemodynamic parameters allow. Heparin infusion is started in ICU when no signs of excessive bleeding, and double antiplatelet therapy is started after drainage system is removed. The second part of the HCR—PCI is performed usually 30 days after MIDCAB procedure and stenting of target non-LAD artery is performed after visualization and assessment of the previously accomplished LIMA-LAD anastomosis (Fig. 7.9).

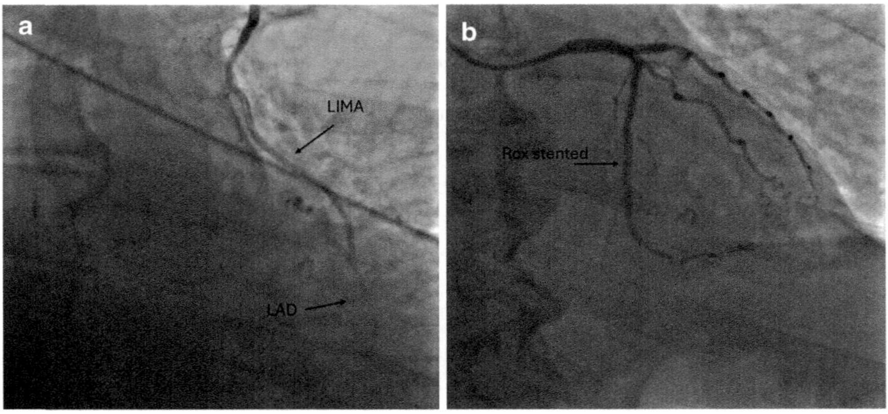

Fig. 7.9 Second stage of HCR—PCI. (**a**) assessment of LIMA-LAD performed bypass. (**b**) PCI on RCx coronary artery

Strategies for HCR

Three possible timing strategies are being considered in hybrid coronary revascularization:

- Staged procedure
  - MIDCAB first, followed by PCI
  - PCI first, followed by MIDCAB
- Simultaneous MIDCAB and PCI, or "One stop" hybrid procedure

The choice what kind of staged procedure or "One stop" hybrid procedure to be performed depends extremely on the individual coronary anatomy and the clinical manifestation of the patient, and final decision-making role has consensus reached in the heart-team [9, 13, 15, 19].

CABG followed by PCI is the preferred staged procedure in patients with stable coronary artery disease with a delay between the initially performed MIDCAB procedure and second-stage PCI from 24 hours to 60 days [4, 9, 11, 15, 19–22]. This sequence of staged hybrid procedure has the advantage of executing the surgical procedure without risk of perioperative bleeding, due to discontinued antiplatelet therapy prior surgical intervention, has the possibility to assess the functionality of the performed LIMA-LAD anastomosis with the potential of interventional treatment if narrowing of anastomotic site is detected, and a very useful advantage is the protected anterior wall of the heart during the stenting process of non-LAD arteries [9, 11]. Panoulas et al. point out a high-risk surgical reintervention like disadvantage in case of failure of PCI procedure [12].

PCI followed by CABG, also known as reverse hybrid coronary revascularization (RHCR), is the procedure of choice when the patient is presented with acute coronary syndrome and the culprit artery is different than LAD artery [11, 12, 22]. Aljamal et al. and Zhang et al. report their results in planned RHCR in series of 60 and 111 patients respectively [4, 23]. This supports the fact that the choice of sequence in HCR is in the hands of the heart-team. The procedure allows us to evaluate the quality of LIMA and gives lower surgical risk of ischemia in the second procedure when partial revascularization of the heart is previously performed [12]. Disadvantages of the PCI followed by MIDCAB sequence are the elevated risk of stent thrombosis or post-surgical bleeding in terms of too soon discontinuation of antiplatelet therapy before MIDCAB, or surgical intervention is performed on antiplatelet therapy [11, 23].

Simultaneous or "One stop" HCR is very specific and costly procedure because it needs a hybrid operative theater, where two different teams have to be accommodated. The procedure is performed with its surgical part first, followed by PCI. The advantages of the procedure are the reduced hospital stay because of the single complete revascularization procedure and the performed LIMA-LAD anastomosis that can be assessed immediately before stent implantation [16]. Disadvantages of the procedure include the need of hybrid operative theater, the elevated risk of stent thrombosis due to protamine administration, inflammatory response to surgery, and increased risk of bleeding related with double antiplatelet therapy [11].

Clinical Outcomes

The late outcomes achieved with established and safe CABG and PCI procedures in specific patient groups for each procedure, along with the lack of strong evidence that HCR provides comparable results, have some consequences. First, there is no identified HCR target group of patients and second, the hybrid procedure is not largely adopted. In a study from the Society of Thoracic Surgeons (STS) Adult Cardiac Database for a period of 2 years, among 198,622 patients who have undergone isolated coronary surgery, only 950 of them HCR procedure was performed, or only 0.48% of the total CABG interventions for the selected period [24]. There are numerous observational studies and meta-analyses comparing short and mid-term results between HCR, CABG, and PCI. Puskas et al. compare the results over 18 months of 200 patients selected for HCR and 98 patients selected for PCI and found no significant difference in major adverse cardiac and cerebrovascular events (MACCE, the composite of death, stroke and myocardial infarction)—free survival at 12 months (hazard ratio, 1.06; 95% CI, 0.66–1.69) and 18 months (hazard ratio, 0.86; 95% CI, 0.56–1.36) [25]. But at 18 months the MACCE-free survival trends began to diverge in favor of HCR, although no statistical difference was found. Shen et al. share their midterm results in simultaneous HCR with CABG and PCI for the treatment of multivessel coronary artery disease for a period of 3 years [18]. They found a lower MACCE rate in the HCR group than in the PCI group ($p < 0.001$), but similar to that in the CABG group ($p = 0.140$). After stratification by EuroSCORE or SYNTAX score, the cumulative MACCE rates were similar among the 3 groups in low and medium tertiles. But in the high EuroSCORE tertile, patients who underwent simultaneous HCR had a lower MACCE rate than did the groups that underwent CABG ($p = 0.030$) and PCI ($p = 0.006$). Patients with a high SYNTAX score who underwent simultaneous HCR had a MACCE rate lower than did those who underwent PCI ($p = 0.002$), but similar to that of those who underwent CABG

($p = 0.362$). In a randomized controlled trial (RCT) conducted by Tajstra et al. [26], long-term survival after HCR as compared to CABG is reported. For a median follow-up of 12.2 years (10.72–13.42) they found significant lower all-cause mortality in patients after HCR as compared to patients after CABG (20.4% vs. 36.3%; $P = 0.02$, respectively). The rates of myocardial infarction were with no significant difference (13.3% vs. 16.7%; $P = 0.63$), repeat revascularization (45.9% vs. 51.0%; $P = 0.57$), stroke (5.9% vs. 7.1%; $P = 0.72$), and major adverse cardiac and cerebrovascular events (56.1% vs. 68.6%; $P = 0.09$) were observed between HCR and CABG groups. Something worth paying attention to, and could be a factor determining long-term prognosis, is the residual SYNTAX score. In a retrospective study, Basman et al. [27] found that despite a higher baseline SYNTAX score (28.9 ± 10.6) before the procedures, HCR was able to achieve a lower residual SYNTAX score (4.5 ± 4.4) than multivessel PCI ($P = 0.001$). Practically all studies that compare HCR with CABG in the treatment of multivessel coronary disease are solid in the benefits of HCR related to lower need of blood transfusion, a few wound infection complications, shorter hospital stay, short time of mechanical ventilation, reduced periods in intensive care unit, a quick recovery and return to work after hospital discharge [9, 11, 12, 23].

The rationality in HCR can be seen in [7, 13, 18, 28]:

- The use of LIMA graft is probably the best revascularization method to treat LAD disease, considering its long-term patency and the influence of the patient prognosis.
- The use of last-generation DES to non-LAD arteries has comparable results with surgical revascularization with venous grafts.
- Minimally invasive surgical approach with a limited surgical trauma and exclusion of cardiopulmonary bypass.

The evolution and improvement of HCR is a process that will be observed in the future. The idea that the HCR is reserved for very morbid patients as a last chance procedure is not actual. The standard procedure—LIMA-LAD performed with minimally invasive surgical access and PCI to non-LAD arteries will probably be widely upgraded to the use of more than one arterial graft, such as RMIA and radial artery for revascularization of the left coronary artery and PCI for the right coronary artery, something that is not currently the standard of HCR. The technological prerequisites for this are present: endoscopic or robotic methods for arterial grafts harvesting, centers where programs for minimally invasive cardiac surgery development have been established, and especially centers with a working heart-team, where each of the members of this team is well informed what are the capabilities and results of the others and on that basis the strategy for the treatment of a particular patient will be determined. Concepts like Advanced Hybrid Coronary Revascularization (AHCR) or Non-classical HCR [23, 29] are present and indicate the trend for HCR development. Staged hybrid procedures do not require the presence of hybrid operative room. The surgical intsrumentarium is not much different from the standard one which make the hybrid procedure financially not very different from the standard one. This means that in the transition to hybrid procedures the most important thing is the mindset. Secondary is the learning curve, which should not be a reason for surgeons to refuse to adopt a new but promising strategy. More and more studies are trying to gain clarity in identifying the appropriate group of patients who have the indications for hybrid coronary revascularization and to make HCR the third major strategy to treat coronary artery disease. We remain awaiting results from large randomized controlled trials concerning the long-term outcomes of the HCR procedure.

Valvular Interventions. Hybrid Approach to Aortic, Mitral, and Tricuspid Valves

In 1996, Carpentier performed the first video-assisted minimally invasive mitral valve surgery (MIMVS) through a minithoracotomy [30]. The term minimally invasive "hybrid approach" for treatment of combined coronary and structural heart diseases was first introduced by Lawrence H. Cohn group around 2005. A small group of very high-risk patients with aortic stenosis and coronary artery disease (CAD) was treated with staged PCI followed by minimally invasive surgical aortic valve replacement (AVR) via upper partial sternotomy [31]. Since that time minimally invasive cardiac surgery (MICS) has become highly adopted. Today in most of the contemporary cardiac surgery departments minimally invasive access for single valve intervention is the standard approach. Conventional sternotomy for one valve intervention is only for selected patients [32]. In the last decade, the selection of the patient for MICS has been converted and now we make a selection for a sternotomy. The presence of additional significant coronary artery stenosis is one of the limitations to perform the structural heart intervention with a small incision. The risk of myocardial hypoprotection or intraoperative MI are the main issues that have to be taken into account, when CAD is neglected during valve surgery [33]. According to the European and American guidelines [34], concomitant significant coronary artery stenosis has to be treated at the time of the cardiac surgical procedure and the CABG is a type of revascularization. The guidelines do not differentiate between single, double, or triple vessel disease in cases of concomitant valve surgery or between minimally invasive or classic approaches for valve therapy. Single-vessel disease, which can be treated sufficiently endovascularly, is recommended to be treated surgically if concomitant valve surgery is to be performed. Evidences for any survival benefits from PCI in patients with CAD and valvular heart disease (VHD) came from transcatheter valve intervention researches. The REVASC-TAVI registry concludes that in patients with severe aortic stenosis and stable coronary artery disease scheduled for TAVI, performance of PCI after TAVI seems to be associated with improved 2-year clinical outcomes compared with other revascularization timing strategies [35]. NOTION-3 study in patients with PCI before TAVI resulted in a 29% lower relative risk of all-cause mortality, MI, or urgent revascularization after a median of 2 years when compared with medical therapy [36]. The recommendations given for such patients in current guidelines are class II a, but the level of evidence is "C" [37]. Nowadays with the exponentiation growth of minimally invasive valve surgical interventions, CABG is becoming an indication for a sternotomy approach in patients with combined pathology. Other possibility to treat these patients is the "hybrid approach". Recent studies show non-inferiority in short-term results with hybrid approach, compared to the conventional one. One of the largest series is published by Santana O with 94 patients treated with staged PCI and minimally invasive mitral valve intervention. Thirty-day mortality occurred in 4 (4.3%) patients. At a mean follow-up of 15.3 ± 13.2 months, 3 (3.4%) patients required target-vessel revascularization. The survival rate was 89% and 85% at 1 and 3 years, respectively [38]. In a large number of ischemic mitral regurgitation patients, the target coronary vessel has been treated with PCI and stent implantation during the acute MI. These patients are also indicated (Class 2 b) for a correction of the mitral insufficiency if they are symptomatic, despite optimal medical therapy or (Class 2 a) at the time of CABG surgery [34, 37]. In polymorbid frail patient with mitral insufficiency and concomitant coronary artery disease Öner et al. report a hybrid approach performing at first percutaneous mitral valve repair with mitraclip device and at second stage MIDCAB procedure for coronary revascularization with very good results at 2 years of follow-up [39]. In elderly patients with mitral annular calcinosis (MAC) and mitral valve stenosis, the conventional surgical technique can be associated with higher perioperative risk. In these cases, "off-label" procedure can be a hybrid approach—open implantation of catheter-based balloon expandable valve [40, 41]. Not infrequently in elderly, high-risk patients, multivalvular disease can be seen. Oatway et al. present a case of a 94-year-old man suffering from severe aortic stenosis and mitral valve insufficiency, in whom they performed simultaneous hybrid transcatheter aortic valve implantation (TAVI) and minimally invasive, endoscopic mitral valve repair [42].

Preoperative Evaluation

Chest X-ray, ECG, and laboratory tests are standard for hospital admission. Specific studies for MICS patients include evaluation of the coronary artery pathology, evaluation of the structural heart disease, and evaluation of the structures and peripheral vessels for the CPB cannulation and MICS performance. For CAD a fresh coronary angiography should be performed if the last intervention is not within 6 months or if there are any symptoms or clinical data for angina. TTE preoperatively and TEE, during the surgical intervention, are the standard modalities for determining the structural valve pathology and to evaluate its function and severity of deterioration [43, 44]. CT scan with arterial contrast phase is mandatory for MICS surgery. The cannulation strategy is determined by the diameter of the femoral and axillary arteries. Descending aorta pathologies like ulceration, plaques, and stenotic segments can result in areas of malperfusion during retrograde flow. CT scan is important for surgical strategy: position of the ports and thoracic structures can be determined on 3D reconstruction. Lung pathologies, pleural adhesions can also change the course of the intervention and the respiratory management. All other studies are performed only if indicated.

Hybrid Strategies in Heart Valve Pathologies: PCI First Concept

It is crucial to ensure adequate coronary perfusion before the surgery or at least ensure adequate myocardial protection with cardioplegia and avoid periprocedural myocardial infarction because authors publications have demonstrated a higher rate of perioperative myocardial infarctions in patients whose diseased coronary vessels were not addressed [45, 46]. In patients with severe valvular symptoms who were operated on within 1 month of PCI, surgery was performed under DAPT. Analysis did not reveal periprocedural myocardial infarctions or low cardiac output syndrome, which reflect adequate myocardial perfusion and protection. Therefore, we believe that it is advisable to first address the CAD to ensure successful revascularization before surgery and to optimize myocardial protection during surgery.

Hybrid Strategies in Heart Valve Pathologies: Valve Surgery First Concept

Most of the angiographically significant coronary stenosis >70% are not hemodynamically significant on FFR [47, 48]. It might be surgically favorable to perform the surgical procedure before initiating double antiplatelet therapy (DPAT) after endovascular therapy for coronary heart disease, because randomized controlled trials and retrospective studies have demonstrated higher rates of postoperative bleeding in patients on DPAT [49]. Regarding the optimum time frame between PCI and valve surgery, the guideline creators unfortunately did not reach a consensus at the time of performing the procedures. Advances in DES technology and PCI optimization have substantially reduced the risk of target lesion failure and several recent randomized trials have shown that 1–3 months of DAPT can be sufficient [50–52].

Our institutional strategy is to wait at least 30 days after PCI with stent implantation, if the valvular disease is tolerable for this period. If not, we perform the valvular intervention before that. In all cases, we stop DPAT 5 days before surgery, protecting the stent with ASA 100 mg and low molecular heparin in therapeutic dose.

Type of Minimally Invasive Surgery

The term MICS has a very wide meaning: from every access smaller than sternotomy to close chest endoscopic approach. According to the visualization, minimally invasive approach can be under direct vision, video-assisted, or totally endoscopic 2D/3D. It could be performed with conventional instruments with traction and approximation of the target structure or with less traction—in situ, with long endoscopic or robotic instruments. According to the access site, it can be through partial sternotomy or thoracotomy. The important thing in MICS surgery is that the quality of the heart intervention shouldn't be sacrificed because of the approach. The visualization should be perfect, the access with the instruments has to be free, and the traction of the structures has to be tolerable by the tissues. In endoscopic surgery, the whole procedure is endoscopically guided. Any attempt to work under direct vision in such a set-up could be dangerous. Compromised light delivery led to forced movement associated with inability of the surgeon to visualize confidently tiny structures and tip of the instruments. In all cases the quality of the procedure is a function of visualization.

Aortic Valve Intervention

Our main surgical approaches to the aortic valve are upper partial “J” sternotomy and endoscopic approach with access port in second or third intercostal space or right anterior thoracotomy. In our institution, the thoracoscopic approach and partial upper sternotomy are the main approaches to the aortic valve.

For partial sternotomy approach the anesthesia management is the same like in conventional valve surgery, we do a median incision 6–8 cm, starting 2 cm under the jugulum. The sternotomy is performed toward the third intercostal space (ICS) in “J” fashion. The arterial cannulation is in the upper ascending aorta, just below the brachiocephalic trunk. Venous canulation is direct in the right atrium with a triple-stage cannula. The course of the operation does not differ from the conventional one. The sternum is closed with three or four wires. For the endoscopic approach single lung ventilation anesthesia is preferable, but not mandatory. The CPB is achieved with surgical femoral arterial and venous, TEE-guided cannulation. The valve intervention is performed using ports: one working port 3–4 cm with soft tissue retractor in the second or third ICS on the mid-clavicular line, one 5 mm port in the second ICS in the anterior axillary line for the 30° endoscope. One 5 mm port in the fourth or fifth ICS in the anterior axillary line for the left vent line. One port in the first ICS in the mid-clavicular line for the Chitwood clamp. For myocardial protection single shot of antegrade Custodiol (Histidine-Tryptophan-Ketoglutarate) is a good solution, giving 2 hours of safe cross-clamping time [53]. The intervention on the valve is endoscopically guided and does not differ from the conventional intervention. At the end of the procedure after weaning from CPB the pericardium is closed over a silicone drain inside, exteriorized through the vent port. And all incisions are closed.

Mitral and Tricuspid Valve Intervention

The surgical access to tricuspid and mitral valve could be under direct vision or endoscopically guided. The endoscopic approach is standardized, and it has some advantages over direct vision intervention. It is performed without metal retractor and rib periosteal damage, gives better visualization and instrumental access to each target structure without any traction of the cardiac structures. The anesthesia and CPB strategy are as described before. Single lung ventilation is not necessary, and the pre-cross clamp set up can be done on CPB. The working port is in the third or fourth ICS. Its position depends on sex, patient constitution, surgeon preferences, position of the heart and the valves. It can be determined by CT scan 3D reconstruction. The principle to determine the position of the working port is to achieve direct instrumental access to the valve with minimum atrial retraction. The 5 mm camera port is in the third ICS on the anterior axillary line. Another 5 mm port in mid-axillary line is used for the vent line. The arm for the left atrial retractor is inserted in the fourth ICS, just parallel to the sternum under thoracoscopic control because of the proximity of the mammary vessels. After initiation of normothermic CPB, the pericardium is opened relatively high, and some stay sutures are put on the right side of the pericardium ant pulled out through the endoscope and vent ports. If right atrium has to be opened SVC and IVC are encircled with teflon stripes. Cardioplegia needle is inserted over tourniquets. Flexible (Sygnet® Peters surgical-France) clamp is used through the working port and 2 l of cold Custodiol is infused into the aortic root. The left atrium is opened in a standard fashion along the inter-atrial groove and the retractor is assembled into the thorax and the atrial septum is retracted just enough to allow free access of the instruments to the valve.

When tricuspid valve has to be corrected it is done after closing the left atrium. It could be done on beating heart. The strips around the IVC and SVC are tightly fixed around the venous cannula. The right atrial retractor is assembled, and the atrial free wall is gently lifted. The suction vent is positioned near the coronary sinus. After finishing the procedure, the pericardium is closed over the drain, before weaning from CPB and lung expansion. Postoperative management does not differ from that in all other cardiac surgery patients.

In MICS patients, minimization of surgical trauma allows diminishing of the ICU stay and early postoperative rehabilitation and home discharge. Patient's outcome depends on preoperative factors like in every conventional surgical patient [54], but surgical trauma is the major intraoperative factor that leads to enhanced recovery [55, 56].

Anticoagulation and antiplatelet therapy in patients with stent implantation and minimally invasive valve correction is according to current guidelines. If the stent is implanted within 1 month, DAPT is resumed as soon as there is no concern over bleeding. Discontinuing of the DAPT in patients treated with oral anticoagulants (OAC) is recommended after 12 months. OAC with vitamin K antagonists are used in every patient with mechanical heart valve, in all patients in sinus rhythm with valve reconstruction or biological valve prosthesis within 90 days. After 90 days patient in AF could be on novel oral anticoagulants (NOACs) plus aspirin or clopidogrel [57].

Hybrid Procedures in Aortic Arch and Thoracoabdominal Aortic Pathology

Hybrid aortic repair procedures combine open surgical techniques with endovascular stent-grafting to treat complex aortic pathologies in a less invasive manner [58]. Over the past two decades, these hybrid approaches continue to evolve as alternatives to conventional open surgery for the aortic arch and thoracoabdominal aorta, aiming to reduce the high morbidity and mortality associated with extensive open repairs [58, 59]. Many patients with aortic arch or thoracoabdominal aneurysms are older or have significant comorbidities that may preclude traditional open surgery—a situation that demands finding an alternative solution. Avoiding prolonged cardiopulmonary bypass and deep hypothermic circulatory arrest in arch cases, or extensive thoracoabdominal incisions in aneurysm cases, hybrid techniques create a viable option for these high-risk patients [58]. This section reviews recent (past 5–10 years) research on hybrid aortic arch and thoracoabdominal repairs, discussing surgical techniques, patient selection criteria, clinical outcomes, innovations in stent-graft technology, and long-term results, with emphasis on findings from contemporary studies and high-impact reviews.

Hybrid Aortic Arch Repair: Technics and Patient Selection

Hybrid aortic arch repair (HAAR) typically involves surgical rerouting of one or more supra-aortic branch vessels (debranching) to create a landing zone, followed by endovascular stent grafting of the arch aneurysm (a thoracic endovascular aortic repair, TEVAR) [58, 60]. Various hybrid arch techniques are classified (Type I, II, III) based on the extent of debranching: from partial debranching of the left subclavian artery (Type I) up to complete arch vessel revascularization (Type II/III) with stent graft coverage of the arch [58, 61]. A notable variant is the "frozen elephant trunk" (FET) procedure, wherein open replacement of the ascending arch is combined with deployment of a stented graft into the descending aorta in the same operation [58]. FET devices were not widely commercially available in some countries until recently and hybrid approach was the only available option. Nowadays with FET an affordable alternative, hybrid arch strategies are generally reserved for patients with high operative risk or challenging anatomy that make conventional open total arch replacement associated with unreasonable risk cumulation. For example, patients of advanced age, frailty, prior sternotomies, or a "porcelain" (severely calcified) aorta are often considered candidates for hybrid repair. Multidisciplinary planning by surgeons experienced in both open and endovascular techniques is recommended to tailor the approach to patient-specific factors [61]. Having a dedicated "aortic team" is a major advantage in developing hybrid aortic strategy in every institution.

Clinical Outcomes

Early outcomes for hybrid arch repair have improved over time as techniques and patient selection have been refined. A 2013 meta-analysis of 956 patients undergoing Type I–III hybrid arch procedures reported a pooled 30-day mortality of 12%, stroke rate of 8%, and permanent paraplegia of 3.6% [61]. These early results established hybrid arch repair as a feasible alternative to open surgery, albeit with significant perioperative risks. More recent series demonstrate better outcomes in high-volume centers. For example, a contemporary single-center study (2005–2022, n = 163) reported operative mortality of 9% at 30 days and stroke of 4%, with only 2% incidence of new permanent neurological deficit [59]. Many of these patients had prior aortic surgery or extensive disease, underscoring that hybrids can be performed with acceptable risk in complex scenarios [59]. Comparisons of hybrid versus open arch repair have shown generally comparable early outcomes in experienced hands. Meta-analyses indicate no significant difference in composite early mortality between open and hybrid arch approaches, although hybrid repair may carry a slightly higher stroke risk in some series [62]. Notably, hybrid arch surgery tends to result in less bleeding and fewer blood transfusions than open arch replacement and has a lower risk of re-operation for bleeding, likely due to avoiding extensive circulatory arrest and anastomoses in a hostile field [62, 63]. Overall, hybrid arch repair has proven to be a safe alternative for appropriately selected patients, offering a path to treat arch aneurysms or dissections that might otherwise be inoperable [59, 63].

The long-term durability and survival after hybrid arch repair are areas of active study. Mid-term results have been encouraging, with acceptable survival and low aortic-related complication rates. In the Duke University series mentioned above, overall survival was 59% at 5 years and 47% at 10 years, while aorta-specific survival (freedom from aortic-related death) remained high as 86% and 84% at 5 and 10 years, respectively [59]. Freedom from major aortic reintervention at 5 and 10 years exceeded 90%, suggesting that once the initial repair is successful, the need for late reintervention is low [59]. Operator experience and advances in technique have markedly improved outcomes over the past decade. Similarly, 5-year survival improved dramatically in the later era (78% vs 45% in the earlier cohort) [59]. Other studies have reported 5-year survival rates ranging from 50% to 80% after hybrid arch repair, reflecting differences in patient profiles and techniques [64]. While long-term survival is often limited by patients' underlying comorbid conditions (common in this high-risk group), hybrid repair provides durable aortic aneurysm exclusion in the majority of cases [59]. Ongoing surveillance is required, as late complications such as endoleaks or degeneration of bypass grafts can occur, though these appear infrequent in recent series [59].

Innovations and Future Directions (Arch)

Innovations in stent-graft technology, especially investigational branched and fenestrated endografts designed for the aortic arch, are currently under investigation [60]. These advances may reduce or eliminate the need for open debranching in the future, potentially enabling totally endovascular arch repairs in a broader patient population [60]. Until dedicated arch devices are widely available, hybrid techniques remain critical, particularly in complex or redo-cases. In-situ fenestration is a very useful and practical alternative to multibranched and fenestrated grafts in achieving totally endovascular or hybrid arch repair. As fenestrations are made after the endograft has already been deployed, in situ fenestration offers more flexibility compared to premade fenestrated or branched endografts. Various options of in-situ fenestrations exist including laser fenestration, radiofrequency needle, needle-based manual fenestration, and balloon-assisted puncture. In this respect, our institution has gained experience with a dedicated catheter system developed by Dr. Quing Fu (Fu Through Device) which has proved to be useful in almost all anatomical situations. Chimney grafts and other adjuncts are no longer expanding concepts and should be reserved for the most inoperable patients. In summary, hybrid arch repair is now a growing technique with improving outcomes, and ongoing innovations—particularly branched stent-grafts promise to further expand options for complex arch disease. Adjunct techniques like carotid-carotid-subclavian bypasses and "chimney" grafts (parallel stents for arch branches) are available in extreme cases but carry higher risk for endoleaks [60].

Hybrid Thoracoabdominal Aortic Repair: Techniques and Patient Selection

Hybrid repair of thoracoabdominal aortic aneurysms (TAAAs) involves a two-part strategy: rerouting of visceral blood flow followed by endovascular exclusion of the aneurysm [58]. This means performing surgical bypasses or re-implantations of vital branch arteries (celiac, mesenteric, renal) to an alternate blood supply and then placing a stent-graft across the diseased thoracoabdominal aortic segment [58]. Visceral revascularization can be done via an open abdominal approach, the endograft is then deployed to seal off the aneurysm [58, 60]. Hybrid TAAA repair can be performed in a single session or staged. Two-stage repair may reduce ischemic complications and 30-day mortality for stable aneurysm patients, but carries interval rupture risk and is mainly for stable cases [58]. Patient selection favors those too high-risk for open surgery (elderly, frail, comorbid, or prior abdominal aortic surgery) or in urgent/rupture cases [58, 59]. Open surgery remains the gold standard for fit patients, with hybrid repair for high-risk, anatomically unsuitable ones [58].

Clinical Outcomes

Early outcomes of hybrid thoracoabdominal repair reflect both the complexity of these aneurysms and the high-risk nature of selected patients. Perioperative mortality for hybrid TAAA repair ranges from about 5% to 15%, with permanent paraplegia rates of 4–11% [58]. Hybrid repair, while less invasive than open, still entails substantial physiological stress and does not eliminate the inherent risks [58, 60]. Five-year survival rates after hybrid TAAA repair are 50–60%, with the caveat that many patients are very high risk and not candidates for open or total endovascular approaches [59]. Lifelong surveillance is required, bearing in mind that freedom from reintervention varies; late events relate to endoleaks or graft stenosis [59]. Recent advances include single-stage hybrid grafts that may reduce ischemic and neurological complications [58, 60].

Advanced Devices and Endovascular Innovations

Branched and fenestrated endografts enable more cases to be performed entirely endovascularly [58, 60]. Investigational dual-branch arch grafts, off-the-shelf branched devices, and evolving techniques will likely further reduce the need for open or hybrid approaches in the future [60].

Hybrid Procedures in Congenital and Structural Heart Disease

The hybrid approach, which integrates conventional surgery with catheter-based interventions in specialized operating rooms, is increasingly recognized as a significant advancement in the management of congenital and structural heart diseases. This strategy is particularly beneficial for neonates at high surgical risk, small children with difficult vascular access, and patients with complex cardiac anatomies. Hybrid procedures represent a transformative paradigm in the treatment of congenital and structural heart diseases, combining the strengths of surgical and interventional cardiology techniques. This approach not only reduces procedural morbidity by avoiding cardiopulmonary bypass in certain scenarios but also expands the therapeutic options for complex or high-risk patients. The evolution of hybrid strategies has been propelled by the synergy between surgical precision and catheter-based minimalism, offering a compelling alternative to traditional management pathways. Although its indications are expanding, the development of standardized protocols and the accumulation of robust long-term outcomes data remain ongoing challenges.

Emerging Applications in Congenital Defect Management

Hybrid Stage I Palliation in Hypoplastic Left Heart Syndrome

The hybrid approach in congenital heart disease (CHD) management has broadened substantially, offering innovative solutions for patients traditionally deemed unsuitable for conventional surgical therapies. One of the most transformative applications is in the treatment of hypoplastic left heart syndrome (HLHS) during Norwood stage I palliation. Initially introduced as an alternative to the traditional Norwood procedure, particularly in high-risk neonates, the "hybrid Norwood" involves a combination of bilateral pulmonary artery banding, ductal stenting, and atrial septostomy, all performed without cardiopulmonary bypass. This technique provides hemodynamic stability while deferring more invasive surgery to a later, potentially safer stage of life [65]. Bacha et al. describe the hybrid Norwood as particularly useful in critically ill neonates, those with low birth weight, prematurity, or unfavorable cardiac anatomy—circumstances under which conventional surgery carries increased risk [66]. Moreover, it offers a feasible option in centers with limited access to neonatal cardiopulmonary bypass or where surgical expertise may be evolving [65]. The hybrid strategy has also proven valuable in resource-limited settings, as demonstrated by successful programs in developing countries, where it has enabled the establishment of sustainable HLHS treatment pathways with outcomes comparable to those in developed nations [67]. Despite its advantages, wide inter-institutional variability exists in the execution and protocols surrounding hybrid Stage I palliation. A 2024 multicenter survey by Zanaboni et al. revealed significant diversity in patient selection criteria, the timing and techniques of atrial septostomy, and interstage monitoring practices among 45 centers in North America actively performing hybrid HLHS palliation [68]. While this hybrid approach reduces the hemodynamic insult associated with neonatal bypass and allows stabilization of fragile physiology, it is not without complications. Uhl et al. and other researchers have identified a risk of pulmonary artery distortion, uneven band placement, and increased right ventricular hypertrophy, potentially complicating subsequent surgical stages [66, 69]. The hybrid approach also shifts some risks to later stages, such as the comprehensive Stage II operation, which often requires complex reconstruction of the aortic arch and pulmonary arteries, as well as management of stented ductal tissue. High rates of reintervention, particularly for branch pulmonary artery interventions (reported at 18–86%, higher than after traditional Norwood), and the risk of sudden death during the interstage period are important considerations, especially in settings where close monitoring is challenging [70]. These findings emphasize the importance of careful anatomical planning, longitudinal imaging follow-up, and multidisciplinary decision-making. In summary, hybrid Stage I palliation for HLHS represents a significant advancement in the tailored management of high-risk neonates with single-ventricle physiology. Its success, however, hinges on rigorous patient selection, collaborative surgical–interventional teamwork, and long-term surveillance to mitigate associated vascular and ventricular complications.

Perventricular Closure of Ventricular Septal Defect (VSD)

Another prominent and increasingly utilized hybrid application in congenital heart surgery is the perventricular closure of ventricular septal defects (VSDs), particularly muscular and in selected perimembranous types. Traditional open surgical closure of VSDs in infants, especially those with multiple or apical defects, remains technically demanding due to the complexity of exposure and the associated need for cardiopulmonary bypass. The hybrid perventricular technique, which involves device delivery through a limited sternotomy directly into the right ventricle, enables occluder deployment under echocardiographic and fluoroscopic guidance, circumventing the need for cardiopulmonary bypass or extensive vascular access [71]. Gupta and Amin report high procedural success rates ranging from 77% to 100%, particularly in muscular and apical VSDs, with low incidence of significant complications. This approach allows precise device positioning and shorter operative times, offering an advantage in hemodynamically unstable or low-weight neonates where traditional approaches are high risk [71]. In a multicenter observational study, patients undergoing perventricular closure exhibited less postoperative discomfort and quicker mobilization, contributing to an overall reduction in morbidity and healthcare resource utilization. Despite its advantages, the success of the hybrid VSD closure technique depends on careful patient selection, particularly related to defect anatomy and patient size. The approach is generally best suited to isolated muscular VSDs, or multiple muscular defects clustered closely together, where percutaneous closure would require multiple vascular access points or be technically unfeasible [65]. Overall, perventricular VSD closure exemplifies the potential of hybrid methods to simplify complex repairs while maintaining safety and efficacy, particularly in fragile patient populations. The technique underscores the value of collaboration between cardiac surgeons and interventional cardiologists, where joint planning and shared procedural execution enhance outcomes and broaden therapeutic possibilities.

Hybrid Pulmonary and Aortic Interventions in Congenital Heart Disease

Hybrid strategies have increasingly expanded to address complex pulmonary and aortic pathologies in congenital heart disease (CHD), particularly in anatomically challenging or high-risk patients. One of the most notable applications involves stenting of branch pulmonary arteries and perventricular interventions for aortic coarctation or valve anomalies, typically performed in dedicated hybrid suites that facilitate real-time imaging and collaborative decision-making [65, 71]. In neonates with interrupted aortic arch, hybrid repair strategies that combine surgical access with interventional stenting have shown promising mid-term outcomes. Uhl et al. reported a 91% survival rate at 3–4 years following such hybrid interventions; however, the authors also observed a notable incidence of pulmonary artery narrowing and increased right ventricular pressure loading, underscoring the need for ongoing surveillance and potential reintervention [69]. Hybrid interventions also serve as key adjuncts in complex biventricular repairs, especially in cases requiring nuanced intracardiac manipulation. Devaney et al. highlighted the use of hybrid strategies in patients with atrioventricular septal defect (AVSD), double-outlet right ventricle (DORV), and common atrioventricular valve, where the hybrid approach facilitated precise anatomical assessment, improved exposure, and coordinated device-surgical maneuvers [72]. Such intricate procedures benefit significantly from the synchronous involvement of interventional cardiologists and cardiac surgeons, optimizing both technical accuracy and procedural efficiency. In the postoperative context, hybrid methods have emerged as critical tools for hemodynamic optimization. Uhl et al. further demonstrated that branch pulmonary artery stenting following biventricular repair led to measurable reductions in right ventricular load and enhanced pulmonary artery growth, contributing to more favorable long-term ventricular remodeling [69]. As hybrid suites become more prevalent and technologies improve, the role of these interventions is expected to grow, minimizing surgical trauma, improving early outcomes, and enhancing precision in anatomically complex cases. However, long-term durability, risk of restenosis, and the optimal timing of hybrid interventions remain active areas of investigation requiring standardized protocols and prospective studies.

Complex Adult Congenital Heart Disease

In adults with previously undiagnosed or complex congenital defects, hybrid techniques may be used to address anatomical challenges or when surgical risk is elevated, such as in the management of patent ductus arteriosus or coarctation of the aorta [73].

Stent Placement in Pulmonary Arteries or Veins

Hybrid techniques facilitate precise stent placement in branch pulmonary arteries or pulmonary veins, addressing recurrent stenosis or coarctation with minimal invasiveness.

Operational Protocols and Practice Variation

Despite the promising outcomes, operational variability remains a challenge. A 2024 survey by Zanaboni et al. involving 54 congenital heart centers, 45 of which actively perform hybrid stage I palliation, revealed that while ductal stenting and bilateral pulmonary artery banding are nearly universal, practices around atrial septostomy, imaging protocols, and interstage monitoring vary significantly. This variability underscores the importance of multicenter collaboration and data sharing to standardize care and refine patient selection criteria [68]. Such variation also reflects differing institutional experiences and expertise, further highlighting the need for continuous professional development and the establishment of national or international hybrid procedural registries.

Advantages of Hybrid Procedures

- Reduced invasiveness: by avoiding or minimizing cardiopulmonary bypass and large incisions, hybrid procedures can shorten recovery times and reduce morbidity [1, 74].
- Expanded treatment options: some complex lesions that are not amenable to surgery or catheter intervention alone can be addressed using a hybrid approach, broadening the therapeutic landscape [73].
- Shorter ICU and hospital stays: patients often experience shorter intensive care and overall hospital stays compared to traditional surgery.
- Synergistic expertise: collaboration between surgeons and interventional cardiologists enables more tailored and effective interventions, especially in anatomically complex cases [1, 75, 76].

Limitations and Challenges

- Complications: while generally safe, hybrid procedures are not without risks, including device-related complications or procedural mishaps that may require immediate surgical correction.
- Need for specialized facilities: successful hybrid interventions require dedicated hybrid operating rooms equipped for both surgical and interventional procedures.
- Long-term outcomes: although early results are promising, questions remain regarding long-term survival, neurocognitive outcomes, and the durability of hybrid interventions compared to traditional approaches.

Collaboration Between Cardiac Surgeons and Interventional Cardiologists

Hybrid procedures represent not only a technological and procedural advancement in adult, congenital and structural heart disease but also a transformation in how multidisciplinary care is delivered. At the core of successful hybrid interventions is the seamless collaboration between pediatric cardiac surgeons and interventional cardiologists, a relationship that has matured into a cohesive and adaptive model of care. This partnership is essential for several reasons:

- Shared expertise: each specialty brings unique skills—surgeons provide direct access and anatomical correction, while interventional cardiologists offer advanced imaging and catheter-based device deployment. Their combined expertise enables the design and execution of complex procedures that would be difficult or impossible for either specialty alone [71].

- Real-time decision-making: hybrid procedures often require rapid intraoperative decisions, such as adjusting the degree of pulmonary artery banding based on angiographic and hemodynamic feedback or determining the optimal site for stent deployment. This dynamic environment benefits greatly from multidisciplinary input [77].
- Personalized patient care: collaboration allows for individualized treatment plans, taking into account the patient's anatomy, comorbidities, and procedural risks. This is especially important in congenital heart disease, where anatomical variations are common and prior surgeries may complicate standard approaches.
- Operational efficiency: hybrid procedures are typically performed in specially equipped hybrid suites, allowing for immediate transition between surgical and interventional steps. Effective teamwork ensures smooth workflow and optimal patient outcomes.

Multidisciplinary Teams and Hybrid Suites

The emergence of hybrid suites, operating rooms equipped with fixed C-arm fluoroscopy, rotational angiography, and in some cases intraoperative MRI, has played a foundational role in this evolution. These facilities allow for real-time integration of imaging, surgical access, and catheter-based therapy. As of 2024, national surveys report a growing recognition of such integrated environments, where anatomical and technical barriers to traditional procedures are actively overcome through intraoperative flexibility and interdisciplinary dialogue [75, 78]. Gil-Jaurena et al. emphasize that hybrid procedures require a shared mental model between specialties. At Hospital Gregorio Marañón, their experience reflects how close cooperation encourages technical innovation, mutual respect, and shared planning for challenging cases. Similarly, Zampi et al. describe how "hybrid teams" significantly improve care for high-risk neonates, with synchronized imaging, surgical access, and interventional methods leading to superior outcomes [75, 79]. Bacha et al. further highlight how the hybrid operating room itself is a physical embodiment of this partnership, where open surgery and catheterization can occur simultaneously or sequentially depending on real-time findings. The hybrid suite also fosters collaboration with anesthesiologists, perfusionists, and imaging specialists, transforming it into a central hub of coordinated care [66].

Educational and Cultural Shifts

The hybrid paradigm necessitates not only procedural innovation but also a cultural and educational shift. Surgeons are increasingly required to interpret fluoroscopic and echocardiographic imaging in real time, while interventional cardiologists must be familiar with surgical anatomy and operative workflow. Gil-Jaurena et al. and Zampi et al. both emphasize the significance of cross-training, joint simulation sessions, and shared decision-making, which contribute to better procedural planning and more cohesive teams [75, 79]. As new generations of cardiac specialists are trained in hybrid methods, educational curricula are adapting to include interdisciplinary modules that bridge the traditional silos of surgery and cardiology. This fosters an institutional culture rooted in collaboration rather than hierarchy, driving improvements in innovation, safety, and outcomes.

Conclusion

Hybrid cardiac procedures are a clinical and institutional evolution. They not only expand therapeutic options for complex coronary artery disease, valvular heart disease, aortic and congenital heart disease but also redefine the relationship between cardiac surgeons and interventional cardiologists. As technologies continue to advance and hybrid suites become standard across high-volume centers, the collaborative ethos at the heart of hybrid care will remain essential. Future progress depends not only on tools and techniques but on the continued integration of expertise, training, and shared purpose.

References

1. Leacche M, Umakanthan R, Zhao DX, Byrne JG. Surgical update: hybrid procedures, do they have a role? Circ Cardiovasc Interv. 2010;3(5):511–8. https://doi.org/10.1161/CIRCINTERVENTIONS.110.957951.
2. Angelini GD, Wilde P, Salerno TA, Bosco G, Calafiore AM. Integrated left small thoracotomy and angioplasty for multivessel coronary artery revascularisation. Lancet. 1996;347(9003):757–8. https://doi.org/10.1016/s0140-6736(96)90107-5.
3. Papakonstantinou NA, Baikoussis NG, Dedeilias P, Argiriou M, Charitos C. Cardiac surgery or interventional cardiology? Why not both? Let's go hybrid. J Cardiol. 2017;69(1):46–56. https://doi.org/10.1016/j.jjcc.2016.09.007.
4. AlJamal YN, Nisivaco S, Bhasin R, Kitahara H, Nathan S, Balkhy HH. Robotic totally endoscopic reverse hybrid coronary revascularization: early and midterm outcomes. Innovations (Phila). 2025:15569845251334117. https://doi.org/10.1177/15569845251334117.
5. Kiaii B, McClure RS, Kostuk WJ, Rayman R, Swinamer S, Dobkowski WB, et al. Concurrent robotic hybrid revascularization using an enhanced operative suite. Chest. 2005;128(6):4046–8. https://doi.org/10.1378/chest.128.6.4046.
6. Melly L, Torregrossa G, Lee T, Jansens JL, Puskas JD. Fifty years of coronary artery bypass grafting. J Thorac Dis. 2018;10(3):1960–7. https://doi.org/10.21037/jtd.2018.02.43.
7. Patel PM, Arrington RL, Jonsson A, Wei JW, Binongo J, Devireddy C, et al. Advancing the treatment paradigm for multivessel coronary artery disease: hybrid coronary revascularization. Innovations (Phila). 2025;20(1):57–64. https://doi.org/10.1177/15569845241311292.
8. Lytle B. Evolution of coronary surgery. Circulation. 2024;150(17):1311–2. https://doi.org/10.1161/CIRCULATIONAHA.124.070918.
9. Elassal AA, Al-Ebrahim K, Makhdoom AM, Fatani M, Ibrahim M. Hybrid coronary revascularization: perspective current state after 25 years of start. Heart Surg Forum. 2021;24(2):E392–401. https://doi.org/10.1532/hsf.3693.

10. Taggart DP. PCI versus CABG in coronary artery disease. Vasc Pharmacol. 2024;155:107367. https://doi.org/10.1016/j.vph.2024.107367.
11. Moreno PR, Stone GW, Gonzalez-Lengua CA, Puskas JD. The hybrid coronary approach for optimal revascularization: JACC review topic of the week. J Am Coll Cardiol. 2020;76(3):321–33. https://doi.org/10.1016/j.jacc.2020.04.078.
12. Panoulas VF, Colombo A, Margonato A, Maisano F. Hybrid coronary revascularization: promising, but yet to take off. J Am Coll Cardiol. 2015;65(1):85–97. https://doi.org/10.1016/j.jacc.2014.04.093.
13. Mishra YK, Yadav J. Hybrid myocardial revascularization. Indian J Thorac Cardiovasc Surg. 2018;34(Suppl 3):310–20. https://doi.org/10.1007/s12055-018-0646-y.
14. Neumann FJ, Hochholzer W, Siepe M. [ESC/EACTS guidelines on myocardial revascularization 2018: the most important innovations]. Herz. 2018;43(8):689–94. https://doi.org/10.1007/s00059-018-4764-5.
15. Fazmin IT, Ali JM. Hybrid coronary revascularisation: indications, techniques, and outcomes. J Clin Med. 2025;14(3):880. https://doi.org/10.3390/jcm14030880.
16. Willard R, Scheinerman J, Pupovac S, Patel NC. The current state of hybrid coronary revascularization. Ann Thorac Surg. 2024;118(2):318–28. https://doi.org/10.1016/j.athoracsur.2024.04.010.
17. Raja SG. New clinical advances in minimally invasive coronary surgery. J Clin Med. 2025;14(9):3142. https://doi.org/10.3390/jcm14093142.
18. Shen L, Hu S, Wang H, Xiong H, Zheng Z, Li L, et al. One-stop hybrid coronary revascularization versus coronary artery bypass grafting and percutaneous coronary intervention for the treatment of multivessel coronary artery disease: 3-year follow-up results from a single institution. J Am Coll Cardiol. 2013;61(25):2525–33. https://doi.org/10.1016/j.jacc.2013.04.007.
19. Halkos ME, Vassiliades TA, Douglas JS, Morris DC, Rab ST, Liberman HA, et al. Hybrid coronary revascularization versus off-pump coronary artery bypass grafting for the treatment of multivessel coronary artery disease. Ann Thorac Surg. 2011;92(5):1695–701; discussion 701-2. https://doi.org/10.1016/j.athoracsur.2011.05.090.
20. Hannan EL, Wu Y, Cozzens K, Sundt TM 3rd, Girardi L, Chikwe J, et al. Hybrid coronary revascularization versus conventional coronary artery bypass surgery: utilization and comparative outcomes. Circ Cardiovasc Interv. 2020;13(10):e009386. https://doi.org/10.1161/CIRCINTERVENTIONS.120.009386.
21. Kaliyamoorthy D, Mohamed Yusuf M, Ramalingam V, Kasha A, Kathiresan M, Suliankatchi Abdulkader R, et al. Comparison of hybrid coronary revascularization versus conventional coronary artery bypass surgery in patients with multi-vessel coronary artery disease in a real-world setting: in-hospital outcomes and medium-term follow-up: COHOS study. Indian Heart J. 2025;77(2):98–104. https://doi.org/10.1016/j.ihj.2025.03.002.
22. Patel NC, Hemli JM, Kim MC, Seetharam K, Pirelli L, Brinster DR, et al. Short- and intermediate-term outcomes of hybrid coronary revascularization for double-vessel disease. J Thorac Cardiovasc Surg. 2018;156(5):1799–807 e3. https://doi.org/10.1016/j.jtcvs.2018.04.078.
23. Zhang S, Li P, Li G, Yan Y, Sun T, Lin J, et al. Generalized hybrid coronary revascularization vs. conventional off-pump coronary artery bypass grafting for multivessel coronary artery disease. Front Cardiovasc Med. 2025;12:1459072. https://doi.org/10.3389/fcvm.2025.1459072.
24. Harskamp RE, Brennan JM, Xian Y, Halkos ME, Puskas JD, Thourani VH, et al. Practice patterns and clinical outcomes after hybrid coronary revascularization in the United States: an analysis from the society of thoracic surgeons adult cardiac database. Circulation. 2014;130(11):872–9. https://doi.org/10.1161/CIRCULATIONAHA.114.009479.
25. Puskas JD, Halkos ME, DeRose JJ, Bagiella E, Miller MA, Overbey J, et al. Hybrid coronary revascularization for the treatment of multivessel coronary artery disease: a multicenter observational study. J Am Coll Cardiol. 2016;68(4):356–65. https://doi.org/10.1016/j.jacc.2016.05.032.
26. Tajstra M, Zembala MO, Gierlotka M, Filipiak K, Gasior M, Hrapkowicz T, et al. Hybrid coronary revascularization in multivessel disease: long-term clinical outcomes of a prospective randomized study. Kardiol Pol. 2024;82(12):1278–80. https://doi.org/10.33963/v.phj.103539.

27. Basman C, Hemli JM, Kim MC, Seetharam K, Brinster DR, Pirelli L, et al. Long-term survival in triple-vessel disease: hybrid coronary revascularization compared to contemporary revascularization methods. J Card Surg. 2020;35(10):2710–8. https://doi.org/10.1111/jocs.14891.
28. Thielmann M, Bonaros N, Barbato E, Barili F, Folliguet T, Friedrich G, et al. Hybrid coronary revascularization: position paper of the European Society of Cardiology Working Group on Cardiovascular Surgery and European Association of Percutaneous Cardiovascular Interventions. Eur J Cardiothorac Surg. 2024;66(2):ezae271. https://doi.org/10.1093/ejcts/ezae271.
29. Balkhy HH, Nisivaco S, Kitahara H, AbuTaleb A, Nathan S, Hamzat I. Robotic advanced hybrid coronary revascularization: outcomes with two internal thoracic artery grafts and stents. JTCVS Tech. 2022;16:76–88. https://doi.org/10.1016/j.xjtc.2022.08.012.
30. Carpentier A, Loulmet D, Carpentier A, Le Bret E, Haugades B, Dassier P, et al. [Open heart operation under videosurgery and minithoracotomy. First case (mitral valvuloplasty) operated with success]. CR Acad Sci III. 1996;319(3):219–23.
31. Brinster DR, Byrne M, Rogers CD, Baim DS, Simon DI, Couper GS, et al. Effectiveness of same day percutaneous coronary intervention followed by minimally invasive aortic valve replacement for aortic stenosis and moderate coronary disease ("hybrid approach"). Am J Cardiol. 2006;98(11):1501–3. https://doi.org/10.1016/j.amjcard.2006.08.010.
32. Ludwig Müller DH, Holfeld J, Hangler H, Bonaros N, Grimm M. Indications and contraindications for minimally invasive mitral valve surgery. J Vis Surg. 2018;4:255. https://doi.org/10.21037/jovs.2018.
33. Catinella FP, Cunningham JN Jr, Spencer FC. Myocardial protection during prolonged aortic cross-clamping. Comparison of blood and crystalloid cardioplegia. J Thorac Cardiovasc Surg. 1984;88(3):411–23.
34. Otto CM, Nishimura RA, Bonow RO, Carabello BA, Erwin JP 3rd, Gentile F, et al. 2020 ACC/AHA guideline for the management of patients with valvular heart disease: a report of the American College of Cardiology/American Heart Association Joint Committee on Clinical Practice Guidelines. J Thorac Cardiovasc Surg. 2021;162(2):e183–353. https://doi.org/10.1016/j.jtcvs.2021.04.002.
35. Rheude T, Costa G, Ribichini FL, Pilgrim T, Amat Santos IJ, De Backer O, et al. Comparison of different percutaneous revascularisation timing strategies in patients undergoing transcatheter aortic valve implantation. EuroIntervention. 2023;19(7):589–99. https://doi.org/10.4244/EIJ-D-23-00186.
36. Lonborg J, Jabbari R, Sabbah M, Veien KT, Niemela M, Freeman P, et al. PCI in patients undergoing transcatheter aortic-valve implantation. N Engl J Med. 2024;391(23):2189–200. https://doi.org/10.1056/NEJMoa2401513.
37. Vahanian A, Beyersdorf F, Praz F, Milojevic M, Baldus S, Bauersachs J, et al. 2021 ESC/EACTS guidelines for the management of valvular heart disease. Eur Heart J. 2022;43(7):561–632. https://doi.org/10.1093/eurheartj/ehab395.
38. Santana O, Xydas S, Williams RF, Mawad M, Heimowitz TB, Pineda AM, et al. Hybrid approach of percutaneous coronary intervention followed by minimally invasive mitral valve surgery: a 5-year single-center experience. J Thorac Dis. 2017;9(Suppl 7):S595–601. https://doi.org/10.21037/jtd.2017.06.29.
39. Oner A, Alozie A, Dohmen PM. Hybrid approach for percutaneous mitral valve repair (MitraClip(R)) followed by minimally invasive direct coronary artery bypass (MIDCAB) in a patient with a high risk constellation. J Card Surg. 2021;36(11):4419–22. https://doi.org/10.1111/jocs.15967.
40. Bagaev E, Ali A, Saha S, Sadoni S, Orban M, Naebauer M, et al. Hybrid surgery for severe mitral valve calcification: limitations and caveats for an open transcatheter approach. Medicina (Kaunas). 2022;58(1):93. https://doi.org/10.3390/medicina58010093.
41. El-Eshmawi A, Tang GHL, Sun E, Alexis SL, Cangut B, Pandis D, et al. Contemporary surgical techniques for mitral valve replacement in extensive mitral annular calcification. JTCVS Tech. 2023;22:1–12. https://doi.org/10.1016/j.xjtc.2023.10.009.

42. Oatway C, Shimamura J, Bagur R, Fujii S, Chu MWA. Simultaneous hybrid transcatheter aortic valve implantation and endoscopic mitral valve repair. CJC Open. 2023;5(3):230–2. https://doi.org/10.1016/j.cjco.2022.12.002.
43. Nicoara A, Skubas N, Ad N, Finley A, Hahn RT, Mahmood F, et al. Guidelines for the use of transesophageal echocardiography to assist with surgical decision-making in the operating room: a surgery-based approach: from the American Society of Echocardiography in Collaboration with the Society of Cardiovascular Anesthesiologists and the Society of Thoracic Surgeons. J Am Soc Echocardiogr. 2020;33(6):692–734. https://doi.org/10.1016/j.echo.2020.03.002.
44. Ender J, Sgouropoulou S. Value of transesophageal echocardiography (TEE) guidance in minimally invasive mitral valve surgery. Ann Cardiothorac Surg. 2013;2(6):796–802. https://doi.org/10.3978/j.issn.2225-319X.2013.10.09.
45. Alamanni F, Dainese L, Naliato M, Gregu S, Agrifoglio M, Polvani GL, et al. On- and off-pump coronary surgery and perioperative myocardial infarction: an issue between incomplete and extensive revascularization. Eur J Cardiothorac Surg. 2008;34(1):118–26. https://doi.org/10.1016/j.ejcts.2008.03.031.
46. Leviner DB, Torregrossa G, Puskas JD. Incomplete revascularization: what the surgeon needs to know. Ann Cardiothorac Surg. 2018;7(4):463–9. https://doi.org/10.21037/acs.2018.06.07.
47. Pijls NH, Fearon WF, Tonino PA, Siebert U, Ikeno F, Bornschein B, et al. Fractional flow reserve versus angiography for guiding percutaneous coronary intervention in patients with multivessel coronary artery disease: 2-year follow-up of the FAME (Fractional Flow Reserve Versus Angiography for Multivessel Evaluation) study. J Am Coll Cardiol. 2010;56(3):177–84. https://doi.org/10.1016/j.jacc.2010.04.012.
48. Tonino PA, Fearon WF, De Bruyne B, Oldroyd KG, Leesar MA, Ver Lee PN, et al. Angiographic versus functional severity of coronary artery stenoses in the FAME study fractional flow reserve versus angiography in multivessel evaluation. J Am Coll Cardiol. 2010;55(25):2816–21. https://doi.org/10.1016/j.jacc.2009.11.096.
49. Karkouti K, Wijeysundera DN. The clinical dilemma of managing patients who are on dual antiplatelet therapy and require major non-cardiac surgery. Br J Anaesth. 2019;122(2):162–4. https://doi.org/10.1016/j.bja.2018.10.002.
50. Giacoppo D, Matsuda Y, Fovino LN, D'Amico G, Gargiulo G, Byrne RA, et al. Short dual antiplatelet therapy followed by P2Y12 inhibitor monotherapy vs. prolonged dual antiplatelet therapy after percutaneous coronary intervention with second-generation drug-eluting stents: a systematic review and meta-analysis of randomized clinical trials. Eur Heart J. 2021;42(4):308–19. https://doi.org/10.1093/eurheartj/ehaa739.
51. Sullivan AE, Nanna MG, Wang TY, Bhatt DL, Angiolillo DJ, Mehran R, et al. Bridging antiplatelet therapy after percutaneous coronary intervention: JACC review topic of the week. J Am Coll Cardiol. 2021;78(15):1550–63. https://doi.org/10.1016/j.jacc.2021.08.013.
52. Valgimigli M, Bueno H, Byrne RA, Collet JP, Costa F, Jeppsson A, et al. 2017 ESC focused update on dual antiplatelet therapy in coronary artery disease developed in collaboration with EACTS: the task force for dual antiplatelet therapy in coronary artery disease of the European Society of Cardiology (ESC) and of the European Association for Cardio-Thoracic Surgery (EACTS). Eur Heart J. 2018;39(3):213–60. https://doi.org/10.1093/eurheartj/ehx419.
53. Petar H, Uzov CMI. Single-dose cold modified Bretschneider solution for myocardial protection in the surgical treatment of patients with aortic valve stenosis and left ventricular hypertrophy. J Biomed Clin Res. 2022;14(2):169–77. https://doi.org/10.2478/jbcr-2021-0021.
54. Sundermann SH, Back C, Bischoff-Ferrari HA, Dehbi HM, Szekely A, Voller H, et al. Preinterventional frailty assessment in patients scheduled for cardiac surgery or transcatheter aortic valve implantation: a consensus statement of the European Association for Cardio-Thoracic Surgery (EACTS) and the European Association of Preventive Cardiology (EAPC) of the European Society of Cardiology (ESC). Eur J Cardiothorac Surg. 2023;64(4). https://doi.org/10.1093/ejcts/ezad181.

55. Goecke S, Pitts L, Dini M, Montagner M, Wert L, Akansel S, et al. Enhanced recovery after cardiac surgery for minimally invasive valve surgery: a systematic review of key elements and advancements. Medicina (Kaunas). 2025;61(3):495. https://doi.org/10.3390/medicina61030495.
56. Sabatino ME, Okoh AK, Chao JC, Soto C, Baxi J, Salgueiro LA, et al. Early discharge after minimally invasive aortic and mitral valve surgery. Ann Thorac Surg. 2022;114(1):91–7. https://doi.org/10.1016/j.athoracsur.2021.07.047.
57. Vahanian A, Beyersdorf F, Praz F, Milojevic M, Baldus S, Bauersachs J, et al. 2021 ESC/EACTS guidelines for the management of valvular heart disease. Eur J Cardiothorac Surg. 2021;60(4):727–800. https://doi.org/10.1093/ejcts/ezab389.
58. Archie MM, Archie MM, Khoynezhand A. Techniques in hybrid repair of aortic arch and thoracoabdominal aortic pathologies. Expert Rev Med Devices. 2025;22(1):23–30. https://doi.org/10.1080/17434440.2024.2442483.
59. Vekstein AM, Jensen CW, Weissler EH, Downey PS, Kang L, Gaca JG, et al. Long-term outcomes for hybrid aortic arch repair. J Vasc Surg. 2024;79(4):711–20 e2. https://doi.org/10.1016/j.jvs.2023.11.032.
60. Xydas S, Mihos CG, Williams RF, LaPietra A, Mawad M, Wittels SH, et al. Hybrid repair of aortic arch aneurysms: a comprehensive review. J Thorac Dis. 2017;9(Suppl 7):S629–S34. https://doi.org/10.21037/jtd.2017.06.47.
61. Moulakakis KG, Mylonas SN, Markatis F, Kotsis T, Kakisis J, Liapis CD. A systematic review and meta-analysis of hybrid aortic arch replacement. Ann Cardiothorac Surg. 2013;2(3):247–60. https://doi.org/10.3978/j.issn.2225-319X.2013.05.06.
62. Zhan Y, Kooperkamp H, Lofftus S, McGrath D, Kawabori M, Chen FY. Conventional open versus hybrid aortic arch repair: a meta-analysis of propensity-matched studies. J Thorac Dis. 2021;13(8):4714–22. https://doi.org/10.21037/jtd-21-183.
63. Chen CW, Hu J, Li YY, Chen GX, Zhang W, Chen XY. The outcomes of aortic arch repair between open surgical repair and debranching endovascular hybrid surgical repair: a systematic review and meta-analysis. J Vasc Surg. 2024;79(6):1510–24. https://doi.org/10.1016/j.jvs.2023.12.025.
64. Ikeno Y, Yokawa K, Matsueda T, Yamanaka K, Inoue T, Tanaka H, et al. Long-term outcomes of total arch replacement using a 4-branched graft. J Thorac Cardiovasc Surg. 2019;157(1):75–85 e3. https://doi.org/10.1016/j.jtcvs.2018.09.118.
65. Bacha EA, Hijazi ZM. Hybrid procedures in pediatric cardiac surgery. Semin Thorac Cardiovasc Surg Pediatr Card Surg Annu. 2005:78–85. https://doi.org/10.1053/j.pcsu.2005.01.001.
66. Bacha EA, Marshall AC, McElhinney DB, del Nido PJ. Expanding the hybrid concept in congenital heart surgery. Semin Thorac Cardiovasc Surg Pediatr Card Surg Annu. 2007:146–50. https://doi.org/10.1053/j.pcsu.2007.01.019.
67. Bitar F, El-Rassi IM, Zareef R, Jassar Y, Abboud J, Bulbul Z, et al. Hybrid stage 1 palliation for HLHS: the experience of a tertiary center in a developing country. Front Cardiovasc Med. 2024;11:1355989. https://doi.org/10.3389/fcvm.2024.1355989.
68. Zanaboni DB, Sower CT, Yu S, Lowery R, Romano JC, Zampi JD. Practice variation using the hybrid stage I procedure in congenital heart disease: results from a national survey. JTCVS Open. 2024;21:248–56. https://doi.org/10.1016/j.xjon.2024.07.020.
69. Uhl S, Grieshaber P, Arnold R, Loukanov T, Gorenflo M. Impact of hybrid procedure on pulmonary arterial dimensions and right ventricular load after biventricular repair. J Cardiothorac Surg. 2023;18(1):65. https://doi.org/10.1186/s13019-023-02162-z.
70. Farias M, Fleishman CE, Nykanen D, DeCampli WM. Clinical update on the hybrid comprehensive stage II operation. JTCVS Open. 2021;7:327–35. https://doi.org/10.1016/j.xjon.2021.04.019.
71. Gupta A, Amin Z. Popular hybrid congenital heart procedures without cardiopulmonary bypass. Front Surg. 2017;4:9. https://doi.org/10.3389/fsurg.2017.00009.
72. Devaney EJ, Lee T, Gelehrter S, Hirsch JC, Ohye RG, Anderson RH, et al. Biventricular repair of atrioventricular septal defect with common atrioventricular valve and double-outlet right

ventricle. Ann Thorac Surg. 2010;89(2):537–42; discussion 42–3. https://doi.org/10.1016/j.athoracsur.2009.10.049.
73. Holoshitz N, Kenny D, Hijazi ZM. Hybrid interventional procedures in congenital heart disease. Methodist Debakey Cardiovasc J. 2014;10(2):93–8. https://doi.org/10.14797/mdcj-10-2-93.
74. Di Bernardo SSN, Mivelaz Y, Fall AL, von Segesser LK, Hurni M. Interventions hybrides et malformations cardiaques congénitales [hybrid procedures in congenital heart disease]. Rev Med Suisse. 2008;150:788–92.
75. Gil-Jaurena JM, Zunzunegui JL, Perez-Caballero R, Pita A, Pardo C, Calle C, et al. Hybrid procedures. Opening doors for surgeon and cardiologist close collaboration. Front Pediatr. 2021;9:687909. https://doi.org/10.3389/fped.2021.687909.
76. Byrne JG, Leacche M, Vaughan DE, Zhao DX. Hybrid cardiovascular procedures. JACC Cardiovasc Interv. 2008;1(5):459–68. https://doi.org/10.1016/j.jcin.2008.07.002.
77. Akintuerk H, Schranz D, Voelkel N. Hybrid procedures for congenital heart disease. Thoracic key: thoracic key.
78. Salavitabar A, Armstrong AK, Carrillo SA. Hybrid interventions in congenital heart disease. Interv Cardiol Clin. 2024;13(3):399–408. https://doi.org/10.1016/j.iccl.2024.02.005.
79. Zampi JD, Sower CT, Lancaster TS, Sood V, Romano JC. Hybrid interventions in congenital heart disease: a review of current practice and rationale for use. Ann Thorac Surg. 2024;118(2):329–37. https://doi.org/10.1016/j.athoracsur.2024.03.001.

Trans-Catheter Interventions for Native Mitral Valve Regurgitation

8

Andrea Marrone and Alfonso Ielasi

Introduction

Mitral regurgitation (MR) is the second most common valvular heart disease in European countries, where approximately 10% of the population over the age of 75 years is affected by this condition [1, 2].

From an etiological standpoint, MR can be divided into two main categories: primary (or organic) and secondary (or functional). This etiological classification is crucial for therapeutic purposes, as different causes require distinctly different treatment strategies [1, 2].

Primary MR (PMR) is characterized by intrinsic lesions affecting one or more components of the mitral valve apparatus. In Western countries, the most common underlying causes are fibroelastic deficiency and Barlow disease, while in developing countries, rheumatic heart disease remains a significant contributor. Infective endocarditis may also be a cause of PMR in both settings [3, 4].

Secondary or functional MR (FMR), on the other hand, may result from left ventricular dilation or systolic dysfunction with associated regional wall motion abnormalities, leading to leaflet tethering (ventricular FMR or V-FMR), or from left atrial dilation causing an "annulus-leaflet area imbalance" and subsequent leaflet tethering (atrial FMR or A-FMR) [5–7].

While adhering to the recommendations outlined in the most recent 2021 European Society of Cardiology and European Association for Cardio-Thoracic Surgery (ESC/EACTS) guidelines for the management of MR [1], the ongoing development and expansion of percutaneous techniques have established and

A. Marrone · A. Ielasi (✉)
Catheterization Laboratory, U.O. Cardiologia Ospedaliera, IRCCS Ospedale Galeazzi Sant'Ambrogio, Milan, Italy

G. Tinică, A. Burlacu (eds.), *Surgical, Hybrid and Minimally Invasive Structural Cardiac Interventions*, https://doi.org/10.1007/978-3-032-16676-0_8

increasingly consolidated a valid alternative to conventional surgery, particularly for patients at high surgical risk or those deemed unsuitable for traditional surgical approaches [8].

Transcatheter Mitral Valve Repair (TMVr)

In the field of TMVr, a range of devices, procedures, and techniques have been developed in order to target the underlying pathophysiological mechanisms of MR, with the aim of achieving a valve repair specifically tailored to the etiology of the disease. These include:

- Indirect annuloplasty: Carillon Mitral Contour System (Cardiac Dimensions Inc., WA, USA), Arto System (MVRx, Inc., Belmont, CA, USA).
- Direct annuloplasty: Cardioband Mitral System (Edwards Lifesciences, Irvine, California), Millipede Transcatheter Mitral Valve Annuloplasty System (Boston Scientific, MA, USA).
- Leaflet's approximation: MitraClip system (Abbott, IL, USA), PASCAL Transcatheter Valve Repair System (Edwards Lifesciences), Dragonfly (Hangzhou Valgen Medtech Co., Ltd.), MyClip (Meril, Vapi, India).
- Chordal repair: HARPOON Beating Heart Mitral Valve Repair System (MVRS; Edwards Lifesciences, CA, USA), *NeoChord Artificial Chordae Delivery System* (NeoChord, Inc., MN, USA).

Indirect Annuloplasty

Annuloplasty has long been one of the main surgical techniques, employed both as a standalone procedure and in combination with other mitral valve repair methods. It is therefore not surprising that some percutaneous approaches have been developed to replicate their surgical counterparts. One of the main challenges of mitral annuloplasty is the intraprocedural visualization and anchoring of a device to the mitral annulus. For this reason, the first annuloplasty devices were "indirect," acting primarily at the level of the coronary sinus (CS) rather than directly on the mitral annulus. This technique is primarily indicated in cases of FMR secondary to annular dilation (Carpentier type I), or in the presence of restricted leaflet motion during systole, whether ischemic or non-ischemic in origin (Carpentier type IIIb). The rationale underlying indirect annuloplasty is based on the anatomical relationship between the CS and the mitral annulus. Anatomically, the CS runs within the atrioventricular groove, in close proximity to the mitral annulus [9]. With the shift from the traditional paradigm—where FMR was considered solely a consequence of left ventricular dilation—to a broader understanding that includes atrial dilation, often associated with supraventricular arrhythmias (such as atrial fibrillation and atrial flutter), it has been demonstrated that in approximately two-thirds of patients with FMR, the distance between the CS and the mitral annulus increases. This results in a flattening of the characteristic "saddle-shaped" morphology of the mitral annulus. Consequently, annular dilation contributes significantly to FMR in more than half of the patients. Therefore, remodeling of the CS can lead to a reduction in the dimensions of the mitral annulus and an improvement in valvular function [10, 11].

The Carillon Mitral Contour System is a CE-approved device for the treatment of FMR via indirect annuloplasty with the aim to improve coaptation of the mitral leaflets. As part of the device system, the sizing catheter is used to estimate the dimensions of the CS and the great cardiac vein (GCV), which are preliminarily assessed by angiography, taking into account both the length and diameter of the CS. The delivery system, advanced through the right internal jugular vein, enables the percutaneous deployment of the device at the implantation site and allows for repositioning or recapture if necessary. The Carillon device consists of a nitinol band with self-expanding anchors at both the proximal and distal ends. The device is available in lengths of 60 mm and 80 mm. Distal anchor diameters range from 7 to 14 mm, while proximal anchor diameters range from 12 to 20 mm. There are 37 different combinations of distal and proximal anchor diameters and device lengths [10, 12]. Procedurally, the distal anchor is positioned as deeply as possible within the CS (extending into the GCV), and tension is then applied to the annulus. The proximal anchor is positioned in the ostium of the CS. The degree of tension to be applied is typically guided by the immediate reduction of MR observed through intraprocedural echocardiographic monitoring. Once optimal tension is achieved, the proximal anchor is deployed. At this stage, performing coronary angiography is essential to assess for potential compromise of the ostium of the left circumflex artery (LCx), as previous studies have shown that the LCx crosses the CS and the mitral annulus in approximately 80% of patients [12–14].

The initial studies evaluating the safety and efficacy of the Carillon system were: AMADEUS (CARILLON Mitral Annuloplasty Device European Union Study) [15], TITAN (Tighten the Annulus Now) [16], and TITAN II trials [17]. AMADEUS was the trial which led to the granting of CE certification. Among 48 patients suffering FMR and left ventricular systolic dysfunction, Carillon was successfully implanted in 30, resulting in a significant reduction in MR and an improvement in NYHA class from 2.9 to 1.8 [15]. The TITAN study enrolled a cohort of 53 symptomatic (NYHA III) patients with severely reduced left ventricle ejection fraction (LVEF). Among these, 36 were successfully treated, while in the remaining 17 the procedure was halted and Carillon was retrieved because of transient coronary compromise in 8 patients and reduction in FMR of less than one grade in 9 patients. In the subgroup of patients successfully treated, a significant improvement in symptoms and a reduction of more than 50% in regurgitant volume, as well as in systolic and diastolic volumes, was reported as compared to the non-implanted group [16]. The TITAN II study was conducted to assess the safety and structural integrity of an updated version of the Carillon, incorporating design modifications aimed at enhancing the device's resistance to mechanical fatigue: mXE2. This study essentially confirmed previous findings, demonstrating improved functional capacity at 1-year follow-up as measured by the 6-minute walk test, along with echocardiographic improvement in MR [17]. More recent randomized data come from the REDUCE-FMR trial, in which 120 patients with severely depressed LVEF were randomized to receive either the Carillon device or medical therapy. At 1-year follow-up, patients in the device group showed a statistically significant reduction in the primary endpoint of regurgitant volume compared to the medical therapy group, along with significant left ventricular reverse remodeling [18]. Currently, the CARILLON randomized trial is ongoing (ClinicalTrials.gov Identifier: NCT03142152), with the aim to compare the device versus medical therapy in a broad population of patients with FMR.

Main limitation of the indirect mitral annuloplasty with Carillon is the distance between the CS and the mitral annulus, which is approximately 1 cm or even more in patients with heart failure, representing a limiting factor in the procedural outcome. Another concern is associated with the potential *ab estrinseco* compression of the LCx or its branches leading to impaired blood flow. In this case, it is necessary to reduce the tension and/or reposition the device; for this reason, continuous coronary arteries monitoring throughout the procedure is essential. Torsional and tensile forces may also lead to device fracture. Carillon implantation is actually not indicated in CRT-D patients [19, 20].

Arto System

The Arto system is an indirect mitral annuloplasty device designed to enhance mitral leaflet coaptation through a bridging mechanism involving the close approximation of magnetically linked MagneCaths positioned in the left atrium (LA) and the great cardiac vein (GCV). This approach enables an anteroposterior reduction of the mitral annulus—posterior to the P2 segment—while offering the advantage of being non-injurious to surrounding tissue. The procedure is performed under transesophageal echocardiographic guidance. The CS is cannulated via the right external jugular vein, and a T-bar is implanted in the lateral wall of the GCV. A left atrial septal implant is then performed via transseptal puncture. A bridging suture is subsequently created between these two components, resulting in a reduction of the anteroposterior diameter of the mitral annulus. The device can be recaptured and repositioned during the procedure [21, 22].

The main data on the use of this device come from the MAVERIC (Mitral Valve Repair Clinical) trial, in which the Arto system was implanted in 45 patients with symptomatic heart failure and FMR. The primary endpoint—a composite of death, stroke, myocardial infarction, device-related surgery, renal failure, and cardiac tamponade—was observed in 4.4% of patients at 30-day and 17.8% at 1-year. The anteroposterior diameter of the mitral annulus decreased from 41.4 mm at baseline to 36.0 mm at 30 days and 35.3 mm at 1-year follow-up. Additionally, patients experienced an improvement in NYHA functional class and a significant reduction in FMR, with only 8% of patients exhibiting grade 3/4+ FMR at 1-year post-procedure [23]. In 2021, the 2-year follow-up results were published, demonstrating that the composite safety outcome was achieved (2 out of 45 adverse events at 30 days), and no device-related deaths were reported at the 2-year mark. These findings were supported by a sustained reduction in functional MR [grade < 2: 21/31 (68%) vs. 0/31 (0%); $P < 0.0001$] and a progressive improvement in symptoms [NYHA class ≤II: 27/34 (80%) vs. 12/34 (36%); $P < 0.0001$] [24].

Direct Annuloplasty

Anatomically, the mitral annulus is a thin, C-shaped structure composed of fibrous tissue, measuring approximately 3 to 5 mm in thickness, that encircles the mitral valve and attaches to the anterior and posterior trigones. The inter-trigonal region—located between the anterior and posterior trigones—represents an even more delicate area, as it is characterized by the direct anatomical contiguity of the aortic root and the base of the anterior mitral leaflet. More recently, in contrast to indirect annuloplasty devices, novel approaches have increasingly focused on direct annuloplasty techniques, which specifically target the mitral annulus itself. Most of these techniques involve the placement of rings or bands directly anchored to the annulus, without involving adjacent structures. Despite procedural complexity—including the need for highly precise placement on a beating heart, the risk of impingement of nearby structures, and the potential for device pull-out—the advantages of these techniques lie in the direct remodeling of the annulus, thereby more closely replicating the traditional surgical approach [25, 26].

Cardioband Mitral System is a percutaneous device delivered under general anesthesia and transesophageal echocardiographic (TEE) guidance via transeptal atrial access with the aim of reducing the mitral annular circumference, thereby improving leaflet coaptation. The system consists of a delivery system covered with a polyester sleeve, featuring radiopaque markers placed every 8 mm. The delivery system is used to implant multiple anchors (ranging from 12 to 17 depending on the device size). The band is implanted on the atrial side of the mitral annulus. Lateral and anterior placement of the first anchor is the initial, critical step. After this, coronary angiography is performed to confirm the patency of the LCx. Subsequent anchors are then deployed sequentially along the mitral annulus until the catheter tip reaches the final anchoring point on the medial side of the annulus. The device does not encompass the entire mitral annulus but is positioned along a partial perimeter. A contraction wire is then connected to a coil designed to apply tension and consequently reduce the annular circumference. Continuous TEE guidance allows real-time assessment of MR reduction.

Various implant sizes are available (Table 8.1); the total device length and number of anchors to be implanted are determined through a computed tomography (CT)-based reconstruction [25, 27, 28]. Initial clinical results were reported in a cohort of 31 patients with moderate-to-severe FMR and reduced LVEF, showing a 100% procedural success rate with no periprocedural mortality. The device

Table 8.1 Cardioband sizing chart

Implant size	Deployment length by CT (mm)	Total anchors required
A	73–80	12
B	81–66	13
C	89–96	14
D	97–104	15
E	105–112	16
F	113–120	17

CT computed tomography

demonstrated a 6-month reduction in septo-lateral annular dimensions from 3.7 ± 0.5 cm at baseline to 2.4 ± 0.4 cm, with the proportion of patients with MR grade ≥ 3 decreasing from 77.4% to 13.6% [29]. Subsequently, *Messika-Zeitoun et al.* reported results from a prospective single-arm study involving 60 patients with similar baseline characteristics. There were two in-hospital deaths unrelated to the device, one stroke, two coronary complications, and one case of cardiac tamponade. Anchor misalignment occurred in 10 patients, and in 5 of these, the device was deemed ineffective. Technical success, device success, and procedural success were: 97%, 72%, and 68%, respectively. At 1 year, MR grade was ≤2+ in 61% of the cohort studied [30].

Overall, the data demonstrate a reasonable safety and efficacy profile, leading to CE mark approval in 2016. Currently, a randomized trial—the ACTIVE trial (ClinicalTrials.gov Identifier: NCT03016975)—is actually enrolling patients who are being randomized to receive either the Cardioband device plus guideline-directed medical therapy (GDMT) or GDMT alone. The MiBAND study (ClinicalTrials.gov Identifier: NCT03600688), instead is a post-market, prospective, single-arm, European post-market study to assess the safety and efficacy of the Cardioband system.

Leaflet's Approximation

The trans-catheter strategies aiming to reduce MR degree by leaflet's approximation mime the surgical mitral valve repair technique known as "edge-to-edge" which was first described by Alfieri et al. [31]. It consists in suturing the central scallops of the anterior and posterior leaflets, thereby creating a double mitral orifice [32]. Several devices are used for percutaneous transcatheter mitral edge-to-edge repair (mTEER) [33] with the aim to approximate the mitral leaflets by grasping one or more scallops by clips.

MitraClip

The MitraClip system received CE mark in 2008 while FDA approval for PMR in 2013, and for FMR in 2019.

The system consists of a stabilizer, a 24Fr steerable guide catheter (SGC), and a clip delivery system (CDS), which includes the clip itself. These components allow for precise maneuverability in both the anteroposterior and mediolateral directions via dedicated control knobs. The MitraClip is composed of two movable rigid arms made of cobalt-chromium alloy and features flexible nitinol grippers equipped with longitudinal frictional elements/hooks for secure leaflet grasping. Since its introduction in the market, several iterations of this device have been provided by the manufacturer.

In 2020, the fourth-generation MitraClip (G4) was released for clinical use. The G4 generation is available in four sizes, differing in the width and length of the clip arms. The NT and XT sizes have a width of 4 mm and arm lengths of 9 mm and 12 mm, respectively. The NTW and XTW versions feature a wider implantation base of 6 mm, while maintaining the same arm lengths as the NT and XT, respectively [34–36].

From a procedural standpoint, the intervention is performed under general anesthesia to allow for continuous TEE guidance. The procedure is carried out via femoral venous access, followed by a transseptal puncture at the fossa ovalis (at a distance of 4–4.5 cm from the leaflet coaptation point). After the puncture, a stiff guidewire is advanced into the left superior pulmonary vein to facilitate the advancement of the SGC (24 Fr) into the left atrium. Once the catheter is in place, the guidewire and dilator are removed, leaving the SGC positioned within the left atrium. Subsequently, the CDS is advanced through the SGC. At this stage, a series of anterior-posterior and medial-lateral rotational maneuvers are performed to align the clip perpendicularly to the mitral valve plane, with the clip arms positioned perpendicular to the coaptation line. Once within the left ventricle, the mitral valve leaflets are grasped by the respective clip arms and grippers, thereby creating the desired dual-orifice configuration. If simultaneous grasping of both leaflets proves challenging, sequential leaflet capture—first one, then the other—can be employed to facilitate the procedure. Before releasing the device, a hemodynamic evaluation must be conducted. Once the assessment of hemodynamics and residual MR is completed, the clip can be deployed. In the event of residual regurgitation or iatrogenic stenosis, the clip may be repositioned [34, 35].

This procedure is generally considered safe, with a low risk of life-threatening complications. Potential complications may be either device-related or procedure-related. Device-related complications include structural failures—such as single leaflet device attachment (1.5–5.1%), device embolization (0.05–0.7%), or leaflet damage (0–2%)—as well as functional impairments, such as residual MR greater than 2+ (reported in up to 17% of cases) or iatrogenic mitral stenosis with a mean gradient >5 mmHg (observed in up to 15% of cases). Procedure-related complications include major vascular events (1.4–4.0%), pericardial effusion (0.5%), and major bleeding requiring blood transfusion (0–17%). Less common, though documented, are thromboembolic complications such as myocardial infarction (0–3%) and stroke (0–1%) [36–39].

One of the most critical steps in determining the outcome of this procedure occurs very early in the clinical pathway and lies in the selection of appropriate candidates. This includes a comprehensive evaluation of the valvular pathology and of the left atrial and ventricular anatomy, with a particular focus on defining anatomical complexity based on specific criteria. Such criteria are essential to exclude patients in whom the procedural risk would outweigh the expected benefit. To fully understand these mechanisms, it is first necessary to distinguish between the treatment of PMR and that of FMR. Regarding PMR, the first available data pertain to first- and second-generation devices. In the EVEREST II trial, 73% of the study population had PMR. Among these patients, 5-year mortality rates were similar between those treated with transcatheter repair and those undergoing surgery (20.8% vs. 26.8%, respectively). When evaluating efficacy in terms of freedom from death, mitral valve surgery, reoperation, and moderate-to-severe MR at 5-year, surgical treatment was shown to be superior to MitraClip (76.2% vs. 45.5%, respectively), primarily due to a higher reintervention rate for residual MR within the first 6-month following MitraClip implantation

[38]. Buzzatti et al. have similarly demonstrated higher reintervention rates after MitraClip compared to surgical repair; however, periprocedural complications and 1-year mortality were significantly lower in the MitraClip cohort [40]. These outcomes may be affected by the limited operator experience and device technology available between 2005 and 2008, when these earlier studies were conducted, and by the exclusive use of first-generation devices. More recently, the EXPAND registry assessed the use of third-generation MitraClip devices (NTR and XTR) in high-risk patients with PMR or mixed etiology, who represented approximately 40% of the enrolled population. At 30 days, the composite event rate—including all-cause mortality, stroke, and myocardial infarction—was significantly lower in the percutaneously treated group compared to the surgical cohort, reinforcing the procedural safety of transcatheter repair [41]. Subsequently, 1-year results from the EXPAND G4 registry, which investigated the use of fourth-generation devices and included a population with 43% PMR, continued to demonstrate sustained MR reduction, low all-cause mortality, and a reduced rate of heart failure-related hospitalizations [42].

Ongoing randomized clinical trials—*REPAIR MR* (Percutaneous MitraClip Device or Surgical Mitral Valve Repair in Patients With Primary Mitral Regurgitation Who Are Candidates for Surgery, ClinicalTrials.gov: NCT04198870), *PRIMARY* (Percutaneous or Surgical Mitral Valve Repair, ClinicalTrials.gov: NCT05051033), and *MITRA-HR* (Multicenter Study of MitraClip Transcatheter Mitral Valve Repair in Patients With Severe Primary Mitral Regurgitation Eligible for High-risk Surgery, ClinicalTrials.gov: NCT03271762)—will aim to compare MitraClip with surgical MV repair in both lower- and high-risk PMR populations.

The two major clinical trials assessing the outcomes of Mitraclip treatment of FMR are the COAPT (*Cardiovascular Outcomes Assessment of the MitraClip Percutaneous Therapy for Heart Failure Patients with Functional Mitral Regurgitation*) [43] and the MITRA-FR (*Percutaneous Repair with the MitraClip Device for Severe Functional/Secondary Mitral Regurgitation*) [44]. The MITRA-FR trial evaluated 302 symptomatic patients with heart failure and reduced ejection fraction (HFrEF) with FMR, defined by an effective regurgitant orifice area (EROA) > 20 mm^2 or a regurgitant volume (RV) > 30 mL. Patients were randomized to either GDM alone or MitraClip in addition to GDMT. The results showed no significant differences between the two groups in the primary endpoint of all-cause mortality or heart failure-related rehospitalizations at 12 and 24 months [44]. The COAPT trial included 614 patients with heart failure and moderately to severely reduced ejection fraction, and with moderate-to-severe or severe FMR defined using a multiparametric approach (i.e., EROA >30 mm^2 or systolic flow reversal in the pulmonary veins). Patients were randomized to receive MitraClip plus GDMT or GDMT alone. The results demonstrated a marked reduction in the primary endpoint of heart failure hospitalizations at 2 years, along with a reduction in all-cause mortality, and improvements in both quality of life and exercise capacity [43].

The seemingly conflicting results of these two trials may be attributed to several factors.

- First, the severity of FMR differed between the studies. Baseline EROA data reveal that FMR was less severe in MITRA-FR compared to COAPT: 52% of patients in MITRA-FR had an EROA <30 mm^2, while only 14% of patients in COAPT had an EROA <20 mm^2. Furthermore, COAPT implemented an upper threshold for left ventricular dimensions (left ventricular end-systolic diameter—LVESD—capped at 70 mm), unlike MITRA-FR. Thus, in MITRA-FR, outcomes may have been more closely associated with the degree of myocardial impairment rather than the actual severity of FMR. As a consequence, COAPT enrolled a larger proportion of patients with so-called "disproportionate" FMR—characterized by a mismatch between left ventricular size and the severity of regurgitation—compared to MITRA-FR.
- Secondly, differences in the heart failure spectrum must be considered. MITRA-FR exclusively enrolled patients with HFrEF (EF 15–40%), whereas COAPT included patients with EF ranging from 20% to 50%. Despite this, the mean EF was similar between the two studies (33.1% in MITRA-FR vs. 31.3% in COAPT). This supports the hypothesis that MITRA-FR enrolled patients with more advanced heart failure, as reflected by a higher prevalence of "proportionate" FMR, typically associated with a larger left ventricular end-diastolic volume (LVEDV).
- Patients in MITRA-FR were not necessarily on maximally optimized medical therapy, and adjustments to medical treatment were permitted during the trial, in contrast to COAPT, where therapy was required to be stable and optimized prior to enrollment.
- Lastly, patients with severe right ventricular dysfunction—and thus likely to have end-stage biventricular heart failure—were excluded from the COAPT trial, whereas no data on right ventricular function were reported in the MITRA-FR study [5, 43–45].

The main difference between these two randomized controlled trials is shown in Table 8.2.

More recently, in 2024, new trial data have been presented. The MATTERHORN trial (*A Multicenter, Randomized, Controlled Study to Assess Mitral Valve Reconstruction for Advanced Insufficiency of Functional or Ischemic Origin*) randomized 210 patients with FMR and symptomatic heart failure (NYHA class $\geq$ II) with a LVEF of at least 20% to receive either surgical treatment (repair or replacement) or mTEER with MitraClip. At 1-year follow-up, mTEER was non-inferior to surgical intervention—whether repair or replacement—with respect to the composite primary endpoint of death, heart failure hospitalization, reintervention, implantation of a mechanical circulatory support device, or stroke. The mTEER strategy was also associated with a favorable safety profile [46]. The RESHAPE-HF2 trial (*A Clinical Evaluation of the Safety and Effectiveness of the MitraClip System in the Treatment of Clinically Significant Functional Mitral Regurgitation*) further demonstrated that, in patients with symptomatic heart failure and moderate-to-severe or severe FMR, mTEER led to a reduction in the composite endpoint of recurrent heart failure hospitalizations or all-cause mortality, as well as a reduction in the incidence

Table 8.2 Differences between MITRA-FR, COAPT and RESHAPE-HF2

	MITRA-FR [44]	COAPT [43, 44]	RESHAPE HF2 [47]
Randomization	MitraClip + GDMT vs GDMT	MitraClip + GDMT vs GDMT	MitraClip + GDMT vs GDMT
Study population	152/152	302/312	250/255
LVEF	15–40%	20–50%	NYHA II: 15–35%. NYHA III/IV: 15–45%
MR grade	EROA > 20 mm^2 RV > 30 ml	EROA ≥ 30 mm^2 RV > 45 ml	EROA > 30 mm^2 RV > 45 ml
LVESD	No LVESD threshold	≤ 70	No LVESD threshold
Baseline GDMT	Not required to be on OMT + variations allowed	OMT and cardiac resynchronization therapy if appropriate	OMT, revascularization and/or cardiac resynchronization therapy if appropriate
NYHA class	II, III, IV	II, III, IVa	II, III, IV
Surgical risk	Not candidate for MV surgery	Not candidate for MV surgery	MV surgery is not the preferred option
Primary endpoint	Composite of death from any cause or HF hospitalization (12 months)	HF hospitalizations (24 months)	First or recurrent HF hospitalization and CV death (24 months), KCCQ-OS (12 months)
Results	54.6% device group 51.3% control group	35.8% device group 67.9% control group	37% device group 58.9% control group

CV cardiovascular, *GDMT* guideline-directed medical therapy, *EROA* effective regurgitant orifice area, *LVEF* left-ventricular ejection fraction, *LVESD* left ventricular end-systolic diameter, *NYHA* New York Heart Association, *MR* mitral regurgitation, *OMT* optimal medical therapy, *RV* regurgitant volume, *KCCS-OS* Kansas City Cardiomyopathy Questionnaire–Overall Summary

of recurrent heart failure hospitalizations over 24 months. These findings are consistent with those of the COAPT trial. Considering the mean EROA value of 0.23 cm^2 in both study arms, patients enrolled in RESHAPE-HF2 appeared to have less severe MR compared to those in COAPT (0.41 cm^2) and MITRA-FR (0.31 cm^2). This may suggest that mTEER provides clinical benefit even in patients with less severe FMR [47].

Although the study did not demonstrate a significant reduction in all-cause mortality, a meta-analysis of these three trials revealed a clear trend toward a beneficial effect of mTEER on mortality or all-cause mortality at 2-year follow-up [48].

Regarding anatomical criteria, the optimal parameters are based on the inclusion criteria of the EVEREST trial, which defined a population of patients with a high pretest probability of a favorable outcome following mTEER. When deviating from these criteria, procedural complexity increases, along with the likelihood of a suboptimal and less durable result, potentially impacting clinical outcomes. Table 8.3 provides a detailed overview of anatomical features associated with high or low procedural complexity [38].

In the EXPAND registry, anatomical complexity was characterized by the following criteria: a wide coaptation gap (≥15 mm), a large flail gap (≥10 mm),

Table 8.3 Anatomical complexity criteria for mitral valve suitability in M-TEER

		Ideal Anatomy	Complex Anatomy	Unsuitable Anatomy
Regurgitant jet	Single (A1-P1/A3-P3), commissural	✓		
	Multiple, commissural		✓	
	Multiple/wide			✓
MVA	>4.0 cm^2	✓		
	3.0–3.5 cm^2		✓	
	<3.0 cm^2			✓
Posterior leaflet	>10 mm/7–10 mm	✓		
	5–7 mm		✓	
	<5 mm			✓
Calcifications	Absent/annular without leaflet involvement	✓		
	Annular with leaflet involvement		✓	
	Concentric MAC with stenosis			✓
	Calcification in the grasping zone			✓
Barlow's disease			✓	
Deep regurgitant cleft				✓
Leaflet perforation				✓
Mean diastolic gradient >5 mmHg				✓

A1/P1 lateral segments of anterior (A1) and posterior (P3) mitral valve leaflets, *A3/P3* medial segments of anterior (A3) and posterior (P3) mitral valve leaflet, *MAC* mitral annular calcification, *MR* mitral regurgitation, *MS* mitral stenosis, *MVA* mitral valve area

regurgitant jets located outside the canonical A2/P2 position, a small mitral valve area (MVA), a calcified landing zone, and minimal leaflet tissue. Patients presenting with at least one of these features were more likely to experience a suboptimal outcome, defined as residual MR $\leq$ 1+ [41]. Other studies have identified annular or leaflet calcifications, leaflet infiltration of $\geq$6 mm, MVA <4 cm^2, a baseline transmitral gradient $\geq$4 mmHg, and multiple regurgitant jets as risk factors for a mean diastolic gradient $\geq$5 mmHg post-mTEER. Severe calcifications within the grasping area, active endocarditis foci, and hemodynamically significant mitral stenosis constitute absolute contraindications to mTEER [36, 49–51].

Pascal Transcatheter Valve Repair System

This mTEER system comprises three components: a 22 Fr steerable guide sheath, a steerable catheter, and a delivery catheter with the device pre-mounted at its distal tip. The PASCAL P10 device consists of two spring-loaded, curved paddles capable of spanning 26 mm when fully opened at 180°, two 10 mm clasps, and a central spacer designed to reduce leaflet tension and to occupy the regurgitant orifice, thereby minimizing MR. A second device, known as the PASCAL Ace, has also become available. While it retains the same technical characteristics as the P10, it features narrower 6 mm paddles, allowing implantation in smaller anatomies.

The steerable catheter is responsible for controlling implant trajectory and positioning, while the delivery catheter manages device orientation and deployment. These three catheters can be operated independently, allowing precise manipulation in all three spatial planes. The procedure is performed under general anesthesia with hemodynamic monitoring, guided by TEE and fluoroscopy. Left atrial access is achieved via transseptal puncture, through which the guide sheath and introducer are advanced over a guidewire already positioned in the left atrium. The delivery catheter is introduced via a loader through the guide sheath, and the steerable catheter is advanced until the device exits the loader. The steerable catheter is then used to advance the delivery system until the device exits through the sheath tip. Manipulation of the steerable catheter allows adjustment of the trajectory and position until the system is aligned perpendicularly to the mitral valve plane, directly above the regurgitant jet. At this stage, the actuation knob on the delivery catheter is rotated to open the paddles into the capture position. The paddles must be aligned perpendicularly to the coaptation line, a process facilitated by rotation of the delivery catheter. The system is then advanced into the left ventricle, with prior identification of anterior and posterior leaflets using clasp positioning. Leaflet grasping can be performed either simultaneously or independently. Prior to device release, a hemodynamic assessment is required to confirm adequate device placement [36, 52–54].

The PASCAL system received CE mark approval and was introduced in 2019 after demonstrating safety and feasibility in the CLASP study, which enrolled patients with functional, degenerative, or mixed MR. This international early feasibility study included 124 patients with primary and secondary MR (31% and 69%, respectively), all treated with the PASCAL P10 (the PASCAL Ace became available in 2020). At 1-year follow-up, overall survival was 92% (89% in FMR and 96% in PMR), with 88% freedom from heart failure hospitalization (80% FMR, 100% PMR). MR ≤1+ was achieved in 82% of patients (79% FMR, 86% PMR), and MR ≤2+ in 100% of patients. Additionally, 88% of patients were classified as NYHA class I or II. At 30-day echocardiographic follow-up, MR was reduced to ≤1+ in 80% of cases (77% FMR, 86% PMR) and to ≤2+ in 96% of cases (96% FMR, 97% PMR). These outcomes were sustained at 2-year follow-up. Overall, the CLASP study demonstrated a low complication rate and high survival, with durable MR reduction and significant improvements in functional status and quality of life at 1 year following Pascal implantation [55].

Dragonfly

In addition to the aforementioned devices, a novel mTEER system known as DragonFly has recently been developed with the aim of addressing several complications commonly associated with the MitraClip and PASCAL systems. These include challenges in leaflet grasping, the need for multiple repositionings, limited anatomical indications, and risks of adverse events such as leaflet or chordal rupture and clip dislodgement. The DragonFly system introduces several innovative design features aimed at improving procedural outcomes in mitral valve repair. First, it incorporates a central filler component with high compressibility and shape-memory capabilities, which enables the clip to close at broader angles. This configuration not only minimizes residual MR but also alleviates leaflet stress and allows dynamic adjustment of post-implantation pressure gradients across the mitral valve, thereby enhancing both efficacy and safety. Second, the clip features a self-locking mechanism that permits mechanical adjustment of the grasping force across a spectrum of closure angles. This adaptability allows the device to accommodate diverse anatomical variations and pathological presentations, thereby mitigating the risk of iatrogenic mitral stenosis. Third, the system includes an independent leaflet capture design, which facilitates more precise and flexible deployment, enhancing procedural simplicity and operator control. Structurally, the DragonFly clip comprises four key components: arms, grippers, a central filler, and a locking mechanism. Both the gripper and the central filler are constructed from a nickel-titanium (nitinol) alloy, leveraging its shape-memory and elasticity properties. Importantly, the device demonstrates a strong ability to prevent structural failure, particularly in avoiding single leaflet device attachment (SLDA)—a condition in which the clip loses its grasp on one mitral leaflet. SLDA is the most frequent mode of device failure in mTEER procedures, often occurring acutely or within the first 24 hours post-intervention, and is primarily attributed to suboptimal leaflet capture. Even when proper grasping is achieved, SLDA may result from mechanical damage such as leaflet tearing or perforation. This complication can lead to the recurrence or worsening of MR, underscoring the need for secure and stable leaflet engagement—a function effectively addressed by the DragonFly system [56].

The *DRAGONFLY-DMR trial* was a prospective, multicenter, single-arm study designed to evaluate the safety and efficacy of the DragonFly system in patients with symptomatic DMR who were considered at prohibitive surgical risk. The primary endpoint was defined as clinical success at 1 year, encompassing freedom from all-cause mortality, mitral valve reintervention, and residual MR greater than 2+. A total of 120 patients were enrolled, and the primary efficacy endpoint was met with a clinical success rate of 87.5% at 1 year (95% CI: 80.1–92.3%). Procedural success was high, with 99.2% of patients successfully implanted. The majority of patients achieved an acute MR reduction to ≤2+ at discharge (100%) and sustained this at 1-year (92.0%). A substantial proportion of patients (approximately 65%) achieved MR ≤1+ early post-procedure, and this effect remained stable over follow-up. Safety outcomes were favorable, with a major adverse event rate of 9.2% and an all-cause mortality of 5.0% at 1 year. The trial also demonstrated improvements in functional status and quality of life [57].

Chordal Repair

Percutaneous mitral chordal repair systems have been developed to treat severe degenerative MR due to flail or prolapse of the anterior, posterior, or both leaflets in the absence of annular dilation and/or left ventricular remodeling. The two systems currently in clinical use are the *NeoChord Artificial Chordae Delivery System* and the *HARPOON Beating Heart Mitral Valve Repair System*. Both techniques require a left lateral thoracotomy and are performed via a transapical, beating-heart, off-pump approach. The key difference compared to conventional surgical repair lies in the fixation point of the neochordae: the distal end is not anchored to the papillary muscle but rather to a pledget located at the apical access site [34].

NeoChord Artificial Chordae Delivery System

The NeoChord system was the first transapical device to be clinically available. The procedure is performed under general anesthesia, off-pump, through a mini-thoracotomy—typically posterolateral—to avoid disrupting the sub-valvular mitral apparatus.

Mitral valve morphology is further classified based on TEE echocardiographic appearance as follows:

- *Type A*: isolated central posterior leaflet prolapse or flail.
- *Type B*: multi-segment posterior leaflet prolapse or flail.
- *Type C*: anterior or bileaflet prolapse or flail.
- *Type D*: para-commissural prolapse/flail or any morphology associated with significant leaflet or annular calcification.

Patients with type A or B anatomy are considered ideal candidates for this procedure. Following thoracotomy, the entry point into the left ventricle is identified approximately 2–3 cm lateral to the true apex and continuously confirmed using TEE guidance. Once positioned, the device jaws are opened, and the leaflet edge is grasped by retracting the device from the left atrium. Leaflet capture is confirmed when all four optical indicators on the fiberoptic monitor switch from red to white, indicating proper jaw closure on the mitral leaflet. A suture loop and girth hitch knot can then be formed on the leaflet. The device may subsequently be reloaded with additional sutures, and the procedure repeated until a sufficient number of neochordae have been implanted—typically at least 3 to 4. The length of each neochordae can be individually adjusted to achieve maximal reduction of the regurgitant jet. Once satisfactory leaflet coaptation is confirmed, the neochordae are anchored to the epicardial pledget [34, 58–60].

The TACT Trial (*Trans-Apical Chordae Tendineae*) was the pivotal study validating this approach and led to CE mark approval in 2012, demonstrating the technical feasibility and safety of the NeoChord system with an overall reduction of MR to ≤2+ in 86.7% of 30 patients [61]. The ongoing *ReChord Trial* (ClinicalTrials.gov: NCT02803957) is currently evaluating the safety and efficacy of off-pump transapical systems versus conventional on-pump surgical techniques. Additionally, the *AcChord Trial* (ClinicalTrials.gov: NCT04190602) is assessing 5-year clinical outcomes of patients treated with the NeoChord DS1000 in a post-marketing surveillance setting.

HARPOON Beating Heart Mitral Valve Repair System

The HARPOON Beating Heart Mitral Valve Repair System is a percutaneous chordal repair device indicated for patients with degenerative MR due to posterior mitral leaflet prolapse. The system consists of two main components: a 12 Fr introducer equipped with a hemostatic valve, and a 9 Fr delivery system that enables the anchoring of expanded polytetrafluoroethylene (ePTFE) cords to the prolapsing leaflet via a percutaneous, beating-heart approach.

The procedure is performed under general anesthesia through a left lateral thoracotomy, typically at the level of the fourth or fifth intercostal space. The introducer is inserted into an area located 2 to 4 cm basal to the true apex of the left ventricle and lateral to the left anterior descending artery. A 3–0 polypropylene horizontal mattress suture is used to secure two pledgets at the apical access site. The delivery system is then advanced through the introducer at an angle of 30° and guided to the ventricular side of the mitral valve under TEE echocardiographic guidance. Once stable contact with the target area on the mitral leaflets is confirmed, the plunger is deployed to create a double-helical knot through the free edge of the leaflet. After the plunger returns to its original position, the suture release mechanism is activated to disengage the ePTFE cords, and the delivery system is withdrawn from the introducer. These steps are repeated for each cord to be implanted, proceeding in a lateral-to-medial way. Once the desired number of chords has been implanted, they are simultaneously anchored to the pledget and tensioned under transesophageal echocardiographic guidance to achieve optimal leaflet coaptation. Upon achieving the appropriate tension, a rubber-shod clamp is applied between the pledget and the tourniquet. The tourniquet is then removed, and each chord is secured with at least 15 alternating knots. Finally, the apical access site on the left ventricle is closed [62, 63].

This device obtained CE marking following the publication of data from the early feasibility study and subsequently the TRACER Trial.

The first-in-human study evaluating the Harpoon system was a prospective, observational investigation [63]. A total of 11 patients with severe MR caused by posterior leaflet prolapse were enrolled. The efficacy and safety of the procedure were assessed at the end of the intervention and at 30-day post-procedure. Procedural success was defined as the implantation of ≥1 ePTFE chord and a reduction in MR severity from severe to moderate, while safety was defined as the absence of major adverse events. The mean follow-up duration was 186 days. Procedural success was achieved in 100% of cases. An average of 3.6 ± 0.7 (range, 3–5) pairs of ePTFE chords were implanted, resulting in an intraoperative MR reduction from severe to none/trivial in 8 patients and too mild in 3 patients. Two in-hospital adverse events occurred: 2 patients required reintervention due to delayed pericardial effusion on postoperative days 5 and 13, respectively, but both were subsequently discharged in good condition. At 1-month follow-up, the average MR grade was mild, with significant reductions in left ventricular end-diastolic volume (from 139 to 107 mL; $p = 0.03$) and left atrial volume (from 118 to 85 mL; $p = 0.04$). MR remained moderate in two patients: one required reintervention, and the other showed a mild residual posterior leaflet prolapse. Favorable reverse remodeling of both the left ventricle and left atrium was also observed.

The TRACER study (Mitral TransApical NeoChordal Echo-Guided Repair) was a multicenter, non-randomized trial involving 30 patients with the same indication

[64]. The primary endpoints were identical to those of the previous study. Technical success was achieved in 27 out of 30 patients (90%), with a mean of 3.9 ± 1 (range, 1 to 5) pairs of chords implanted. Three patients required conversion to conventional open-heart surgery. No deaths, strokes, or permanent pacemaker implantations were reported. At 1-month follow-up, MR was mild or less in 89% (24/27) and moderate in 11% (3/27) of patients. At 6 months, MR remained mild or less in 85% (22/26), moderate in 8% (2/26), and severe in 8% (2/26). Favorable cardiac remodeling at 6 months included reductions in left ventricular end-diastolic volume (from 161 ± 36 mL to 122 ± 30 mL; $p < 0.001$) and left atrial volume (from 106 ± 36 mL to 69 ± 24 mL; $p < 0.001$).

Transcatheter Mitral Valve Replacement (TMVR)

On the other hand, the feasibility of percutaneous native mitral valve replacement (TMVR) is progressively being supported by emerging data, primarily in high-risk patients with FMR. The vast majority of the corresponding devices are currently undergoing clinical evaluation while only one received CE mark. Although the development of these technologies remains largely in progress, their use raises important considerations, such as the potential for these novel procedures to eventually replace more complex valve repair systems. Among the bioprosthesis used for TMVR can be mentioned: Intrepid (Medtronic), Tendyne (Abbott Structural), AltaValve (4C Medical), CardioValve (Venus MedTech), and Innovalve Transcatheter Mitral Valve Replacement System (Innovalve BioMedical Ltd). All of these systems follow a so-called "single-step" implantation approach, distinguishing them from "multi-step" devices such as SAPIEN M3 (Edwards Lifesciences) [65].

At present, the only device to have received CE marking is the *Tendyne*, which is implanted via a transapical approach through thoracotomy on the beating heart under TEE guidance. It comprises three porcine pericardial tissue leaflets sewn onto an internal circular nitinol stent, known as the valve inner, made of a self-expanding, radiopaque nickel-titanium alloy. Surrounding it is an outer nitinol stent, which is covered with porcine pericardium and a polyethylene terephthalate (PET) fabric cuff. This outer stent is D-shaped to optimize positioning within the native annulus, with the elevated edge of the cuff aligned toward the aorto-mitral continuity to facilitate appropriate seating. The combination of the inner and outer stents forms a self-expanding structure that is anchored to a tether composed of ultra-high molecular weight polyethylene. This tether exits through the left ventricular apex and is fixed externally using a polyether ether ketone (PEEK) button. Intra-procedurally, the tether serves to adjust tension and ensure optimal device positioning within the annulus. A specialized "apical pad tool" is used to secure the apical pad and fasten the tether via a locking pin mechanism allowing re-adjustment of tension. Overall, the prosthesis rests against the atrial floor, and the opposing forces generated by the tether help stabilize it, minimizing the risk of ventricular migration and PVL. As for the procedure, after selecting the optimal apical puncture site, a 34 Fr delivery sheath is positioned into the left atrium over a 0.035″ guidewire previously advanced up to the left atrium with a balloon-tipped catheter to make sure the guidewire is not entrapped in the sub-valvular apparatus The device is advanced within the sheath and partially extruded, allowing the outer frame to expand to approximately 85% of its final deployed configuration. Once properly positioned, the apical pad is applied externally, and tension is adjusted through the tether. Final fixation is achieved by inserting a locking pin through the tether using the cam-driven tool. The study that led to CE mark approval was the Global Feasibility Study, which enrolled 100 patients with a mean STS score of 7.8 ± 5.7, the majority of whom (89%) had FMR. The implantation success rate was 97%, with the procedure being abandoned in three patients. One-year all-cause mortality was 26%. Thrombosis and hemolysis represented the main adverse events, occurring in a total of nine patients [66]. More recently, the TENDER Registry evaluated the largest cohort of patients treated with the Tendyne system, demonstrating a high technical success rate of 95%. Cardiovascular mortality was 7% at 30 days and 17% at 1 year, while all-cause mortality was 9% and 29%, respectively. The rate of reintervention or conversion to surgical mitral valve replacement after discharge was 4%. Notably, hospital readmissions for heart failure decreased from 68% in the year prior to the procedure to 25% at 1-year follow-up. More than 98% of patients achieved residual MR of less than 1+, and 83% were in NYHA functional class I or II [67, 68].

The *Intrepid* TMVR system (Medtronic Inc., Minneapolis, MN, USA) comprises a bioprosthetic valve traditionally implanted via the transapical approach, but more recently also via the transfemoral transseptal route. The bioprosthesis consists of a tri-leaflet bovine pericardial valve mounted within a self-expanding nitinol frame featuring a dual-structure design: an inner circular stent housing the valve and an outer fixation ring designed to engage the native mitral annulus. This configuration is specifically intended to accommodate the wide anatomical variability of the native mitral valve apparatus. The internal stent that supports the valve has a diameter of 27 mm and provides an effective orifice area (EOA) of 2.4 cm^2. The outer frame is available in three sizes—43 mm, 46 mm, and 50 mm in outer diameter. A key aspect of this system lies in its anchoring and sealing mechanisms, which are achieved through several structural features. Firstly, the outer fixation ring has a circumference larger than that of the native mitral annulus, thereby providing substantial radial force. The atrial portion of the outer frame is flexible, allowing the device to conform to the annular anatomy, whereas the ventricular portion is stiffer and offers greater resistance to compression. This design enables the atrial segment to deflect inward, aligning the device with the native annulus, while the more rigid ventricular segment maintains the overall structure. The final configuration, with a narrower waist and broader ends, enhances device stability and reduces the risk of migration under systolic pressure. PVL is minimized by a polyester skirt that covers both the inner and outer stent frames. A distinguishing feature of this device is the functional separation between the hemodynamic performance, ensured by the inner circular frame that remains unchanged throughout the cardiac cycle, and the anchoring and sealing function, provided by the outer frame that conforms to the mitral anatomy during the different phases of systole and diastole. The transapical delivery system includes an introducer with its dilator and a delivery catheter. The valve is crimped to 33 Fr and loaded into the delivery capsule, then advanced to the target site under transesophageal echocardiographic guidance. Once positioned in the left atrium, the brims are expanded and the valve aligned with the mitral annulus. The capsule is then retracted, and the device is gradually released through a self-expanding mechanism [69].

The initial data derive from the Intrepid Global Pilot Study by Bapat et al., in which 50 patients were enrolled (72% with FMR and a mean STS score of 6.4 ± 5.5). The device success rate was 98%, with no reported cases of device malfunction or thrombosis. At 30-day follow-up, the mortality rate was 14%, and the rate of rehospitalization for heart failure was 8%. At a median follow-up of 3.5 years, residual MR was no more than mild, with sustained improvement in symptoms and quality of life [70]. More recent data come from Zahr et al., who evaluated 33 patients, 60.6% of whom had PMR, with a mean STS score of 5.3%. At 30-day follow-up, no deaths or strokes were reported. Eight patients experienced major vascular complications, none of which required surgical intervention. Four cases of venous thromboembolism were recorded, all effectively managed, and one patient underwent repeat mitral intervention due to severe left ventricular outflow tract obstruction (LVOTO). At 1-year follow-up, the mortality rate was 6.7%, and echocardiographic assessment showed no more than mild residual MR and no evidence of PVL in any patient. Clinical outcomes were favorable, with sustained improvement in symptoms and quality of life [71].

Recently, a 35-Fr delivery system specifically designed for transfemoral transseptal implantation has been developed to allow for a less invasive approach. This system was initially evaluated in a pilot study that demonstrated the safety and efficacy of the device [72], and later validated by the results of the study by Zahr et al., which confirmed the benefits of transfemoral Intrepid implantation even at 1-year follow-up. These benefits included low rates of mortality and reintervention, and near-complete elimination of MR, all achieved with a favorable safety profile and promising device durability [71].

The *Cardiovalve system* (Valtech Cardio Ltd., Or Yehuda, Israel) is a self-expanding device composed of a bovine pericardial valve mounted on a nitinol frame, specifically designed for transfemoral–transseptal implantation (28 Fr). The system also includes a steerable catheter to facilitate coaxial deployment. Three valve sizes are currently available: medium, large, and extra-large. The medium size is designed for annulus diameters between 36 and 43 mm, the large for diameters between 42 and 48 mm, and the extra-large for diameters ranging from 47 to 53 mm. The low-profile design of the valve reduces the risk of LVOTO by limiting ventricular protrusion and enables multi-directional maneuverability at both the atrial and ventricular levels, allowing for improved alignment and leaflet grasping.

The Cardiovalve system is an investigational device and is not currently commercially available in Europe or the United States. It does not have CE marking and is not approved by the FDA; however, it has been successfully tested in preclinical animal studies and bench testing, confirming its safety and performance. The AHEAD study aims to evaluate the safety and performance of the Cardiovalve system. Data collected in this clinical trial will include 30-day device and delivery system safety and performance, as well as long-term clinical outcomes over a 3-year period. The study is currently ongoing, although preliminary data regarding technical success are promising [73].

The *Sapien M3* system consists of two main components: the docking system and the valve. The implantation process is divided into two stages: the placement of the anchoring ring, followed by the deployment of the valve to achieve complete mitral valve replacement. The anchoring ring encircles the mitral leaflets, drawing them along with the chordae tendineae toward the center, thereby approximating the papillary muscles. This creates a stable and uniform anchoring zone for valve deployment. Specifically, the dock is composed of a nitinol structure coated with polytetrafluoroethylene (PTFE), designed to envelop the chordae tendineae below the mitral annulus through a dual-turn configuration. The first turn, with a larger diameter (37 mm), surrounds the chordae, while the second, smaller turn (25.5 mm), acts as an anchoring point for the valve. The PTFE coating is intended to reduce the risk of valve migration and embolization.

In terms of sizing, the Sapien M3 shares the same dimensions as the 29 mm Sapien 3 trans-catheter heart (aortic) valve. However, a key difference lies in the external covering: the M3 features a polyethylene terephthalate (PET) wrap that covers the entire surface of the valve frame. The system can be implanted via the transfemoral route using a 20 Fr introducer. Procedurally, it shares several features with the Sapien 3 used in treating degenerated mitral bioprostheses, including a balloon-expandable mechanism and the need for rapid pacing during deployment [74].

The initial clinical data were reported by Webb et al., who presented outcomes from 10 patients, achieving a technical success rate of 90% (9 out of 10 cases). The single unsuccessful case was due to the development of a pericardial effusion during docking. At 30-day follow-up, there were no reported deaths, and the implanted valves demonstrated good functional performance [74]. An ongoing early feasibility study in the United States and Canada has also shown promising results. Among the first 35 patients, the technical success rate was 88.6%, with no procedural deaths and a stroke incidence of 8.6% [75]. The ongoing ENCIRCLE trial (NCT04153292) aims to establish the safety and effectiveness of the SAPIEN M3 System in adult patients with symptomatic, at least 3+ MR, who are considered unsuitable for commercially available surgical or transcatheter treatment options due to clinical, anatomical, or technical considerations.

The *Innovalve* transcatheter mitral valve replacement system (........) is a prosthetic valve composed of a cylindrical frame housing three bovine pericardial cusps, an atrial skirt that forms a funnel- or cone-shaped configuration, and six arms that extend radially into the sub-valvular mitral apparatus. From a procedural standpoint, implantation is performed via a 32 Fr transeptal delivery system. Once positioned, the arms are gradually rotated to engage the native sub-valvular chordae through multiple fixation mechanisms. This design ensures a robust anchoring and sealing of the valve, effectively minimizing the risk of PVL. Simultaneously, it displaces the anterior mitral leaflet away from the LVOT, thereby reducing the risk of obstruction. The TWIST-GE pilot study evaluated the safety and feasibility of the

Innovalve Transcatheter Mitral Valve Replacement System in 10 high-surgical-risk patients with moderate-to-severe or severe MR. Conducted in Georgia, all patients underwent successful device implantation with no procedural mortality or major complications. At 30 days, there were no deaths, strokes, myocardial infarctions, or LVOTO. PVL was mild or less in most cases, and no transvalvular leaks were observed. Functional outcomes improved significantly, with better KCCQ-12 scores and increased 6-minute walk distances. The findings demonstrate that the Innovalve system offers a safe and effective transcatheter option for mitral valve replacement, providing stable anchoring and reducing the risk of PVL and LVOTO [76, 77].

The *AltaValve system* (4C Medical Technologies, MN, USA) is a novel transcatheter mitral valve replacement device characterized by a supra-annular fixation mechanism, designed to reduce contact with the left ventricle or subvalvular apparatus. This unique approach aims to reduce the risk of LVOTO, PVL, and annular sizing constraints commonly encountered in other TMVR systems. The device consists of a self-expanding nitinol frame housing a 27 mm bovine pericardial tissue valve. Fixation is achieved by oversizing the atrial frame relative to the left atrium, complemented by a polyester skirt at the annular level to promote hemostasis. Annular ring sizes include 40 mm, 46 mm, and 54 mm, selected based on gated cardiac CT imaging with systolic measurements. Patient selection relies on strict anatomical criteria including a left atrial dimension <85 mm, mitral annular diameter between 29–51 mm, and atrial volume variation <20%. Pre-procedural planning involves advanced 3D imaging, MAC burden quantification, and evaluation of aorto-mitral angle and anterior leaflet length. Initially delivered via a transapical approach (34 Fr), a transseptal delivery system (29 Fr) has since been developed, offering a less invasive alternative. Notably, rapid ventricular pacing and balloon valvuloplasty are not required. Device positioning is guided by fluoroscopy and TEE. In some cases, an intra-aortic balloon pump or atrial septal defect closure may be employed. Anticoagulation following implantation includes a 6-month regimen with warfarin or a non-vitamin K oral anticoagulant. Across studies, the mean transvalvular gradient post-implantation remains consistently low (~2 mmHg), and valve seating is stable. The shift toward fully percutaneous transseptal access represents a major advancement in procedural safety and patient eligibility [78, 79]. Clinical evidence for the AltaValve system derives from case reports, single-center experiences, multicenter studies, and the early feasibility study. Across cohorts, the device demonstrated high technical success rates (97–100%), consistent MR reduction, and favorable safety outcomes with no reported valve embolization, structural failure, or clinically significant thrombosis [79]. In the first-in-human case, complete MR resolution was achieved with no complications over 16 months. Another early US case confirmed technical success, though the patient died of unrelated causes (amyloidosis); valve positioning was confirmed post-mortem as optimal [80]. A single-center experience with three patients reported successful transseptal implantations in high-risk patients with secondary MR. All showed marked NYHA improvement (to class I–II), stable valve function, low gradients (0.7–1.0 mmHg), and no device-related adverse events over 6 months [81]. In a separate multicenter series of 14 patients with atrial secondary MR, AltaValve achieved MR elimination in all cases, with 91% maintaining trace/no MR at 30 days. NYHA class improved in all survivors; mean mitral gradient increased to 5 mmHg without inducing stenosis or LVOTO [82]. The AltaValve early feasibility study enrolled 30 patients unsuitable for surgery or TEER. MR was reduced to none/trace in all cases, and 86% improved to NYHA I–II. Significant gains were observed in 6-minute walk distance and KCCQ scores, with no strokes, valve thrombosis, or device failures at 6 months [78]. Collectively, these results underscore the system's potential to provide safe and effective MR reduction in high-risk populations, especially those ineligible for conventional mitral therapies. Long-term data and randomized studies are awaited to validate durability and comparative outcomes.

What is important to understand, in conclusion, is that both transcatheter mitral valve repair and replacement have distinct advantages and limitations. In general, repair strategies are more respectful of the native anatomy and physiology of the mitral valve and subvalvular apparatus, which is inherently complex. Valve repair also preserves normal flow hemodynamics, whereas replacement creates a non-physiological inflow pattern that may lead to increased left ventricular wall stress and a potential reduction in effective cardiac workload. Additional drawbacks of replacement compared to repair include the potential loss of mitro-aortic continuity and impaired basal left ventricular contraction due to prosthesis fixation within the mitral apparatus. Conversely, the key advantages of replacement lie in its greater procedural versatility and reproducibility, with more consistent elimination of MR and the possibility of applying a single device across a broader range of anatomies. Considering these pros and cons, it becomes increasingly evident that TMVr and TMVR should be viewed as complementary, rather than competing, approaches in the evolving field of percutaneous mitral valve therapy [83].

References

1. Vahanian A, Beyersdorf F, Praz F, Milojevic M, Baldus S, Bauersachs J, et al. 2021 ESC/EACTS guidelines for the management of valvular heart disease. Eur Heart J. 2022;43(7):561–632.
2. Iung B, Delgado V, Rosenhek R, Price S, Prendergast B, Wendler O, et al. Contemporary presentation and management of valvular heart disease: the EUrobservational research programme valvular heart disease II survey. Circulation. 2019;140(14):1156–69.
3. Dziadzko V, Dziadzko M, Medina-Inojosa JR, Benfari G, Michelena HI, Crestanello JA, et al. Causes and mechanisms of isolated mitral regurgitation in the community: clinical context and outcome. Eur Heart J. 2019;40(27):2194–202.
4. Kingué S, Ba SA, Balde D, Diarra MB, Anzouan-Kacou JB, Anisubia B, et al. The VALVAFRIC study: a registry of rheumatic heart disease in Western and Central Africa. Arch Cardiovasc Dis. 2016;109(5):321–9.
5. Bartko PE, Hülsmann M, Hung J, Pavo N, Levine RA, Pibarot P, et al. Secondary valve regurgitation in patients with heart failure with preserved ejection fraction, heart failure with mid-range ejection fraction, and heart failure with reduced ejection fraction. Eur Heart J (Oxford University Press). 2020;41:2799–810.
6. Deferm S, Bertrand PB, Verbrugge FH, Verhaert D, Rega F, Thomas JD, et al. Atrial functional mitral regurgitation: JACC review topic of the week. J Am Coll Cardiol. 2019;73(19):2465–76.

7. Brugiatelli L, Rolando M, Lofiego C, Fogante M, Capodaglio I, Patani F, et al. Transcatheter mitral valve intervention: current and future role of multimodality imaging for device selection and periprocedural guidance. Medicina (Lithuania) (Multidisciplinary Digital Publishing Institute (MDPI)). 2024;60:1082.
8. Mirabel M, Iung B, Baron G, Messika-Zeitoun D, Détaint D, Vanoverschelde JL, et al. What are the characteristics of patients with severe, symptomatic, mitral regurgitation who are denied surgery? Eur Heart J. 2007 Jun;28(11):1358–65.
9. Habib A, Lachman N, Christensen KN, Asirvatham SJ. The anatomy of the coronary sinus venous system for the cardiac electrophysiologist. Europace. 2009;11(Suppl 5):v15–21.
10. Krishnaswamy A, Kapadia SR. Indirect mitral annuloplasty using the Carillon device. Front Cardiovasc Med (Frontiers Media S.A.). 2020;7:576058.
11. Choure AJ, Garcia MJ, Hesse B, Sevensma M, Maly G, Greenberg NL, et al. In vivo analysis of the anatomical relationship of coronary sinus to mitral annulus and left circumflex coronary artery using cardiac multidetector computed tomography. Implications for percutaneous coronary sinus mitral annuloplasty. J Am Coll Cardiol. 2006;48(10):1938–45.
12. Nagaraja V, Kapadia SR. Transcatheter mitral annuloplasty: Carillon device. Interv Cardiol Clin. 2024;13(2):249–55.
13. Rottländer D, Degen H, Haude M. The Carillon: strategies for optimal patient selection and optimised results. EuroIntervention. 2016;12:Y64–6.
14. Goldberg SL, Lipiecki J, Sievert H. The CARILLON mitral contour transcatheter indirect mitral valve annuloplasty system. EuroIntervention (Europa Group). 2015;11:W64–6.
15. Schofer J, Siminiak T, Haude M, Herrman JP, Vainer J, Wu JC, et al. Percutaneous mitral annuloplasty for functional mitral regurgitation. Circulation. 2009;120(4):326–33.
16. Siminiak T, Wu JC, Haude M, Hoppe UC, Sadowski J, Lipiecki J, et al. Treatment of functional mitral regurgitation by percutaneous annuloplasty: results of the TITAN trial. Eur J Heart Fail. 2012;14(8):931–8.
17. Lipiecki J, Siminiak T, Sievert H, Müller-Ehmsen J, Degen H, Wu JC, et al. Coronary sinus-based percutaneous annuloplasty as treatment for functional mitral regurgitation: the TITAN II trial. Open Heart. 2016;3(2):e000411.
18. Witte KK, Lipiecki J, Siminiak T, Meredith IT, Malkin CJ, Goldberg SL, et al. The REDUCE FMR trial: a randomized sham-controlled study of percutaneous mitral Annuloplasty in functional mitral regurgitation. JACC Heart Fail. 2019;7(11):945–55.
19. Tops LF, Van De Veire NR, Schuijf JD, De Roos A, Van Der Wall EE, Schalij MJ, et al. Noninvasive evaluation of coronary sinus anatomy and its relation to the mitral valve annulus: implications for percutaneous mitral annuloplasty. Circulation. 2007;115(11):1426–32.
20. Lansac E, Di Centa I, Al Attar N, Messika-Zeitoun D, Raffoul R, Vahanian A, et al. Percutaneous mitral annuloplasty through the coronary sinus: an anatomic point of view. J Thorac Cardiovasc Surg. 2008;135(2):376–81.
21. Rogers JH, Macoviak JA, Rahdert DA, Takeda PA, Palacios IF, Low RI. Percutaneous septal sinus shortening. Circulation. 2006;113(19):2329–34.
22. Erglis A, Thomas M, Morice MC, Narbute I, Zabunova M, Hovasse T, et al. The Arto transcatheter mitral valve repair system. EuroIntervention. 2015;14(W):W47–8.
23. Worthley S, Redwood S, Hildick-Smith D, Rafter T, Whelan A, De Marco F, et al. Transcatheter reshaping of the mitral annulus in patients with functional mitral regurgitation: one-year outcomes of the MAVERIC trial. EuroIntervention. 2021;16(13):1106–13.
24. Patterson T, Gregson J, Erglis A, Joseph J, Rajani R, Wilson K, et al. Two-year outcomes from the MitrAl ValvE RepaIr Clinical (MAVERIC) trial: a novel percutaneous treatment of functional mitral regurgitation. Eur J Heart Fail. 2021;23(10):1775–83.
25. Rogers JH, Bolling SF. Transseptal direct complete annuloplasty: early experience. Ann Cardiothorac Surg. 2021;10(1):57–65.
26. Matos J, Kronzon I, Panagopoulos G, Perk G. Mitral annular plane systolic excursion as a surrogate for left ventricular ejection fraction. J Am Soc Echocardiogr. 2012;25(9):969–74.

27. Feldman T, Guerrero M. Transcatheter direct mitral valve annuloplasty: a brief review. EuroIntervention (Europa Group). 2015;11:W53–7.
28. Testa L, Latib A, Montone RA, Bedogni F. Transcatheter mitral valve regurgitation treatment: State of the art and a glimpse to the future. J Thorac Cardiovasc Surg (Mosby Inc.). 2016;152:319–27.
29. Nickenig G, Hammerstingl C, Schueler R, Topilsky Y, Grayburn PA, Vahanian A, et al. Transcatheter mitral Annuloplasty in chronic functional mitral regurgitation 6-month results with the Cardioband percutaneous mitral repair system. JACC Cardiovasc Interv. 2016;9:2039.
30. Messika-Zeitoun D, Nickenig G, Latib A, Kuck KH, Baldus S, Schueler R, et al. Transcatheter mitral valve repair for functional mitral regurgitation using the Cardioband system: 1 year outcomes. Eur Heart J. 2019;40(5):466–72.
31. Alfieri O, Maisano F, De Bonis M, Stefano PL, Torracca L, Oppizzi M, et al. The double-orifice technique in mitral valve repair: a simple solution for complex problems. J Thorac Cardiovasc Surg. 2001;122(4):674–81.
32. Alfieri O, De Bonis M, Lapenna E, Regesta T, Maisano F, Torracca L, et al. 'Edge-to-edge' repair for anterior mitral leaflet prolapse. Semin Thorac Cardiovasc Surg. 2004;16(2):182–7.
33. Feldman T, Wasserman HS, Herrmann HC, Gray W, Block PC, Whitlow P, et al. Percutaneous mitral valve repair using the edge-to-edge technique: six-month results of the EVEREST phase I clinical trial. J Am Coll Cardiol. 2005;46(11):2134–40.
34. Taramasso M, Feldman T, Maisano F. Transcatheter mitral valve repair: review of the clinical evidence. EuroIntervention. 2018;14(AB):AB91–100.
35. Grasso C, Baldus S. The MitraClip transcatheter mitral valve repair system. EuroIntervention (Europa Group). 2015;11:W45–6.
36. Hausleiter J, Stocker TJ, Adamo M, Karam N, Swaans MJ, Praz F. Mitral valve transcatheter edge-to-edge repair. EuroIntervention. 2023;18(12):957–76.
37. Schnitzler K, Hell M, Geyer M, Kreidel F, Münzel T, Stephan Von Bardeleben R. Complications following MitraClip implantation. Available from: https://doi.org/10.1007/s11886-021-01553-9.
38. Feldman T, Foster E, Glower DD, Kar S, Rinaldi MJ, Fail PS, et al. Percutaneous repair or surgery for mitral regurgitation. N Engl J Med. 2011;364(15):1395–406.
39. Otto CM, Nishimura RA, Bonow RO, Carabello BA, rwin JP, Gentile F, et al. 2020 ACC/AHA guideline for the Management of Patients with Valvular Heart Disease: executive summary: a report of the American College of Cardiology/American Heart Association Joint Committee on Clinical Practice Guidelines. Circulation (Lippincott Williams and Wilkins). 2021;143:E35–71.
40. Buzzatti N, Van Hemelrijck M, Denti P, Ruggeri S, Schiavi D, Scarfò IS, et al. Transcatheter or surgical repair for degenerative mitral regurgitation in elderly patients: a propensity-weighted analysis. J Thorac Cardiovasc Surg. 2019;158(1):86–94.e1.
41. Kar S, von Bardeleben RS, Rottbauer W, Mahoney P, Price MJ, Grasso C, et al. Contemporary outcomes following transcatheter edge-to-edge repair: 1-year results from the EXPAND study. JACC Cardiovasc Interv. 2023;16(5):589–602.
42. von Bardeleben RS, Mahoney P, Morse MA, Price MJ, Denti P, Maisano F, et al. 1-year outcomes with fourth-generation mitral valve transcatheter edge-to-edge repair from the EXPAND G4 study. JACC Cardiovasc Interv. 2023;16(21):2600–10.
43. Stone GW, Lindenfeld J, Abraham WT, Kar S, Lim DS, Mishell JM, et al. Transcatheter mitral-valve repair in patients with heart failure. N Engl J Med. 2018;379(24):2307–18.
44. Obadia JF, Messika-Zeitoun D, Leurent G, Iung B, Bonnet G, Piriou N, et al. Percutaneous repair or medical treatment for secondary mitral regurgitation. N Engl J Med. 2018;379(24):2297–306.
45. Grayburn PA, Sannino A, Packer M. Proportionate and disproportionate functional mitral regurgitation: a new conceptual framework that reconciles the results of the MITRA-FR and COAPT trials. JACC Cardiovasc Imaging (Elsevier Inc.). 2019;12:353–62.
46. Baldus S, Doenst T, Pfister R, Gummert J, Kessler M, Boekstegers P, et al. Transcatheter repair versus mitral-valve surgery for secondary mitral regurgitation. N Engl J Med. 2024;391:1787.

47. Anker SD, Friede T, von Bardeleben RS, Butler J, Khan MS, Diek M, et al. Transcatheter valve repair in heart failure with moderate to severe mitral regurgitation. N Engl J Med. 2024;391(19):1799–809.
48. Gupta A, Packer M, Makkar R, Grayburn P. A volume-based framework reconciling COAPT, MITRA-FR and RESHAPE-HF2. J Am Coll Cardiol. 2024;84:2376.
49. Oguz D, Padang R, Rashedi N, Pislaru SV, Nkomo VT, Mankad SV, et al. Risk for increased mean diastolic gradient after transcatheter edge-to-edge mitral valve repair: a quantitative three-dimensional transesophageal echocardiographic analysis. J Am Soc Echocardiogr. 2021;34(6):595–603.e2.
50. Thaden JJ, Malouf JF, Nkomo VT, Pislaru SV, Holmes DR, Reeder GS, et al. Mitral valve anatomic predictors of hemodynamic success with transcatheter mitral valve repair. J Am Heart Assoc. 2018;7(2):e007315.
51. Lesevic H, Karl M, Braun D, Barthel P, Orban M, Pache J, et al. Long-term outcomes after MitraClip implantation according to the presence or absence of EVEREST inclusion criteria. Am J Cardiol. 2017;119(8):1255–61.
52. Schneider L, Markovic S, Mueller K, Felbel D, Gerçek M, Friedrichs K, et al. Mitral valve transcatheter edge-to-edge repair using MitraClip or PASCAL: a multicenter propensity score–matched comparison. JACC Cardiovasc Interv. 2022;15(24):2554–67.
53. Praz F, Windecker S, Kapadia S. PASCAL: a new addition to the armamentarium of Transcatheter repair systems for mitral leaflet approximation. JACC Cardiovasc Interv (Elsevier Inc.). 2019;12:1379–81.
54. Praz F, Spargias K, Chrissoheris M, Büllesfeld L, Nickenig G, Deuschl F, et al. Compassionate use of the PASCAL transcatheter mitral valve repair system for patients with severe mitral regurgitation: a multicentre, prospective, observational, first-in-man study. Lancet. 2017;390(10096):773–80.
55. Webb JG, Hensey M, Szerlip M, Schäfer U, Cohen GN, Kar S, et al. 1-year outcomes for transcatheter repair in patients with mitral regurgitation from the CLASP study. JACC Cardiovasc Interv. 2020;13(20):2344–57.
56. Zhang T, Zhang W, Zhen X, Luo R, Yang L, Zhang X, et al. A transcatheter mitral valve clip with a central filler for mitral valve regurgitation. Biomaterials. 2025;321:123317.
57. Wang J, Liu X, Pu Z, Chen M, Fang Z, Jin J, et al. Safety and efficacy of the DragonFly system for transcatheter valve repair of degenerative mitral regurgitation: one-year results of the DRAGONFLY-DMR trial. EuroIntervention. 2024;20(4):e239–49.
58. Colli A, Adams D, Fiocco A, Pradegan N, Longinotti L, Nadali M, et al. Transapical NeoChord mitral valve repair. Ann Cardiothorac Surg. 2018;7(6):812–20.
59. Colli A, Manzan E, Zucchetta F, Bizzotto E, Besola L, Bagozzi L, et al. Transapical off-pump mitral valve repair with Neochord implantation: early clinical results. Int J Cardiol. 2016;204:23–8.
60. Fatehi Hassanabad A, Kent WDT, Adams C. Review of transapical off-pump mitral valve intervention with NeoChord implantation. Curr Opin Cardiol. 2021;36(2):130–40.
61. Seeburger J, Rinaldi M, Nielsen SL, Salizzoni S, Lange R, Schoenburg M, et al. Off-pump transapical implantation of artificial neo-chordae to correct mitral regurgitation: the TACT trial (Transapical Artificial Chordae Tendinae) proof of concept. J Am Coll Cardiol. 2014;63(9):914–9.
62. Gerosa G, D'Onofrio A, Besola L, Colli A. Transoesophageal echo-guided mitral valve repair using the Harpoon system. Eur J Cardiothorac Surg. 2018;53(4):871–3.
63. Gammie JS, Wilson P, Bartus K, Gackowski A, Hung J, D'Ambra MN, et al. Transapical beating-heart mitral valve repair with an expanded polytetrafluoroethylene cordal implantation device. Circulation. 2016;134(3):189–97.
64. Gammie JS, Bartus K, Gackowski A, D'Ambra MN, Szymanski P, Bilewska A, et al. Beating-heart mitral valve repair using a novel ePTFE Cordal implantation device a prospective trial. 2018.
65. Urena M, Lurz P, Sorajja P, Himbert D, Guerrero M. Transcatheter mitral valve implantation for native valve disease. EuroIntervention. 2023;19(9):720–38.

66. Sorajja P, Moat N, Badhwar V, Walters D, Paone G, Bethea B, et al. Initial feasibility study of a new transcatheter mitral prosthesis: the first 100 patients. J Am Coll Cardiol. 2019;73(11):1250–60.
67. Hell MM, Wild MG, Baldus S, Rudolph T, Treede H, Petronio AS, et al. Transapical mitral valve replacement: 1-year results of the real-world Tendyne European experience registry. JACC Cardiovasc Interv. 2024;17(5):648–61.
68. Hensey M, Brown RA, Lal S, Sathananthan J, Ye J, Cheung A, et al. Transcatheter mitral valve replacement: an update on current techniques, technologies, and future directions. JACC Cardiovasc Interv. 2021;14(5):489–500.
69. Meredith I, Bapat V, Morriss J, McLean M, Prendergast B. Intrepid transcatheter mitral valve replacement system: technical and product description. EuroIntervention. 2016;12(Y):Y78–80.
70. Bapat V, Weiss E, Bajwa T, Thourani VH, Yadav P, Thaden JJ, et al. 2-year clinical and echocardiography follow-up of transcatheter mitral valve replacement with the transapical intrepid system. JACC Cardiovasc Interv. 2024;17(12):1440–51.
71. Zahr F, Song HK, Chadderdon S, Gada H, Mumtaz M, Byrne T, et al. 1-year outcomes following transfemoral transseptal transcatheter mitral valve replacement: intrepid TMVR early feasibility study results. JACC Cardiovasc Interv. 2023;16(23):2868–79.
72. Bapat V, Rajagopal V, Meduri C, Farivar RS, Walton A, Duffy SJ, et al. Early experience with new transcatheter mitral valve replacement. J Am Coll Cardiol. 2018;71(1):12–21.
73. Yasmin F, Najeeb H, Fareed Siddiqui H, Hamayl Zeeshan M, Mehdi A, Sohaib Asghar M, et al. Current practices and considerations for transcatheter mitral valve implantation based on risk stratification among patients with mitral valve regurgitation. Curr Probl Cardiol. 2023;48(1):101413.
74. Webb JG, Murdoch DJ, Boone RH, Moss R, Attinger-Toller A, Blanke P, et al. Percutaneous transcatheter mitral valve replacement. J Am Coll Cardiol. 2019;73(11):1239–46.
75. Webb J. Transseptal SAPIEN M3: device, results, and ongoing studies. Presented at: TVT 2019: Structural heart summit.
76. Mangieri A, Cannata F, Cozzi O, Monti L, Regazzoli D, Guetta V, et al. A fully percutaneous transeptal transcatheter mitral valve replacement with a novel device. JACC Cardiovasc Interv. 2023;16(16):2050–2.
77. Meerkin D, Guetta V, Shaburishvili T, Gogorishvili I, Kipiani Z, Orlov B, et al. Early experience with the innovalve transcatheter mitral valve replacement system. JACC Cardiovasc Interv. 2024;17(5):712–4.
78. Généreux P, Wróbel K, Rinaldi MJ, Modine T, Bapat V, Ninios V, et al. AltaValve atrial fixation system for the treatment of severe mitral regurgitation and mitral annular calcification. Struct Heart. 2024;8(3):100294.
79. Penteris M. The AltaValve system for transcatheter mitral valve replacement: a narrative review of early safety and efficacy data Cardiovasc Revasc Med (Elsevier Inc.); 2025.
80. Goel SS, Zuck V, Christy J, Nallamothu N, Jagtap P, Gao J, et al. Transcatheter mitral valve therapy with novel supra-annular AltaValve. JACC Case Rep. 2019;1(5):761–4.
81. Ninios V, Ninios I, Ranard LS, Vahl TP, Wróbel K. Transcatheter transseptal treatment of patients with severe mitral regurgitation using an atrial fixation mitral valve replacement technology. Cardiovasc Revasc Med. 2024;58:25–30.
82. Saxon JT, Genereux P, Ninios V, Waggoner T, Tahirkheli N, Grygier M, et al. Transcatheter mitral valve replacement with atrial fixation for treatment of atrial functional mitral regurgitation. Circ Cardiovasc Interv. 2025;18(4):e014985.
83. Cohen DJ, Ludwig S, Piazza N. Transcatheter mitral valve replacement will remain a niche therapy: pros and cons. EuroIntervention. 2023;18(15):1222–5.

Transcatheter Interventions for Aortic Valve

9

Andrei Țăruș, Alberto Bacușcă, and Grigore Tinică

Introduction

Aortic valve disease is a major cause of morbidity and mortality in the elderly, with aortic stenosis (AS) being the most prevalent valvular heart disease in older adults [1]. The prevalence of severe calcific AS increases with age, affecting approximately 3–4% of individuals over 75 years old in developed countries [1]. This burden is expected to grow as populations age, making AS a significant public health concern [1]. By contrast, pure aortic regurgitation (AR) is a less common primary lesion in the elderly; it often arises from different etiologies (e.g., congenital or rheumatic disease) and has a distinct epidemiology. Once AS becomes symptomatic, the prognosis without intervention is extremely poor—historical data indicate that over half of patients die within 2–3 years if left untreated [2]. In these patients, timely aortic valve replacement is critical to improve survival and quality of life [2]. Severe AR can also be life-threatening, but its pathophysiology (often a non-calcified annulus) has made transcatheter therapy more challenging; as a result, surgical valve replacement remains the standard for AR, and transcatheter solutions for AR are still under investigation [3].

A. Țăruș (✉) · A. Bacușcă
Faculty of Medicine, University of Medicine and Pharmacy "Grigore T Popa", Iasi, Romania

Institute of Cardiovascular Diseases "Prof. Dr. George I.M. Georgescu", Iasi, Romania

G. Tinică
Cardiovascular Surgery, Cardiovascular Diseases Institute, Iași & Grigore T. Popa University of Medicine and Pharmacy, Iași, Romania
e-mail: grigore.tinica@umfiasi.ro

G. Tinică, A. Burlacu (eds.), *Surgical, Hybrid and Minimally Invasive Structural Cardiac Interventions*, https://doi.org/10.1007/978-3-032-16676-0_9

Historical Background

For decades, surgical aortic valve replacement (SAVR) has been the definitive treatment for severe symptomatic AS, with a track record dating back to the 1960s and well-established long-term outcomes [4, 5]. SAVR reliably relieves obstruction and improves survival, but it requires open-heart surgery with cardiopulmonary bypass and carries substantial operative risk in elderly or comorbid patients [5]. Many frail patients with severe AS were historically deemed "inoperable" or very high-risk for surgery due to advanced age or medical comorbidities. This unmet need provided the rationale for developing less invasive transcatheter techniques that could deliver a new valve without open surgery [5]. In the 1980s, balloon aortic valvuloplasty emerged as an initial catheter-based palliative treatment for AS. Alain Cribier and colleagues first performed percutaneous balloon valvuloplasty in 1986, temporarily improving valve area in elderly AS patients [6]. However, balloon valvuloplasty benefits were short-lived due to high rates of restenosis, underscoring the need for a more durable percutaneous solution [6].

The concept of transcatheter aortic valve replacement (TAVR) was born out of these efforts to treat high-risk patients less invasively. After years of animal research and prototypes, the first-in-human TAVR procedure was accomplished by Cribier in April 2002, when a crimped balloon-expandable bioprosthetic valve was successfully implanted percutaneously in an elderly patient with calcific AS [5]. This landmark case demonstrated the feasibility of replacing the aortic valve via a catheter, ushering in a new era of transcatheter aortic interventions [5]. In the following years, procedural refinements and device innovations rapidly advanced the field. Early TAVR approaches used an antegrade trans-septal route, but soon the retrograde transfemoral approach became preferred for its relative simplicity and lower invasiveness. By 2004–2005, self-expanding TAVR devices were introduced (first implanted by E. Grube), and multiple vascular access routes (transfemoral, transapical, subclavian, etc.) were developed to accommodate different patient anatomies [7]. Over time, improvements in valve design (e.g., lower-profile delivery systems, sealing skirts to reduce paravalvular leak) and accumulating operator experience greatly enhanced the safety and efficacy of TAVR procedures.

Transcatheter techniques offered a fundamentally different treatment paradigm compared to surgery. TAVR is performed via peripheral arterial access (commonly the femoral artery) and deployed on a beating heart, removing the need for sternotomy, cardiopulmonary bypass, or general anesthesia in many cases [5, 8]. This minimally invasive nature allows for shorter hospital stays and faster recovery, which appealed to patients and physicians alike [8]. Initially, TAVR was used as a last resort in patients who had "no other option," but as the technology matured, it began to challenge SAVR even in patients who could undergo surgery. Notably, despite its less invasive approach, TAVR was shown in trials to provide hemodynamic relief equivalent to surgical valves, while avoiding the substantial surgical trauma of open-heart surgery [8]. These advantages, combined with favorable clinical outcomes, have made TAVR a disruptive innovation in cardiology—analogous to how stenting revolutionized coronary disease treatment decades earlier [8].

Landmark Trials Establishing TAVR

The clinical adoption of TAVR has been driven by a series of pivotal randomized trials that established its efficacy relative to SAVR. The first landmark trial was PARTNER 1, which had two cohorts. In PARTNER 1B (2010), patients with severe AS deemed inoperable were randomized to TAVR vs. medical therapy (including ballon aortic valvuloplasty); TAVR conferred a dramatic survival benefit, reducing one-year mortality by ~20% (31% vs 51%) compared to conservative management [9]. This was the first demonstration that transcatheter therapy could improve outcomes in AS, leading to regulatory approval for TAVR in inoperable patients [9]. PARTNER 1A (2011) then tested TAVR against SAVR in high-risk surgical candidates (STS score ~ 11%); the results showed that TAVR was non-inferior to surgery in terms of mortality at 1 year (24.2% vs 26.8%), meeting the criterion for equivalence [10]. Although concerns were noted about stroke and paravalvular regurgitation with early-generation TAVR devices, the overall finding that TAVR could match surgical outcomes in high-risk patients was transformative [10]. Around the same time, the CoreValve U.S. Pivotal Trial (2014) tested a self-expanding transcatheter valve in high-risk patients and actually found superior outcomes for TAVR: at 1 year, all-cause mortality was significantly lower with TAVR (14.2%) than with SAVR (19.1%). This was the first trial to show a survival advantage of TAVR over surgery in any population [11].

Buoyed by these successes, investigators moved to broader populations. The PARTNER 2A trial (2016) extended the comparison to intermediate-risk patients (STS ~5–6%). In this cohort, TAVR was again non-inferior to SAVR for the primary endpoint (death or disabling stroke), and in a transfemoral-access subgroup analysis, TAVR showed a slight mortality/stroke benefit over surgery at 2 years [12]. Similarly, the SURTAVI trial (2017), which also enrolled intermediate-risk patients, found no significant difference in survival between TAVR and SAVR at 2 years, with TAVR showing a trend toward fewer strokes [12, 13]. These trials cemented TAVR's role as an alternative to surgery in intermediate-risk patients. Most recently, studies have focused on low-risk patients, who are younger and generally have fewer comorbidities. The PARTNER 3 trial (2019) examined TAVR vs. SAVR in low-risk patients (STS ~1.9%, mean age 73) and reported that TAVR was not only non-inferior but actually superior to surgery for the composite endpoint of death, stroke, or rehospitalization at 1 year (occurring in 8.5% of TAVR patients vs 15.1% of SAVR patients) [14].

Patient Selection and Indications for TAVR

Current ACC/AHA and ESC/EACTS guidelines concordantly endorse TAVR for most patients with severe symptomatic AS (Fig. 9.1), with decisions guided by age, comorbidity, and surgical risk [15, 16]. The 2020 ACC/AHA guidelines recommend a Heart Team–based decision for symptomatic AS in patients aged 65–80, allowing either SAVR or transfemoral TAVR (Class I) [16]. In practice, TAVR is preferred in those >80 years or with limited life expectancy (<10 y), whereas SAVR is favored in younger patients (<65 y) or those expected to outlive 20 years [16]. Notably, symptomatic patients at high or prohibitive surgical risk should receive TAVR if

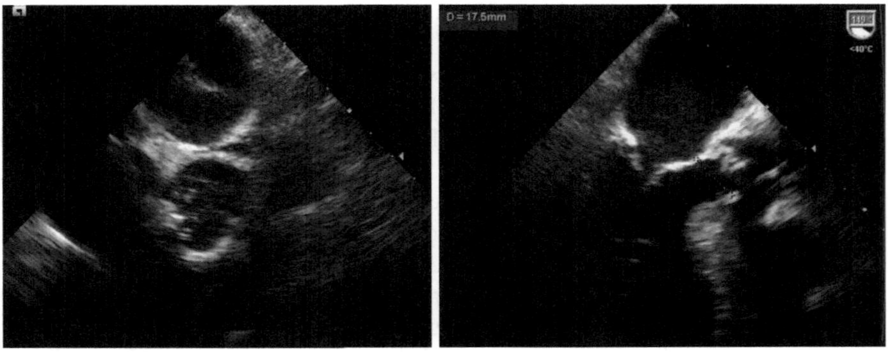

Fig. 9.1 Transthoracic echocardiography in severe aortic stenosis

Table 9.1 Surgical risk categories by STS-PROM and EuroSCORE II

Risk category	STS-PROM	EuroSCORE II	Notes
Low risk	<4%	<4%	TAVI and SAVR both acceptable
Intermediate risk	4–8%	~4–8%	Heart Team preference based on anatomy/comorbidity
High risk	>8%	>8%	TAVI generally preferred if feasible
Prohibitive risk	–	–	Defined by >50% 1-yr mortality risk or severe frailty

their projected ≥1-year survival and quality of life justify intervention [16]. The 2021 ESC/EACTS guidelines apply similar criteria: SAVR is recommended in younger, low-risk patients (<75 years and STS/EuroSCORE II <4%), while TAVR is Class I in older or high-risk patients (age ≥ 75 or STS/EuroSCORE II >8%) [15]. All guidelines emphasize intervention for symptomatic severe AS (high gradient or low-flow severe AS with contractile reserve), and generally reserve therapy in asymptomatic AS for those with adverse features (e.g., LV dysfunction, abnormal exercise response, rapidly rising gradients) [15, 16].

Surgical Risk Stratification

Formal risk scores and clinical judgment are both integral to choosing SAVR versus TAVR. The Society of Thoracic Surgeons Predicted Risk of Mortality (STS-PROM) and EuroSCORE II calculators are validated tools to estimate surgical mortality [17]. By convention, STS-PROM <4% denotes low risk, 4–8% intermediate risk, and > 8% high risk [17]. Similar thresholds are often applied to EuroSCORE II (though EuroSCORE II tends to run slightly higher); ESC guidelines explicitly use EuroSCORE II <4% for low risk and > 8% for high risk [15] (Table 9.1). Patients with prohibitive risk have expected mortality and morbidity >50% at 1 year or multiple major comorbidities (severe frailty, end-organ failure) [17]. Crucially, these scores are adjuncts: the Heart Team must integrate factors beyond the scores (frailty, hostile chest, porcelain aorta, prior surgeries, chest radiation, advanced age, or dementia) in defining operative risk and viability [17].

Multidisciplinary Heart Team

Both American and European guidelines mandate that Heart Teams assess all candidates for valve intervention [15, 16]. This team—comprising interventional cardiologists, cardiac surgeons, imaging specialists, anesthesiologists, and geriatricians—jointly reviews the patient's clinical status, comorbidities, and anatomy. The Heart Team context ensures balanced consideration of SAVR versus TAVR, incorporating patient values, life expectancy, frailty, and procedural feasibility. Notably, current guidance states that TAVR and SAVR decisions should hinge on symptom status, age/life expectancy, surgical risk, and anatomical suitability for transfemoral access. In practice, any severe AS case referred for valve therapy is discussed by a Heart Valve Center team before finalizing the treatment strategy.

Anatomical Considerations

Critical anatomical factors determine the suitability and planning of TAVR. Aortic annulus size and morphology must be carefully measured by multi-detector CT or 3D echo. Annular dimensions outside the device-specific range (too small or too large) can preclude secure valve anchoring [18]. Undersizing risks significant paravalvular regurgitation, whereas oversizing raises rupture risk (Fig. 9.2); accurate annular sizing is therefore essential. Valve morphology also matters: bicuspid aortic valves (BAV) are common in younger patients but pose challenges (eccentric calcification, elliptical annulus, and concomitant aortopathy). The 2020 ACC/AHA guideline explicitly favors SAVR for bicuspid AS (especially with ascending aorta dilation), noting TAVR in bicuspid anatomy is reserved for prohibitive-risk patients [16]. The ESC/EACTS guidelines similarly note that SAVR is usually more appropriate for BAV with aortopathy, as no specific class I recommendation for TAVR exists in this subgroup. With evolving evidence, TAVR in selected bicuspid cases may be considered, but only after rigorous imaging and Heart Team review. Vascular access is another key consideration. Transfemoral access is preferred, but requires adequate iliofemoral diameter (usually ≥6–7 mm) and minimal tortuosity or calcification [18]. Severe peripheral calcification, small vessels, or excessive tortuosity may necessitate alternative approaches (trans-subclavian, transapical) or render TAVR unfeasible. Leaflet and annular calcification burden influences risk of complications: heavy, asymmetric calcification in the annulus or leaflets predisposes to paravalvular leak and annular injury. While mild calcific AS may reduce prosthesis anchoring, excessive calcification (especially below the annulus) is strongly linked to residual leak after TAVR [18]. Finally, coronary artery height and sinus anatomy must be assessed. Low coronary ostia (<10–12 mm above the annulus) or narrow sinuses of Valsalva can risk coronary obstruction when the bulky bioprosthetic

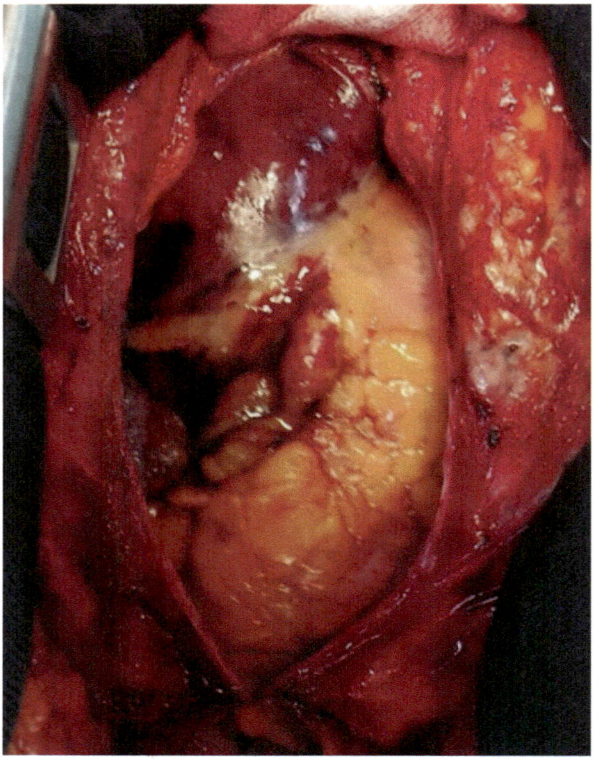

Fig. 9.2 Aortic annular rupture and acute dissection of the ascending aorta are rare but life-threatening complications that may occur following TAVR

leaflets are displaced by the TAVR valve [18]. Such findings may prompt coronary protection strategies or favor SAVR if obstruction cannot be safely mitigated.

Devices and Delivery Systems

Major Valve Platforms

Edwards SAPIEN family (XT, S3, S3 Ultra) are balloon-expandable bovine pericardial valves mounted on cobalt–chromium frames (Fig. 9.3). They have demonstrated excellent acute hemodynamic performance and low rates of paravalvular leak (PVL), even though with a moderate pacemaker implantation (PPI) risk (3–12%) and requirement for rapid pacing during deployment [12].

Medtronic CoreValve/Evolut series (R, PRO, PRO+) (Fig. 9.4), self-expanding nitinol-based supra-annular valves, offer larger effective orifice areas and lower gradients, but higher PPI rates (10–20%) than balloon-expandable valves [11, 19]. Their repositionable design (Evolut PRO+) allows adjustments after deployment, minimizing PVL.

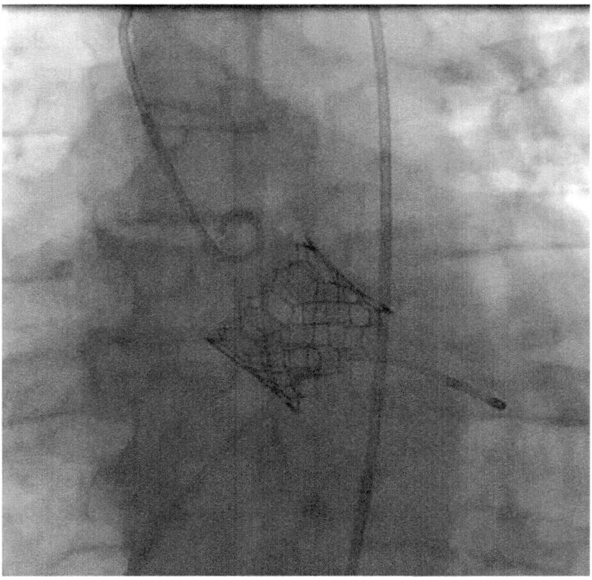

Fig. 9.3 Deployment of a balloon-expandable Edwards SAPIEN 3 valve under rapid ventricular pacing

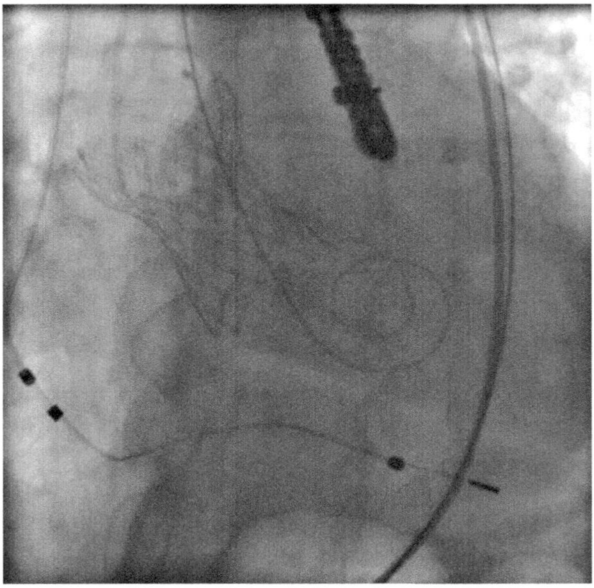

Fig. 9.4 Deployment of a self-expandable Medtronic Evolut R valve

Boston Scientific Acurate Neo, a self-expanding nitinol valve, features an upper stabilization crown and limited radial force. Initial trials show low stroke rates and quick deployment, but moderate PVL and higher PPI compared to competitor devices [20, 21].

Abbott Portico and Navitor systems (self-expanding intra-annular valves) offer key advantages in retrievability and intra-procedural repositioning. Navitor adds an anti-leak skirt and low-profile delivery aimed at reducing PVL [22, 23].

Technological Advancements (Table 9.2)

- *Sealing Skirts* (e.g., SAPIEN 3 Ultra, Evolut PRO+, Navitor): designed to minimize PVL by expanding at the annulus to seal leaks.
- *Repositionability/Recapturability:* Evolut PRO+, Portico/Navitor allow repositioning during deployment, reducing malposition and PVL, although adding technical complexity.
- *Low-Profile Delivery Systems:* Requiring smaller access sheaths (14–16 Fr), modern TAVR devices reduce vascular complications and extend transfemoral eligibility to patients with smaller vessels.
- *Enhanced Imaging Compatibility:* New systems are optimized for fluoroscopic and CT-based implantation, improving alignment and valve positioning.

Procedural Techniques

Access Routes

TF access is the preferred route for TAVR, being the least invasive and associated with faster recovery and fewer complications [24]. The procedure involves percutaneous femoral artery puncture, retrograde advancement of the delivery system through the iliac and aortic vasculature, and deployment of the transcatheter heart valve under fluoroscopic and echocardiographic guidance [25].

When transfemoral access is not feasible due to small-caliber, heavily calcified, tortuous, or diseased iliofemoral vessels, alternative access routes are considered [26]. These include:

- *Transapical:* a direct approach via left mini-thoracotomy and puncture of the left ventricular apex. It provides coaxial alignment with the aortic valve and is commonly used for balloon-expandable valves [27].
- *Transaortic:* involves a mini-sternotomy or right thoracotomy and direct cannulation of the ascending aorta, typically in patients with hostile peripheral vasculature [28].
- *Transsubclavian/axillary:* allows retrograde access via the left or right subclavian/axillary arteries. It is often performed using a surgical cutdown or percutaneously, with favorable outcomes in patients with suitable anatomy [29].
- *Transcaval:* involves intentional puncture of the inferior vena cava into the adjacent abdominal aorta, with closure of the aortocaval fistula after valve deployment. This approach is reserved for patients without other viable access [30].

Table 9.2 Characteristics of modern TAVR devices

Device platform	Frame/valve type	Delivery profile	Sealing skirt	Repositionable	PVL rate	PPI rate	Advantages	Disadvantages
SAPIEN 3 / ultra	Balloon-expandable, intra-annular	14–16 Fr	Yes	No	Low (1–3%)	~10%	Low PVL, broad evidence base, excellent imaging alignment	Requires rapid pacing, non-recapturable
Evolut PRO / PRO+	Self-expanding, supra-annular	14–18 Fr	Yes (PRO+)	Yes (PRO+)	Low–moderate	15–20%	Repositionable, large EOA, excellent durability	High PPI rate, potential coronary access challenges
Acurate neo / Neo2	Self-expanding, supra-annular	18 Fr	Yes (Neo2)	Partial	Moderate	~15%	Easy positioning, short frame, Neo2 improves PVL	PVL higher than others (neo), limited data vs next-gen valves
Portico / Navitor	Self-expanding, intra-annular	14–18 Fr	Yes (Navitor)	Yes	Moderate	~12–14%	Fully repositionable, flexible design	Less clinical experience, annulus sizing range narrower

EOA effective orifice area, *PVL* paravalvular leak, *PPI* permanent pacemaker implantation

Pre-procedural Planning

Thorough pre-procedural planning is critical to ensuring procedural success and minimizing complications. Multidetector CT is the gold standard for TAVR planning. It provides accurate measurements of the aortic annulus, coronary ostia height, leaflet calcification, sinotubular junction, and vascular access [31].

The *aortic annulus* is typically elliptical rather than circular in severe calcific aortic stenosis, requiring assessment of perimeter-derived diameters and cross-sectional areas for appropriate valve sizing [32]. Incorrect sizing increases the risk of paravalvular leak (PVL), annular rupture, or device embolization [33].

Coronary ostia height is measured from the annular plane to each coronary artery (Fig. 9.5). Heights <10–12 mm may predispose to coronary obstruction during valve deployment, particularly in balloon-expandable systems [34]. *Sinus of Valsalva* width and height are also evaluated to assess space for displaced native leaflets and prosthesis.

Valve calcification is assessed quantitatively and qualitatively. Extensive, asymmetric calcification can affect valve expansion, sealing, and conduction tissue interaction [35]. Non-contrast CT may also be used for calcium scoring using the Agatston method [36].

Iliofemoral anatomy is assessed to confirm adequate diameter (generally ≥5.5–6.0 mm for low-profile systems) and to exclude severe tortuosity or concentric calcification, which may complicate transfemoral delivery [37] (Figs. 9.5 and 9.6).

Echocardiography complements CT by confirming severity of aortic stenosis, LV systolic function, valve morphology (e.g., bicuspid vs. tricuspid), and identifying concomitant valvular disease (e.g., mitral regurgitation) [15]. Transesophageal echocardiography (TEE) or intracardiac echocardiography (ICE) may be used for more detailed pre-procedural evaluation when TTE is inconclusive.

Intra-Procedural Imaging and Guidance

Intra-procedural imaging is essential for valve positioning, deployment, and functional assessment. *Fluoroscopy* remains the primary modality, used to guide

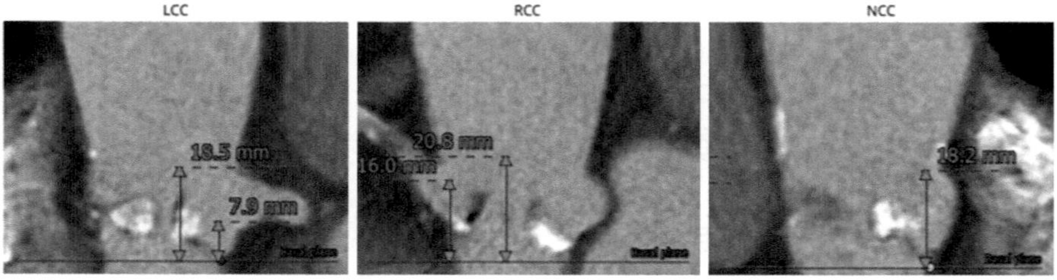

Fig. 9.5 Evaluation of coronary ostial height as part of pre-procedural planning for TAVR

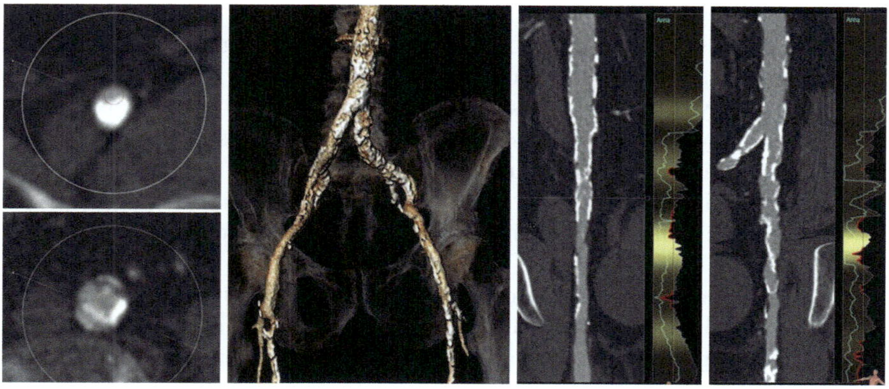

Fig. 9.6 Pre-procedural assessment of the iliofemoral arterial axis is a critical step in planning TAVR, particularly for determining the feasibility of transfemoral access

vascular access, valve positioning, and deployment. Optimal fluoroscopic projection (coplanar view) is derived from pre-procedural CT reconstructions to align with the aortic annulus and minimize parallax [38].

Transesophageal echocardiography (TEE) is commonly used during general anesthesia to assess prosthesis positioning, evaluate aortic regurgitation post-deployment, and guide interventions such as balloon post-dilation [39]. TEE is also critical in detecting complications such as pericardial effusion, aortic root injury, or valve malposition.

Intracardiac echocardiography (ICE) is gaining popularity, especially in conscious sedation protocols, offering real-time imaging of the valve, annulus, and surrounding structures without the need for general anesthesia [40]. *Fusion imaging* technology overlays CT-derived 3D models on live fluoroscopy to assist in precise prosthesis positioning and orientation [41].

Valve Deployment and Hemodynamic Assessment

The technique of valve deployment depends on the type of transcatheter valve used:

Balloon-Expandable Valves

- The valve is crimped onto a balloon catheter and positioned across the native valve annulus using fluoroscopic landmarks and contrast injections.
- *Rapid ventricular pacing* is initiated to reduce cardiac motion and output, thereby stabilizing the valve position during balloon inflation.
- The balloon is inflated for 3–5 seconds, expanding the valve, and then deflated. The system is withdrawn, and pacing is stopped.

Self-Expanding Valves

- These devices use nitinol frames and are deployed by gradually retracting a delivery sheath, allowing the valve to self-expand.
- Partial deployment permits assessment of alignment and function before full release. Many modern systems allow recapture and repositioning before final deployment, increasing procedural control.
- No rapid pacing is required for valve deployment, though it may be used briefly in some systems to stabilize hemodynamics during positioning.

Post-deployment, hemodynamic evaluation includes an aortic root angiogram to assess valve position, sealing, and coronary flow. TEE or TTE is used to evaluate for paravalvular regurgitation, central aortic insufficiency, or new wall motion abnormalities.

Balloon post-dilation may be performed if there is under-expansion, paravalvular leak, or malposition, particularly in heavily calcified or elliptical annuli.

Periprocedural Management

Antithrombotic Strategy

During TAVR, patients are systemically anticoagulated with intravenous unfractionated heparin, targeting an activated clotting time (ACT) of 250–300 seconds. Post-procedural antithrombotic regimens have evolved: current guidelines support single antiplatelet therapy with aspirin in most patients unless otherwise indicated [42]. Dual antiplatelet therapy is reserved for patients with recent coronary interventions. Patients with atrial fibrillation may resume oral anticoagulation alone, without added antiplatelet therapy, after TAVR [43].

Cerebral Embolic Protection

Cerebral embolic protection devices (e.g., Sentinel) are designed to capture or deflect aortic debris during valve deployment. These devices are deployed in the brachiocephalic and left common carotid arteries via the radial or brachial route [44]. Although meta-analyses have shown mixed results, some studies demonstrate reduced volume of cerebral emboli on diffusion-weighted MRI and fewer periprocedural strokes in selected high-risk patients [45].

Contrast and Renal Protection

Contrast-induced nephropathy is a major concern in patients with chronic kidney disease (CKD). Strategies to minimize risk include:

- Use of *low-volume contrast protocols.*
- Contrast-sparing imaging techniques (e.g., pre-CT planning with lower kVp, higher pitch).
- *Intra-procedural echo guidance* to reduce contrast use during valve positioning.

- *Peri-procedural hydration,* preferably with isotonic saline and hemodynamic monitoring.
- Avoidance of nephrotoxic agents and prolonged hypotension during rapid pacing.

Outcomes and Evidence

Procedural Success

TAVR has demonstrated consistently high procedural success rates, particularly with newer-generation devices and increasing operator experience. According to data from the French FRANCE-TAVI registry, device success—defined by the Valve Academic Research Consortium (VARC) criteria—was achieved in over 96% of cases [46]. The STS/ACC TVT Registry in the United States similarly reports device success exceeding 95% across centers [47].

Short- and Long-Term Mortality

Short-term (30-day) mortality after TAVR has declined markedly. A contemporary analysis of over 100,000 patients in the STS/ACC TVT Registry showed a 30-day all-cause mortality rate of 2.2% [47]. In longer-term follow-up, one-year mortality varies by surgical risk group. For example, the NOTION trial (low-risk patients) reported a 1-year mortality of 4.9% [48], while the PARTNER 1 trial (high-risk cohort) reported 1-year mortality of 24.2% [49]. Meta-analyses confirm that 1-year mortality ranges from 5% to 25% depending on patient risk profile [50].

At 5 years, outcomes are influenced by patient frailty and comorbidities. A large systematic review found pooled 5-year survival after TAVR to be approximately 48% in predominantly high-risk patients [51]. In the SURTAVI trial (intermediate-risk patients), 5-year all-cause mortality was 30% [52], and in the Evolut Low Risk trial, mortality was 10.7% at 2 years [53].

Functional Improvement (NYHA Class, 6MWT)

Functional status improves substantially after TAVR. Across multiple trials and registries, patients experience an average improvement of 1–2 NYHA classes within 30 days to 6 months [54]. In a pooled analysis, the 6-minute walk distance (6MWT) increased by approximately 50–70 meters at 30 days, with sustained benefit over 1 year [55]. These improvements reflect both relief of obstruction and improved cardiac output following valve implantation.

Quality of Life (QoL) Outcomes

TAVR is associated with large and rapid improvements in health-related quality of life (HRQoL), especially as measured by the Kansas City Cardiomyopathy Questionnaire (KCCQ). In the STS/ACC TVT Registry, KCCQ overall summary scores increased by 27.6 points at 30 days and 31.9 points at 1 year compared to baseline—a change considered highly clinically significant [56]. Additional improvements in general QoL metrics such as SF-12 and EQ-5D have also been reported, particularly in physical function domains [55].

Special Scenarios and Expanding Indications

Low Surgical Risk Patients With accumulating evidence, TAVR is now an established option even in patients deemed low risk by STS scores. Landmark trials (PARTNER 3 and Evolut Low Risk) randomized low-risk patients (mean STS ≈ 1–2%, mean age ~ 74 y) to TAVR versus SAVR [57]. At 1 year, TAVR with contemporary devices met noninferiority (and in PARTNER 3 even superiority) for the composite of death, stroke, or rehospitalization (e.g., 8.5% vs 15.1% in PARTNER 3) [57]. These studies showed similar mortality and stroke rates with lower perioperative morbidity after TAVR. For truly low-risk patients <65 without other concerns, a shared decision is advised: TAVR may be reasonable, but long-term data on valve durability are still maturing.

Bicuspid Aortic Valves As above, bicuspid AS has unique anatomy. TAVR in bicuspid valves is feasible but technically more complex. Because bicuspid valves often have elliptical annuli, asymmetric calcification, and larger ascending aortas, SAVR is generally preferred in younger patients. Current guidelines reserve TAVR in bicuspid AS for selected high-risk or inoperable cases, emphasizing thorough CT assessment of leaflet and aortic dimensions [16]. Ongoing studies suggest improving outcomes with newer-generation valves in bicuspid AS, but no guideline change has been made beyond recognizing SAVR as standard for most bicuspid presentations.

Valve-in-Valve (ViV) TAVR Patients with failing surgical bioprosthetic aortic valves may undergo a transcatheter ViV procedure rather than repeat surgery (Fig. 9.7). ViV TAVR is now an accepted alternative in high-risk redo cases. Studies show that ViV TAVR yields 30-day and 1-year survival comparable to native-valve TAVR in similar-risk cohorts [58]. The Heart Team must evaluate prior valve type, inner diameter, and coronary height: some small surgical valves or stentless designs portend higher gradients or coronary obstruction after ViV. Careful CT planning (including virtual valve implantation to assess coronary clearance) is critical [58].

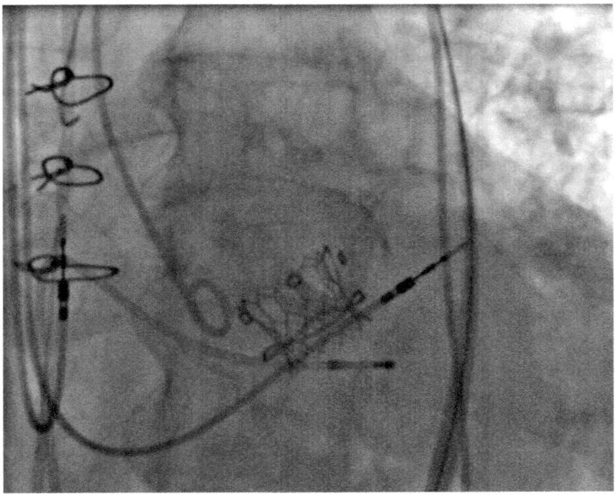

Fig. 9.7 Valve-in-valve TAVR is an established treatment option for patients with failing surgical bioprosthetic aortic valves who are at high surgical risk

In sum, ViV TAVR can safely treat degenerated bioprostheses in suitable candidates, expanding indications beyond native AS.

Frail or Elderly Patients Frailty and advanced age profoundly affect TAVR candidacy and outcomes. Guidelines emphasize that biological age and frailty—more than chronological age—guide therapy. For patients >80 years or with limited life expectancy (<10 y), TAVR's less invasive nature is often favored [16]. However, frailty itself predicts poor outcomes; severe frailty (e.g., slowness, weakness, or inability to perform daily activities) may render even TAVR futile. The ACC expert consensus defines prohibitive risk to include severe frailty or multi-organ compromise [17]. Multidimensional frailty assessment (mobility, gait speed, nutrition, cognitive function) is now recommended in pre-TAVR evaluation. Elderly patients often have multiple comorbidities (pulmonary disease, renal failure, cerebrovascular disease) that heighten procedural risk [15]. Thus, TAVR in the elderly is justified when symptoms are severe and quality-of-life gains are expected; if frailty or comorbidity is too extreme (predicted survival <1 year or < 25% chance of 2-year benefit), palliation may be preferred.

Lifetime Management of Valvular Heart Disease

As TAVR moves into younger and lower-risk populations, the concept of lifetime valve management has become a core principle. Decisions must anticipate not only the index procedure but future coronary access, re-intervention, and durability. This includes:

- *Device selection:* Choosing valve types that allow optimal coronary access and facilitate future valve-in-valve therapy.
- *Coronary re-access planning:* Supra-annular valves may obstruct coronary access in repeat procedures. Techniques such as commissural alignment and high implantation can help preserve access.
- *Aortic root management:* Younger patients may benefit from annular enlargement during SAVR to optimize future TAVR options.
- *Patient-specific strategy:* In some cases, SAVR may be the preferred initial therapy to preserve future TAVR options. In others, an initial TAVR with a high-positioned valve and preserved coronary access may be optimal.

Conclusion

TAVR has evolved from a niche therapy for inoperable patients into a frontline treatment for aortic stenosis across all surgical risk groups. Its integration into routine clinical practice has been driven by consistent results from pivotal randomized controlled trials such as PARTNER, CoreValve, SURTAVI, and Evolut Low Risk, which demonstrated non-inferiority—and in some subgroups, superiority—of TAVR compared to SAVR in terms of mortality, stroke, and functional improvement. Registry data such as from the STS/ACC TVT and FRANCE-TAVI registries confirm that these outcomes translate well into real-world populations, including the elderly and frail.

The core pillars of contemporary TAVR practice include careful patient selection, high-resolution anatomical imaging, and collaborative heart team decision-making. Proper assessment of annular size, valve morphology, coronary height, and vascular access is critical to minimize complications and maximize procedural success. Device selection must be tailored not only to anatomy but also to long-term strategy, with newer-generation valves offering enhanced sealing, repositionability, and coronary access preservation.

Despite these advancements, key challenges remain. Long-term valve durability—especially in younger patients—is still being evaluated, although early- and mid-term data suggest that transcatheter valves may be at least comparable to surgical bioprostheses up to 8–10 years. Coronary access after TAVR, especially in cases of future TAVR-in-TAVR, presents significant technical barriers, particularly with certain self-expanding valve designs. Lifetime management strategies are increasingly emphasized, requiring clinicians to consider how today's valve choice and implant technique will impact future reintervention options.

Looking forward, the role of transcatheter therapies is expected to expand further—not only for aortic stenosis, but also for conditions such as bicuspid valve disease, failed bioprostheses (valve-in-valve), pure aortic regurgitation, and high-risk redo operations. In parallel, innovation in valve design and delivery systems is expected to improve outcomes and extend indications. Ultimately, TAVR has redefined the therapeutic landscape of structural heart disease, and its continued evolution represents a paradigm shift toward less invasive, highly personalized cardiovascular care.

References

1. Osnabrugge RL, Mylotte D, Head SJ, Van Mieghem NM, Nkomo VT, LeReun CM, et al. Aortic stenosis in the elderly: disease prevalence and number of candidates for transcatheter aortic valve replacement: a meta-analysis and modeling study. J Am Coll Cardiol. 2013;62(11):1002–12.
2. Vavilis G, Back M, Barany P, Szummer K. Epidemiology of aortic stenosis/aortic valve replacement (from the Nationwide Swedish Renal Registry). Am J Cardiol. 2022;163:58–64.
3. Poletti E, De Backer O, Scotti A, Costa G, Bruno F, Fiorina C, et al. Transcatheter aortic valve replacement for pure native aortic valve regurgitation: the PANTHEON International Project. JACC Cardiovasc Interv. 2023;16(16):1974–85.
4. Cribier A, Savin T, Berland J, Rocha P, Mechmeche R, Saoudi N, et al. Percutaneous transluminal balloon valvuloplasty of adult aortic stenosis: report of 92 cases. J Am Coll Cardiol. 1987;9(2):381–6.
5. Cribier A, Eltchaninoff H, Bash A, Borenstein N, Tron C, Bauer F, et al. Percutaneous transcatheter implantation of an aortic valve prosthesis for calcific aortic stenosis: first human case description. Circulation. 2002;106(24):3006–8.
6. de Jaegere P, de Ronde M, den Heijer P, Weger A, Baan J. The history of transcatheter aortic valve implantation: The role and contribution of an early believer and adopter, the Netherlands. Neth Heart J. 2020;28(Suppl 1):128–35.
7. Leon MB, Smith CR, Mack M, Miller DC, Moses JW, Svensson LG, et al. Transcatheter aortic-valve implantation for aortic stenosis in patients who cannot undergo surgery. N Engl J Med. 2010;363(17):1597–607.
8. Smith CR, Leon MB, Mack MJ, Miller DC, Moses JW, Svensson LG, et al. Transcatheter versus surgical aortic-valve replacement in high-risk patients. N Engl J Med. 2011;364(23):2187–98.
9. Adams DH, Popma JJ, Reardon MJ, Yakubov SJ, Coselli JS, Deeb GM, et al. Transcatheter aortic-valve replacement with a self-expanding prosthesis. N Engl J Med. 2014;370(19):1790–8.
10. Leon MB, Smith CR, Mack MJ, Makkar RR, Svensson LG, Kodali SK, et al. Transcatheter or surgical aortic-valve replacement in intermediate-risk patients. N Engl J Med. 2016;374(17):1609–20.
11. Reardon MJ, Van Mieghem NM, Popma JJ, Kleiman NS, Sondergaard L, Mumtaz M, et al. Surgical or transcatheter aortic-valve replacement in intermediate-risk patients. N Engl J Med. 2017;376(14):1321–31.
12. Mack MJ, Leon MB, Thourani VH, Makkar R, Kodali SK, Russo M, et al. Transcatheter aortic-valve replacement with a balloon-expandable valve in low-risk patients. N Engl J Med. 2019;380(18):1695–705.
13. Popma JJ, Deeb GM, Yakubov SJ, Mumtaz M, Gada H, O'Hair D, et al. Transcatheter aortic-valve replacement with a self-expanding valve in low-risk patients. N Engl J Med. 2019;380(18):1706–15.
14. Braghiroli J, Kapoor K, Thielhelm TP, Ferreira T, Cohen MG. Transcatheter aortic valve replacement in low risk patients: a review of PARTNER 3 and Evolut low risk trials. Cardiovascular diagnosis and therapy. 2020;10(1):59–71.
15. Vahanian A, Beyersdorf F, Praz F, Milojevic M, Baldus S, Bauersachs J, et al. 2021 ESC/EACTS Guidelines for the management of valvular heart disease. EuroIntervention. 2022;17(14):e1126–e96.
16. Otto CM, Nishimura RA, Bonow RO, Carabello BA, Erwin JP 3rd, Gentile F, et al. 2020 ACC/AHA Guideline for the Management of Patients With Valvular Heart Disease: Executive

Summary: A Report of the American College of Cardiology/American Heart Association Joint Committee on Clinical Practice Guidelines. Circulation. 2021;143(5):e35–71.
17. Otto CM, Kumbhani DJ, Alexander KP, Calhoon JH, Desai MY, Kaul S, et al. 2017 ACC Expert Consensus Decision Pathway for Transcatheter Aortic Valve Replacement in the Management of Adults With Aortic Stenosis: A Report of the American College of Cardiology Task Force on Clinical Expert Consensus Documents. J Am Coll Cardiol. 2017;69(10):1313–46.
18. Bax JJ, Delgado V, Bapat V, Baumgartner H, Collet JP, Erbel R, et al. Open issues in transcatheter aortic valve implantation. Part 1: patient selection and treatment strategy for transcatheter aortic valve implantation. European heart journal. 2014;35(38):2627–38.
19. Ahmed M, Ahsan A, Tabassum S, Tariq I, Zulfiqar E, Raja MF, et al. Hemodynamic and clinical outcomes with balloon-expandable valves versus self-expanding valves in patients with small aortic annulus undergoing transcatheter aortic valve replacement: a meta-analysis of randomized controlled trials and propensity score matched studies. IJC Heart Vasc. 2024;55:101542.
20. Kooistra NH, Intan-Goey VMP, Ziviello F, Leenders GE, Kraaijeveld AO, Doevendans PA, et al. Comparison of the Sapien 3 versus the ACURATE neo valve system: a propensity score analysis. Catheter Cardiovasc Interven. 2021;97(4):e597–606.
21. Ooms JF, Cornelis K, Wijeysundera HC, Vandeloo B, Van Der Heyden J, Kovac J, et al. Safety and feasibility of early discharge after transcatheter aortic valve implantation with ACURATE Neo-the POLESTAR trial. Clin Res Cardiol. 2025;114(3):341–9.
22. Reardon MJ, Chehab B, Smith D, Walton AS, Worthley SG, Manoharan G, et al. 30-day clinical outcomes of a self-expanding transcatheter aortic valve: the International PORTICO NG Study. JACC Cardiovasc Interv. 2023;16(6):681–9.
23. Sondergaard L, Walton AS, Worthley SG, Smith D, Chehab B, Manoharan G, et al. Thirty-day and one-year outcomes of the Navitor transcatheter heart valve in patients with aortic stenosis: the prospective, multicentre, global PORTICO NG Study. EuroIntervention. 2023;19(3):248–55.
24. Webb JG, Wood DA. Current status of transcatheter aortic valve replacement. J Am Coll Cardiol. 2012;60(6):483–92.
25. Piazza N, de Jaegere P, Schultz C, Becker AE, Serruys PW, Anderson RH. Anatomy of the aortic valvar complex and its implications for transcatheter implantation of the aortic valve. Circulation Cardiovascular interventions. 2008;1(1):74–81.
26. Hayashida K, Lefèvre T, Chevalier B, Hovasse T, Romano M, Garot P, et al. Transfemoral aortic valve implantation new criteria to predict vascular complications. JACC Cardiovasc Interv. 2011;4(8):851–8.
27. Himbert D, Descoutures F, Al-Attar N, Iung B, Ducrocq G, Détaint D, et al. Results of transfemoral or transapical aortic valve implantation following a uniform assessment in high-risk patients with aortic stenosis. J Am Coll Cardiol. 2009;54(4):303–11.
28. Biasco L, Ferrari E, Pedrazzini G, Faletra F, Moccetti T, Petracca F, et al. Access sites for TAVI: patient selection criteria, technical aspects, and outcomes. Front Cardiovasc Med. 2018;5:88.
29. Muensterer A, Mazzitelli D, Ruge H, Wagner A, Hettich I, Piazza N, et al. Safety and efficacy of the subclavian access route for TAVI in cases of missing transfemoral access. Clin Res Cardiol. 2013;102(9):627–36.
30. Greenbaum AB, O'Neill WW, Paone G, Guerrero ME, Wyman JF, Cooper RL, et al. Caval-aortic access to allow transcatheter aortic valve replacement in otherwise ineligible patients: initial human experience. J Am Coll Cardiol. 2014;63(25 Pt A):2795–804.
31. Blanke P, Weir-McCall JR, Achenbach S, Delgado V, Hausleiter J, Jilaihawi H, et al. Computed tomography imaging in the context of transcatheter aortic valve implantation (TAVI) /transcatheter aortic valve replacement (TAVR): An expert consensus document of the Society of Cardiovascular Computed Tomography. J Cardiovasc Comput Tomograph. 2019;13(1):1–20.
32. Chiocchi M, Forcina M, Morosetti D, Pugliese L, Cavallo AU, Citraro D, et al. The role of computed tomography in the planning of transcatheter aortic valve implantation: a retrospective analysis in 200 procedures. J Cardiovasc Med (Hagerstown). 2018;19(10):571–8.
33. Ribeiro HB, Webb JG, Makkar RR, Cohen MG, Kapadia SR, Kodali S, et al. Predictive factors, management, and clinical outcomes of coronary obstruction following transcath-

eter aortic valve implantation: insights from a large multicenter registry. J Am Coll Cardiol. 2013;62(17):1552–62.
34. Dvir D, Leipsic J, Blanke P, Ribeiro HB, Kornowski R, Pichard A, et al. Coronary obstruction in transcatheter aortic valve-in-valve implantation: preprocedural evaluation, device selection, protection, and treatment. Circ Cardiovasc Interven. 2015;8(1)
35. Milhorini Pio S, Bax J, Delgado V. How valvular calcification can affect the outcomes of transcatheter aortic valve implantation. Expert Rev Med Device. 2020;17(8):773–84.
36. Flores-Umanzor E, Keshvara R, Reza S, Asghar A, Rashidul Anwar M, Cepas-Guillen PL, et al. A systematic review of contrast-enhanced computed tomography calcium scoring methodologies and impact of aortic valve calcium burden on TAVI clinical outcomes. J Cardiovasc Comput Tomograph. 2023;17(6):373–83.
37. Pontes ÍCM, Guimarães C, Fonseca E, Silva MMA, Sasdelli Neto R, Ishikawa WY. Computed tomography angiography in the planning of transcatheter aortic valve replacement: a step-by-step approach. Radiologia brasileira. 2022;55(6):373–9.
38. Litmanovich DE, Ghersin E, Burke DA, Popma J, Shahrzad M, Bankier AA. Imaging in Transcatheter Aortic Valve Replacement (TAVR): role of the radiologist. Insights into imaging. 2014;5(1):123–45.
39. Zamorano J, Gonçalves A, Lancellotti P, Andersen KA, González-Gómez A, Monaghan M, et al. The use of imaging in new transcatheter interventions: an EACVI review paper. European heart journal. Cardiovasc Imag. 2016;17(8):835-af.
40. Bartel T, Müller S, Biviano A, Hahn RT. Why is intracardiac echocardiography helpful? Benefits, costs, and how to learn. Eur Heart J. 2014;35(2):69–76.
41. Melillo F, Ancona F, Romano V, Ingallina G, Capogrosso C, Stella S, et al. [Fusion imaging in structural heart interventions]. Giornale italiano di cardiologia (2006). 2020;21(4 Suppl 2):34s–41s.
42. Brouwer J, Nijenhuis VJ, Delewi R, Hermanides RS, Holvoet W, Dubois CLF, et al. Aspirin with or without clopidogrel after transcatheter aortic-valve implantation. N Engl J Med. 2020;383(15):1447–57.
43. Hindi MN, Akodad M, Nestelberger T, Sathananthan J. Antithrombotic therapy after transcatheter aortic valve replacement: an overview. Struct Heart. 2022;6(5):100085.
44. Kapadia SR, Makkar R, Leon M, Abdel-Wahab M, Waggoner T, Massberg S, et al. Cerebral embolic protection during transcatheter aortic-valve replacement. N Engl J Med. 2022;387(14):1253–63.
45. Reddy RK, Ahmad Y, Arnold AD, Howard JP. Cerebral embolic protection devices during transcatheter aortic valve replacement: a meta-analysis of randomized controlled trials. J Soc Cardiovasc Angiograph Interven. 2023;2(5):None
46. Didier R, Le Breton H, Eltchaninoff H, Cayla G, Commeau P, Collet JP, et al. Evolution of TAVI patients and techniques over the past decade: the French TAVI registries. Archives of cardiovascular diseases. 2022;115(4):206–13.
47. Bansal K, Rawlley B, Majmundar V, Beale R, Shah M, Kosinski AS, et al. Out-of-hospital 30-day mortality after mitral TEER: insights from the STS/ACC TVT registry. JACC Cardiovasc Interv. 2025;18(7):882–94.
48. Jørgensen TH, Thyregod HGH, Ihlemann N, Nissen H, Petursson P, Kjeldsen BJ, et al. Eight-year outcomes for patients with aortic valve stenosis at low surgical risk randomized to transcatheter vs. surgical aortic valve replacement. Eur Heart J. 2021;42(30):2912–9.
49. Mack MJ, Leon MB, Smith CR, Miller DC, Moses JW, Tuzcu EM, et al. 5-year outcomes of transcatheter aortic valve replacement or surgical aortic valve replacement for high surgical risk patients with aortic stenosis (PARTNER 1): a randomised controlled trial. Lancet (London, England). 2015;385(9986):2477–84.
50. Siontis GC, Praz F, Pilgrim T, Mavridis D, Verma S, Salanti G, et al. Transcatheter aortic valve implantation vs. surgical aortic valve replacement for treatment of severe aortic stenosis: a meta-analysis of randomized trials. Eur Heart J. 2016;37(47):3503–12.

51. Chakos A, Wilson-Smith A, Arora S, Nguyen TC, Dhoble A, Tarantini G, et al. Long term outcomes of transcatheter aortic valve implantation (TAVI): a systematic review of 5-year survival and beyond. Ann Cardiothoracic Surg. 2017;6(5):432–43.
52. Van Mieghem NM, Deeb GM, Søndergaard L, Grube E, Windecker S, Gada H, et al. Self-expanding transcatheter vs surgical aortic valve replacement in intermediate-risk patients: 5-year outcomes of the SURTAVI randomized clinical trial. JAMA Cardiol. 2022;7(10):1000–8.
53. Yakubov SJ, Adams DH, Watson DR, Reardon MJ, Kleiman NS, Heimansohn D, et al. 2-year outcomes after iliofemoral self-expanding transcatheter aortic valve replacement in patients with severe aortic stenosis deemed extreme risk for surgery. J Am Coll Cardiol. 2015;66(12):1327–34.
54. Kodali SK, Williams MR, Smith CR, Svensson LG, Webb JG, Makkar RR, et al. Two-year outcomes after transcatheter or surgical aortic-valve replacement. N Engl J Med. 2012;366(18):1686–95.
55. Kim CA, Rasania SP, Afilalo J, Popma JJ, Lipsitz LA, Kim DH. Functional status and quality of life after transcatheter aortic valve replacement: a systematic review. Ann Intern Med. 2014;160(4):243–54.
56. Arnold SV, Spertus JA, Vemulapalli S, Li Z, Matsouaka RA, Baron SJ, et al. Quality-of-life outcomes after transcatheter aortic valve replacement in an unselected population: a report from the STS/ACC transcatheter valve therapy registry. JAMA Cardiol. 2017;2(4):409–16.
57. Narayan P. Transcatheter aortic valve replacement in low-risk patients: superiority or shifting goalposts and statistical crystal-gazing? Ind J Thoracic Cardiovasc Surg. 2019;35(4):596–8.
58. Perdoncin E, Paone G, Byku I. Valve-in-valve transcatheter aortic valve replacement for failed surgical valves and adjunctive therapies. US Cardiol. 2022;16:e09.

Transcatheter Interventions for Tricuspid and Pulmonary Valve

10

Carina Ureche, Igor Nedelciuc, and Alexandru Burlacu

Introduction

The past two decades have dramatically reshaped structural heart disease treatment, with interventional cardiology now addressing pathologies of the right heart. Historically overlooked due to perceived lower hemodynamic impact and high surgical risk, tricuspid (TV) and pulmonary valve (PV) diseases are now recognized for their significant morbidity and mortality burden. Chronic tricuspid regurgitation (TR) leads to right ventricular dysfunction and heart failure, while pulmonary regurgitation (PR) post-congenital repair can cause RV dilation and arrhythmias.

This chapter explores the rapidly evolving field of transcatheter TV and PV interventions. We will examine the unique anatomy and physiology of these valves, detail the innovative repair and replacement devices, and review the latest clinical evidence on their safety and efficacy. Key procedural considerations—access routes and imaging guidance—along with essential patient care will be discussed.

Finally, we will address current limitations, future technological advancements, refined patient selection, and the vital role of the heart team, as transcatheter therapies for the right heart promise to transform management and improve outcomes for a previously underserved patient population.

C. Ureche (✉)
Department of Cardiology, Institute for Cardiovascular Diseases, "Prof. Dr. George I. M. Georgescu"; Faculty of Medicine, University of Medicine and Pharmacy "Grigore T Popa", Iasi, Romania

I. Nedelciuc
Department of Interventional Cardiology, Institute for Cardiovascular Diseases "Prof. Dr. George I. M. Georgescu", Iași, Romania

A. Burlacu
Interventional Cardiology, Cardiovascular Diseases Institute, Iași & Grigore T. Popa University of Medicine and Pharmacy, Iași, Romania
e-mail: alexandru.burlacu@umfiasi.ro

G. Tinică, A. Burlacu (eds.), *Surgical, Hybrid and Minimally Invasive Structural Cardiac Interventions*, https://doi.org/10.1007/978-3-032-16676-0_10

Transcatheter Tricuspid Valve Interventions

Anatomy and Pathophysiology

The tricuspid valve apparatus is a complex three-dimensional structure comprising several components working in synchrony to ensure unidirectional blood flow. The TV is typically characterized by three leaflets: the anterior (largest), posterior, and septal leaflets. However, anatomical variations, including the presence of two or four leaflets, are not uncommon. These thin, yet resilient, flaps of tissue are central to the valve's opening and closing mechanism. The tricuspid annulus is represented by a fibrous ring that serves as the anchoring point for the valve leaflets. Unlike the more rigid mitral annulus, the tricuspid annulus is less fibrous and more muscular, making it susceptible to significant dilation, particularly in response to right ventricular pressure or volume overload. Its normal shape is saddle-like and elliptical. Additionally, several chordae tendineae are delicate, string-like cords that originate from the papillary muscles and attach to the free margins and ventricular surfaces of the tricuspid leaflets. They prevent the leaflets from prolapsing into the right atrium during ventricular contraction. The valve is anchored by three papillary muscles—anterior, posterior, and septal papillary muscles, although their number and location can vary. They contract during ventricular systole, pulling on the chordae and maintaining leaflet coaptation [1, 2].

Causes of Tricuspid Regurgitation

Tricuspid regurgitation is a condition characterized by the abnormal backflow of blood from the right ventricle into the right atrium during ventricular systole due to incomplete closure of the tricuspid valve. While mild or trace TR is often benign and found in a significant portion of the population (65–85%), moderate to severe TR can lead to increased right atrial and ventricular pressures, right ventricular volume overload, and eventually right heart failure, significantly impacting patient prognosis. TR is primarily classified into two categories based on its etiology: primary and secondary.

Primary TR involves a structural abnormality of the tricuspid valve apparatus itself (leaflets, chordae, papillary muscles, or annulus). The main causes of primary TR are congenital (Ebstein's anomaly, tricuspid valve hypoplasia, clefts, double orifice valve), infective endocarditis, pacemaker/defibrillator leads, rheumatic heart disease, carcinoid syndrome, traumatic injury, drug-induced (fenfluramine, pergolide), myxomatous degeneration, and systemic disease (lupus erythematosus, sarcoidosis).

Secondary TR, also known as functional TR, is the most common form of TR. In this type, the tricuspid valve leaflets are structurally normal, but the valve becomes incompetent due to underlying right heart chamber dilation and/or increased pulmonary pressures, leading to leaflet malcoaptation and tethering. The key mechanisms involved are right ventricular dilation and dysfunction (ventricular TR) due to:

left-sided heart disease (the most common cause of secondary TR), pulmonary hypertension or intrinsic RV disease, and right atrial enlargement due to atrial fibrillation (atrial TR) [2].

Challenges of Imaging and Access

Accurate and comprehensive imaging of the tricuspid valve is crucial for diagnosis, quantification of TR severity, and procedural planning, particularly for transcatheter interventions. However, several inherent anatomical and technical factors make tricuspid valve imaging more challenging compared to the left-sided valves.

The tricuspid valve's anterior position in the chest makes it inherently more difficult to visualize adequately with standard transthoracic echocardiography (TTE). The tricuspid annulus has a complex, saddle-shaped, and highly dynamic 3D geometry and when it dilates, it can become more planar and circular. This complex geometry makes accurate 2D imaging challenging. The number of leaflets can vary (2–4), and the subvalvular apparatus (papillary muscles and chordae) is also highly variable and often smaller and more widely separated than in the mitral valve. The right ventricular wall is thinner and more heavily trabeculated compared to the left, complicating imaging quality and potentially affecting device anchoring [3].

While TEE provides excellent views of the mitral valve, its position in the esophagus is further away from the more anteriorly located tricuspid valve. This distance, coupled with the TV's geometry, can limit the availability of optimal imaging windows, making it harder to assess leaflet coaptation and pathology comprehensively. The tricuspid valve operates in a low-pressure, high-flow environment, leading to lower jet velocities compared to left-sided regurgitation which makes quantitative assessment of TR severity (e.g., using PISA—proximal isovelocity surface area—or Doppler methods) less accurate and more variable, especially as TR severity can fluctuate with respiratory cycle and preload changes. The presence of transvenous pacemaker or defibrillator leads crossing the tricuspid valve is common in patients with TR. These leads can create significant acoustic shadowing on echocardiography, obscuring direct visualization of the leaflets and making it difficult to assess their function and integrity [4].

Due to these limitations, a multi-modality imaging approach is frequently necessary for a thorough evaluation of the tricuspid valve. Both TTE for initial assessment and TEE for detailed morphology, with increasing reliance on intracardiac echocardiography (ICE) during transcatheter procedures for direct, real-time visualization from within the heart [5]. Cardiac computed tomography (CT) provides excellent anatomical detail of the annulus, surrounding structures (like the right coronary artery, conduction system), and leaflet morphology in 3D. It is particularly useful for pre-procedural planning and device sizing. Cardiovascular magnetic resonance (CMR) offers comprehensive assessment of right ventricular size, function, and accurate quantification of regurgitant volume, often considered the gold standard for these parameters.

The growing interest in transcatheter tricuspid valve interventions (TTVI) for severe TR has highlighted specific challenges related to accessing and maneuvering devices within the right heart. Vascular access considerations include large sheath caliber (transcatheter tricuspid valve replacement (TTVR often requires large-bore access sheaths (up to 45 Fr), which are significantly larger than those used for mitral or aortic interventions), access routes (the preferred access routes are typically transjugular or transfemoral), and venous anatomy (patients with severe TR often have dilated vena cavae, which can make device delivery less straightforward. Small vein size can also pose a challenge for large-bore sheath insertion) [6].

Another important point is the anatomical proximity to critical structures, since the tricuspid annulus is in close proximity to several vital cardiac structures that are at risk of injury during intervention—conduction system (the atrioventricular (AV) node and His bundle are located in the triangle of Koch, close to the postero-septal portion of the tricuspid annulus. Interventions carry a risk of damaging the conduction system, potentially leading to new-onset heart block requiring a permanent pacemaker), right coronary artery (annuloplasty procedures, or device implantation, risk compression, kinking, or occlusion of the RCA, particularly if it is located very close to the valve hinge points) and coronary sinus ostium (located near the postero-septal annulus) [3].

Additionally, the right ventricle's thin and highly trabeculated wall can complicate transapical approaches (though less common for tricuspid interventions) and make device anchoring more challenging. The presence of transvenous leads is a significant challenge. Leads can physically obstruct device delivery, interfere with leaflet grasping during edge-to-edge repair, or complicate valve replacement. While many transcatheter procedures are feasible with leads in place, careful planning and technique adjustment are crucial. Lead extraction or repositioning may be considered in challenging cases [7].

Last but not least, patients referred for tricuspid valve interventions often present at an advanced stage of right heart failure, are elderly, and have multiple comorbidities. This makes them high-risk surgical candidates and contributes to the reluctance to perform isolated tricuspid valve surgery. The late referral for intervention means that the right ventricle may already be severely dysfunctional, which can limit the potential benefit of valve repair or replacement and impact post-procedural outcomes [8].

Indications and Patient Selection

The decision to intervene on the tricuspid valve, particularly for severe TR, involves careful consideration of clinical criteria, thorough risk stratification, and a comprehensive imaging workup. Guidelines from major cardiology societies, such as the European Society of Cardiology (ESC) and the American College of Cardiology/American Heart Association (ACC/AHA), provide frameworks for decision-making [2, 9].

Clinical Criteria for Intervention

Intervention for TR is generally considered in patients with severe TR who meet specific clinical criteria:

- *Symptomatic severe TR:* For patients with severe TR who remain symptomatic (e.g., New York Heart Association (NYHA) functional class III or IV) despite optimal guideline-directed medical therapy (GDMT), intervention can be considered. Symptoms often include fatigue, weakness, peripheral edema, ascites, and abdominal discomfort due to venous congestion.
- *Progressive RV dilation and dysfunction:* In asymptomatic or minimally symptomatic patients with severe primary or secondary TR, intervention may be considered if there is evidence of progressive RV dilation and/or dysfunction, or progressive kidney dysfunction, in an effort to prevent irreversible myocardial damage and improve long-term outcomes.
- *Concomitant left-sided heart surgery. Severe TR:* Surgical repair or replacement of the tricuspid valve is recommended for patients with severe TR undergoing concomitant left-sided heart surgery (e.g., mitral valve surgery, aortic valve surgery, or coronary artery bypass grafting). *Moderate TR or mild TR with annular dilation:* Intervention may also be considered in patients with moderate TR, or even mild TR with significant tricuspid annular dilation (e.g., >40 mm or >21 mm/m^2 by echo), if they are undergoing left-sided heart surgery. This is due to the recognition that even milder TR can progress after left-sided surgery and impact prognosis.
- *Specific primary TR etiologies:* For certain primary TR etiologies, such as severe Ebstein's anomaly or significant symptomatic pacemaker lead-induced TR, surgical or transcatheter intervention may be indicated regardless of concomitant left-sided disease.

Risk Stratification

Careful risk stratification and a detailed imaging workup are essential steps before considering tricuspid valve intervention.

Patients with severe TR often present with advanced disease, frailty, and multiple comorbidities, making them high-risk candidates for surgery. It is crucial to assess the overall surgical or procedural risk, taking into account factors such as age, renal function, liver function, prior cardiac surgeries, and the severity of right heart failure. Specific risk scores, such as the TRI-SCORE, which incorporates clinical and imaging parameters, can help predict in-hospital mortality following isolated tricuspid surgery and assist in shared decision-making. A significant challenge is that many patients are referred late, when they have advanced right heart failure and significant end-organ damage (e.g., cardiac cirrhosis), which increases procedural risk and may limit the benefit of intervention [6, 10].

Imaging Workup

A multi-modality imaging approach is pivotal for a comprehensive assessment of the tricuspid valve and right heart, guiding patient and device selection, and facilitating procedural success.

TTE is the first step for the initial assessment of TR severity, right atrial and ventricular size and function, pulmonary artery pressures, and overall cardiac function. TEE provides more detailed anatomical and functional assessment of the tricuspid valve leaflets, coaptation gap, presence of vegetations, and interaction with pacemaker leads. It is crucial for intra-procedural guidance. ICE is increasingly used during transcatheter procedures for direct, real-time visualization of the valve, enabling precise device positioning and deployment while avoiding acoustic shadowing from the TEE probe [1, 11].

Cardiac CT provides excellent 3D anatomical detail of the tricuspid annulus, its precise dimensions and shape, and its spatial relationship to surrounding structures like the right coronary artery, conduction system, and great veins. It is essential for pre-procedural planning, accurate device sizing (especially for valve replacement), and assessing venous access routes [6].

CMR is considered to be the gold standard for accurate, non-invasive quantification of right ventricular volumes, ejection fraction, and TR severity (regurgitant volume and fraction). It provides detailed tissue characterization, which can be important in assessing RV myocardial fibrosis or other pathologies [6].

Right heart catheterization may be performed to directly measure pulmonary artery pressures, right heart pressures, and cardiac output, providing crucial hemodynamic data, especially if there is uncertainty from non-invasive imaging or to assess the reversibility of pulmonary hypertension.

Device Technologies and Techniques

The landscape of transcatheter tricuspid valve intervention is rapidly evolving, offering less invasive treatment options for patients with severe TR, particularly those deemed high-risk for conventional surgery. These technologies can broadly be categorized into repair strategies and replacement strategies.

Transcatheter Edge-to-Edge Repair

Transcatheter edge-to-edge repair aims to reduce tricuspid regurgitation by coapting the leaflets, similar to a surgical "Alfieri stitch." This technique creates a double-orifice valve, improving leaflet coaptation and reducing regurgitant flow. There are two devices available at the moment: The TriClip system and the PASCAL system.

The TriClip system is a transcatheter clip delivery system adapted from the MitraClip device used for mitral regurgitation. It involves grasping the free edges of the tricuspid leaflets (typically the anterior and septal leaflets) and clipping them together to reduce the regurgitant orifice area. Studies like the TRILUMINATE Pivotal trial have demonstrated its safety and effectiveness in reducing TR severity and improving patient symptoms and quality of life in patients with moderate or greater TR. The device is delivered via a transfemoral venous approach under echocardiographic and fluoroscopic guidance [3].

The PASCAL system is another transcatheter repair device that uses a similar edge-to-edge repair concept. It features independent leaflet grasping capabilities and a spacer that helps fill the coaptation gap, potentially offering advantages in complex anatomies or large coaptation gaps. Clinical data from studies like TriCLASP have shown promising results in reducing TR and improving quality of life [12, 13].

Both TriClip and PASCAL have shown similar safety profiles and procedural success rates, with TriClip demonstrating superior efficacy in reducing vena contracta width in some comparative analyses [8].

Annuloplasty Devices

These devices target the tricuspid annulus to reduce its dilation, which is a primary mechanism of functional TR. By cinching or remodeling the annulus, they aim to improve leaflet coaptation. There are two devices available at the moment: The Cardioband system and the Trialign system.

The Cardioband system is a direct annuloplasty device that consists of a Dacron band with multiple anchors that are implanted along the atrial side of the tricuspid annulus. Once anchored, the band can be cinched to reduce the annular circumference, effectively reshaping the annulus and improving leaflet coaptation. The procedure is performed via a transfemoral venous approach and requires careful pre-procedural CT imaging to assess annular dimensions and proximity to the right coronary artery. Early studies suggest its safety and efficacy in reducing TR and improving symptoms in high-risk patients [14].

The Trialign system performs a percutaneous suture annuloplasty, mimicking a surgical bicuspidization technique. It involves delivering pledgeted sutures transannularly from the ventricle to the atrium, typically in the posterior annulus, and then cinching them together to plicate the tissue and reduce annular size. Access is typically gained via the right internal jugular vein. Early data indicate it is safe and feasible, leading to TR reduction and quality-of-life improvements [15].

Caval Valve Implantation (CAVI)

CAVI is a heterotopic valve implantation strategy that does not directly target the tricuspid valve itself. Instead, it involves implanting self-expanding prosthetic valves in the inferior vena cava (IVC) and/or superior vena cava (SVC) at their junctions with the right atrium. The rationale behind CAVI is to prevent the backflow of blood into the systemic venous circulation, thereby alleviating congestive symptoms such as ascites, peripheral edema, and liver congestion, even if the tricuspid regurgitation at the native valve persists. TricValve is a device specifically designed for CAVI, often involving bicaval implantation (both IVC and SVC) [16].

CAVI is a relatively technically simpler procedure and may be an option for patients with severe TR who are deemed unsuitable for direct tricuspid valve intervention due to severe coaptation defects, complex anatomy, or the presence of pacemaker leads. It does not preclude future direct tricuspid valve interventions. The main limitation is the requirement for appropriate cava size, as current valve technology has sizing constraints. While CAVI improves symptoms and quality of life, its impact on overall survival in the long term still requires further investigation [16].

Orthotopic Tricuspid Valve Replacement (TTVR)

Orthotopic TTVR involves implanting a prosthetic valve directly within the native tricuspid annulus, replacing the dysfunctional tricuspid valve. This approach aims for complete elimination or significant reduction of TR.

The most commonly used device for TTVR is the Evoque system, a transcatheter tricuspid valve replacement therapy designed for patients with symptomatic severe TR who are high-risk for surgery. It is implanted orthotopically, meaning it replaces the native tricuspid valve. Clinical trials, such as the TRISCEND II trial, have shown that orthotopic TTVR with the EVOQUE valve can lead to dramatic improvements in TR severity, symptoms, and quality of life compared to medical therapy alone [17]. The procedure requires a large-caliber delivery system and careful pre-procedural CT planning to ensure anatomical suitability and avoid complications related to pacemaker leads or surrounding cardiac structures. While effective in reducing TR, TTVR with devices like EVOQUE may be associated with higher risks of bleeding and the need for new permanent pacemaker implantation compared to medical therapy.

Several other orthotopic TTVR devices are under investigation in clinical trials, including NaviGate, Intrepid, Trisol, and LUX-Valve, highlighting the rapid advancement in this field.

Procedural Considerations

The success of any transcatheter TV intervention hinges upon a well-orchestrated approach that integrates strategic access, precise imaging, and diligent patient management.

Access Routes

The choice of access route for tricuspid valve interventions is primarily dictated by the specific device being used, the patient's anatomy, and the operator's experience. The vast majority of TV interventions are performed via a transfemoral venous approach, leveraging the direct and relatively straightforward path to the right heart.

Transfemoral venous access is the workhorse access for most tricuspid valve interventions, including tricuspid valve repair (e.g., edge-to-edge repair devices like TriClip/PASCAL) and transcatheter tricuspid valve replacement systems (e.g., EVOQUE, Intrepid, tricuspid Tendyne). The right common femoral vein is typically preferred due to its direct course to the inferior vena cava and right atrium (RA). Large-bore sheaths are often required, ranging from 18F to 28F, depending on the device delivery system. Meticulous Seldinger technique is crucial to prevent complications such as vascular injury, hematoma, or retroperitoneal bleeding. Ultrasound guidance is highly recommended for venous access to visualize the vessel, confirm patency, and avoid inadvertent arterial puncture.

While less common as a primary access for TV interventions, the internal jugular vein can be used in specific circumstances, particularly if femoral access is challenging (e.g., severe peripheral vascular disease, thrombosed femoral veins) or for certain specialized devices. However, the more acute angle of approach to the tricuspid valve may make device manipulation more challenging.

In highly selected cases where transfemoral access is not feasible for large-bore devices, and transseptal puncture from the left atrium is not an option, direct transcaval access has been explored. This involves puncturing the IVC from an arterial access site (usually femoral artery) and then advancing the device through the IVC directly into the right heart. This is a complex technique reserved for experienced operators due to the increased risk of vascular complications [18].

Imaging Guidance

Comprehensive and real-time imaging is indispensable for all phases of tricuspid valve interventions, from initial assessment and device sizing to precise deployment and post-procedure evaluation. A multi-modality imaging approach, combining fluoroscopy, TEE, and ICE, provides the necessary spatial orientation and detailed anatomical visualization.

Fluoroscopy provides real-time X-ray visualization of guidewires, catheters, and device delivery systems. It is essential for navigating the venous anatomy, positioning the guidewire across the tricuspid valve, and confirming the gross position of the device. Biplane fluoroscopy or C-arm angulation is frequently used to obtain orthogonal views and minimize foreshortening, crucial for accurate device positioning, especially during leaflet grasping in repair procedures or frame expansion in replacement procedures. Angiography can be used to delineate the right heart chambers and assess the severity of tricuspid regurgitation before and after intervention.

TEE is the cornerstone of imaging guidance for most transcatheter tricuspid valve interventions. It offers high-resolution, real-time visualization of the tricuspid valve leaflets, annulus, chordae, and subvalvular apparatus. TEE is critical for guiding guidewire and catheter advancement across the valve, assessing leaflet grasping during edge-to-edge repair, confirming device position and orientation, and evaluating TR reduction immediately post-deployment. Identifying complications such as leaflet damage, chordal rupture, or paravalvular leak is another main use of TEE. Additionally, it can guide adjustments to device position for optimal TR reduction and leaflet coaptation. Multiple TEE views (e.g., mid-esophageal 4-chamber, RV inflow-outflow, deep esophageal views) are utilized to provide comprehensive anatomical assessment. 3D TEE is increasingly valuable for precise device placement and visualization of complex valve morphology [1].

ICE offers a valuable alternative or adjunct to TEE, particularly for operators who prefer to perform the procedure under conscious sedation without the need for general anesthesia. The ICE catheter is advanced into the right atrium or right ventricle, providing direct visualization of the tricuspid valve from within the cardiac chambers. Key advantages of ICE include: operator control, real-time visualization, reduced need for general anesthesia, and potential for reduced radiation exposure. While ICE can be highly effective, it typically provides a more limited field of view compared to TEE and may require greater operator experience to interpret the images effectively. Hybrid approaches combining ICE for certain steps and TEE for others are also employed [5, 11].

Anticoagulation and Post-procedure Care

Careful management of anticoagulation and comprehensive post-procedure care are crucial for preventing thrombotic and bleeding complications and ensuring long-term success. The specific anticoagulation regimen varies depending on the device used, the patient's underlying rhythm (e.g., atrial fibrillation), and the individual thrombotic and bleeding risk.

Intraprocedural anticoagulation with unfractionated heparin is typically administered to achieve an activated clotting time (ACT) between 250 and 350 s, minimizing the risk of device thrombosis or thrombus formation within the cardiac chambers.

Post-procedural antithrombotic regimen depends on patient characteristics and the type of device that was implanted. For patients undergoing a tricuspid valve repair (e.g., TriClip/PASCAL), a dual antiplatelet therapy (DAPT) regimen with aspirin and a P2Y12 inhibitor (e.g., clopidogrel) is recommended for 1–3 months, followed by lifelong aspirin. For patients with pre-existing indications for oral anticoagulation (e.g., atrial fibrillation with high CHA2DS2-VASc score), oral anticoagulation (OAC) with a direct oral anticoagulant (DOAC) or warfarin is continued, often in combination with aspirin for a short period. In case of transcatheter tricuspid valve replacement, given the larger metallic surface area of TTVR prostheses, there is a higher theoretical risk of thrombosis. Current recommendations often involve a period of OAC (DOACs or warfarin) for 3–6 months, possibly in combination with an antiplatelet agent, followed by lifelong OAC or antiplatelet therapy depending on the specific device and patient characteristics. Data on optimal anticoagulation for TTVR are still evolving, and clinical trial protocols provide specific guidance [2, 3].

A thorough assessment of bleeding risk (e.g., using HAS-BLED score) is essential before and after the procedure to tailor the anticoagulation strategy and minimize adverse events.

Post procedural care involves vascular access site management, with a meticulous hemostasis at the access site that is paramount, especially given the large-bore sheaths often used. Pressure dressings, closure devices, or surgical repair may be necessary. Patients require close monitoring for hematoma, pseudoaneurysm, or arteriovenous fistula formation. Continuous electrocardiographic monitoring is essential to detect arrhythmias, particularly new-onset atrial fibrillation or heart block, which can occur following manipulation within the right heart. A transthoracic echocardiogram is typically performed within 24–48 h post-procedure to assess residual TR, evaluate device function, and screen for potential complications such as pericardial effusion or new-onset valvular dysfunction. Further TTEs are recommended at regular intervals (e.g., 1 month, 6 months, 1 year) to monitor long-term device performance and TR severity. Careful management of fluid status is important, particularly in patients with pre-existing right heart failure, to optimize cardiac output and prevent volume overload. All medications, especially diuretics and heart failure medications, should be reviewed and adjusted as needed based on the patient's post-procedural status. Comprehensive patient education regarding warning signs of complications, medication adherence, and the importance of follow-up appointments is crucial for successful long-term outcomes. For many patients, particularly those with significant pre-existing symptoms, cardiac rehabilitation may be beneficial to improve functional capacity and quality of life [3, 6].

Clinical Outcomes and Evidence

The landscape of transcatheter tricuspid valve interventions has rapidly evolved, moving from early feasibility studies to pivotal randomized controlled trials, providing a growing body of evidence regarding their safety and efficacy.

Safety and Efficacy Data

Initial data from various devices demonstrate that transcatheter TV interventions are generally safe in high-risk patient populations, with acceptable rates of procedural complications.

Major adverse cardiovascular event rates, including procedural mortality, stroke, and major bleeding, have been reported to be relatively low. For tricuspid transcatheter edge-to-edge repair (T-TEER), procedural mortality is typically in the low single digits (around 1–3%), and major bleeding events, while present, are manageable. Transcatheter tricuspid valve replacement (TTVR) may carry a slightly higher risk of device-related complications, such as new permanent pacemaker implantation (due to proximity to the conduction system) or lead-related issues in patients with pre-existing cardiac implantable electronic devices (CIEDs). However, overall safety profiles are generally favorable, especially when compared to the high surgical risk of many of these patients [12, 13, 15].

The primary efficacy endpoint for both repair and replacement therapies is a significant reduction in tricuspid regurgitation severity. Both T-TEER and TTVR have demonstrated significant and sustained reduction in TR severity. T-TEER typically achieves a reduction to moderate or less TR in a high proportion of patients (often >80–90%), while TTVR often results in minimal or no residual TR, given it's a complete valve replacement. A consistent and robust finding across multiple studies is a significant improvement in symptoms and quality of life (QoL) as measured by validated tools like the Kansas City Cardiomyopathy Questionnaire (KCCQ) and an improvement in New York Heart Association (NYHA) functional class. Patients report substantial relief from right-sided heart failure symptoms such as peripheral edema, ascites, and dyspnea [13, 14, 19].

Evidence is emerging that transcatheter TV interventions can reduce the rate of heart failure hospitalizations. This is a critical outcome, reflecting an improvement in the patient's overall clinical stability and a reduction in healthcare burden. While significant improvements in QoL and reduction in TR have been consistently observed, a definitive mortality benefit for transcatheter TV interventions over optimal medical therapy (OMT) alone is still being rigorously evaluated and has not been conclusively demonstrated across all trials, particularly for repair therapies. However, procedural success has been associated with improved 1-year survival. For TTVR, early data suggest no difference in mortality compared to OMT [14–17].

Trials and Registries (TRILUMINATE and TRISCEND II)

The TRILUMINATE Pivotal trial is a landmark randomized controlled trial investigating the safety and efficacy of tricuspid transcatheter edge-to-edge repair using the TriClip device in patients with severe, symptomatic TR. The trial randomized patients with severe, symptomatic TR to either T-TEER plus medical therapy or medical therapy alone. At one year, TRILUMINATE Pivotal demonstrated that T-TEER was safe and led to sustained improvements in quality of life and functional status compared to medical therapy alone. While there was no significant difference in all-cause mortality, patients in the T-TEER group experienced significant improvements in KCCQ scores and a reduction in heart failure symptoms. Longer-term data from TRILUMINATE Pivotal continue to reinforce these findings. At two years, T-TEER was associated with a significantly lower annualized rate of recurrent heart failure hospitalizations compared to the control group. The benefits in TR reduction and improved health status persisted. Rates of all-cause mortality and tricuspid valve surgery were similar between groups, but freedom from all-cause mortality, tricuspid valve surgery, and tricuspid valve intervention was significantly higher with T-TEER, largely driven by more crossover to device treatment in the control arm. The majority of patients in the device group maintained moderate or less TR, and the strong safety profile was consistent with no cases of device embolization, thrombosis, or new conduction disturbances requiring permanent pacing [3].

Another significant trial is TRISCEND II, evaluating orthotopic TTVR using the Edwards EVOQUE valve. This trial also randomized patients with severe symptomatic TR to TTVR plus medical therapy versus medical therapy alone. The results indicated that TTVR with Evoque was superior to medical therapy alone in improving cardiovascular outcomes, primarily driven by improvements in symptoms and quality of life, with dramatic reductions in TR (less than 5% had residual moderate or greater TR at 1 year). Similar to TRILUMINATE, no significant difference in mortality or heart failure hospitalization rates was observed, but TTVR was associated with higher rates of severe bleeding and new permanent pacemaker implantation [19].

Numerous national and international registries (e.g., TriValve, German TR Registry) have collected real-world data on a broader range of patients and devices. These registries complement the trial data by providing insights into device performance in diverse clinical settings, identifying trends, and generating hypotheses for future research.

Limitations and Gaps

Despite the promising advancements, several limitations and gaps in the current evidence base need to be addressed. Firstly, while 1- and 2-year data are becoming available, robust long-term outcomes (beyond 2–3 years) are still limited for most transcatheter TV devices. Durability of repair and replacement devices, especially in the challenging right heart environment, remains a key question. As noted, a consistent mortality benefit over OMT has not been definitively established across all transcatheter TV interventions. This might be due to the complex nature of TR, the advanced disease state of enrolled patients, or the relatively short follow-up periods of some trials.

Optimal patient selection criteria are still evolving. Identifying which patients will derive the greatest benefit from intervention versus medical management alone, or who might benefit more from repair versus replacement, is crucial. Factors like right ventricular (RV) function, pulmonary hypertension, and the etiology of TR (atrial vs. ventricular secondary TR) significantly influence outcomes.

Moreover, there is a lack of head-to-head comparative trials between different repair devices (e.g., TriClip vs. PASCAL) or between repair and replacement strategies. Such trials would provide valuable insights for tailoring therapy. While some studies show signals of favorable RV reverse remodeling, the extent and clinical significance of these changes, and their impact on long-term outcomes, require further investigation. The optimal integration of transcatheter interventions with guideline-directed medical therapy for heart failure and TR needs further refinement. Many patients are still undertreated with medical therapy before considering intervention.

Further research is needed in specific subgroups, such as patients with concomitant severe left-sided heart disease, those with isolated primary TR, or patients with previous cardiac surgery or CIEDs, although some data are emerging for the latter.

Future Directions

The field of transcatheter tricuspid valve interventions is rapidly evolving, with significant advancements expected in the coming years.

Next Gen Devices

The pipeline for novel TV devices is robust, addressing current limitations and expanding treatment options. While edge-to-edge repair is established, next-generation repair devices may offer greater versatility, easier navigation, improved leaflet grasping capabilities, or address different anatomical challenges (e.g., larger coaptation gaps, more severe tethering). Devices focusing on direct or indirect annuloplasty (e.g., tricuspid annuloplasty rings delivered percutaneously) are also under investigation, aiming to replicate surgical principles in a less invasive manner [6].

TTVR is also gaining traction, and next-generation valves are being designed for easier delivery, improved conformability to the native annulus, enhanced anchoring mechanisms, and reduced profiles to minimize vascular complications. Specific designs might also better accommodate pre-existing CIED leads.

Devices implanted in the vena cava (caval valve implantation, CAVI) offer a simpler approach for selected patients, particularly those with severe right ventricular dysfunction who may not tolerate orthotopic valve replacement. While they do not directly address the TV, they reduce venous congestion. Future devices may improve on this concept [18].

Also, the possibility of combining different transcatheter techniques (e.g., annuloplasty with edge-to-edge repair) to achieve more comprehensive TR reduction is an area of active development.

Patient Selection Improvements

Refining patient selection is crucial to ensure that the right therapy is delivered to the right patient at the optimal time. More sophisticated use of multimodality imaging (3D TEE, cardiac CT, CMR) will enable a more precise characterization of TV anatomy, TR mechanism, and RV function. This will allow for better prediction of procedural success and long-term outcomes, aiding in individualized device selection. Distinguishing between atrial and ventricular functional TR, for instance, may guide specific interventional strategies.

Moreover, development and validation of novel biomarkers (e.g., related to right heart function, fibrosis, or inflammation) may help identify patients who will benefit most from early intervention and those at highest risk for adverse outcomes. Improved risk stratification tools, potentially integrating clinical, imaging, and biomarker data, will be essential.

There is a growing consensus that intervening earlier in the disease process, before irreversible RV dysfunction or severe end-organ damage occurs, might lead to better long-term outcomes. Future research will focus on identifying optimal timing for intervention, moving beyond current "last resort" scenarios.

Integration with Heart Team Approach

The multidisciplinary heart team approach, already central to transcatheter aortic and mitral valve interventions, is equally, if not more, critical for TV therapies. The complexity of TR pathophysiology and the varying anatomical and clinical presentations necessitate a comprehensive evaluation by a dedicated heart team. This team typically includes interventional cardiologists, cardiac surgeons, imaging specialists (echocardiographers, cardiac CT/MRI experts), heart failure specialists, and anesthesiologists. Their collective expertise ensures a holistic assessment of the patient's condition, weighing the risks and benefits of all available therapeutic options (medical, surgical, transcatheter). Development of standardized institutional protocols for patient evaluation, procedural planning, and post-procedure care will enhance consistency and improve outcomes. As TV interventions become more widespread, specialized training programs and experience-sharing initiatives will be vital to ensure high-quality care and safe adoption of these complex procedures across centers.

The heart team approach fosters a patient-centered philosophy, considering not only the TR itself but also the patient's overall health, comorbidities, frailty, and quality of life goals. This collaborative model is essential for navigating the nuanced decision-making involved in this evolving field.

In summary, transcatheter tricuspid valve interventions have demonstrated significant clinical benefits, primarily in improving symptoms and quality of life for high-risk patients with severe TR. While ongoing research continues to build the evidence base, particularly regarding long-term outcomes and mortality, the future promises even more sophisticated devices, refined patient selection strategies, and an increasingly integrated heart team approach to deliver optimal care for this previously underserved patient population.

Transcatheter Pulmonary Valve Interventions

Anatomy and Pathophysiology

Pulmonary Valve and Right Ventricular Outflow Tract (RVOT)

The pulmonary valve (PV) and the right ventricular outflow tract (RVOT) form a critical anatomical and functional unit responsible for directing deoxygenated blood from the right ventricle into the pulmonary artery, ensuring efficient pulmonary circulation. Understanding their intricate anatomy and the pathophysiological consequences of their dysfunction, particularly in the context of congenital heart disease (CHD), is paramount for successful transcatheter interventions.

The pulmonary valve is a semilunar valve, typically composed of three delicate, crescent-shaped cusps (anterior, right, and left) that meet at their free edges during diastole to prevent the backflow of blood into the right ventricle. Unlike the aortic valve, the pulmonary valve is not directly supported by a fibrous annulus. Instead, its leaflets are attached to the muscular wall of the RVOT and the fibrous tissue that forms the proximal pulmonary artery. This lack of a well-defined fibrous annulus, coupled with the variability in RVOT morphology, presents unique challenges for valve replacement.

The RVOT itself is a muscular, tunnel-shaped structure extending from the main body of the right ventricle to the pulmonary valve. Its muscular nature is a key differentiating factor from the more fibrous left ventricular outflow tract. The infundibular septum, a muscular structure, separates the RVOT from the main body of the right ventricle. The geometry of the RVOT is highly variable and can be significantly altered by various congenital heart defects or prior surgical interventions.

There are some key anatomical considerations for transcatheter pulmonary valve interventions. While not a true fibrous annulus, the pulmonary "annulus" refers to the narrowest portion of the RVOT at the level of the valve leaflets. Its size and shape are crucial for device sizing and anchoring. The RVOT Morphology is important, since it can be short, long, conical, or cylindrical. It may be entirely muscular or feature significant patches of fibrous tissue or surgical patches from previous repairs.

Another important point is the proximity to coronary arteries, since the right and left main pulmonary arteries can lie in close proximity to the RVOT and the intended landing zone for a transcatheter valve. Pre-procedural imaging must meticulously map the coronary artery origins and their relationship to the RVOT to prevent coronary compression during device deployment.

While less common than with aortic or tricuspid valve interventions, there is a theoretical risk to the right bundle branch, particularly in patients with pre-existing conduction abnormalities or extensive RVOT scarring. In addition, the distance from the valve plane to the bifurcation is important, as a valve that extends too far distally could obstruct the branch pulmonary arteries [20].

Congenital Heart Disease (Tetralogy of Fallot) Implications

The vast majority of patients requiring transcatheter pulmonary valve interventions are young adults or adolescents with congenital heart disease (CHD). Among these, tetralogy of Fallot (ToF) is the most common underlying condition. ToF is a complex congenital heart defect characterized by four primary anomalies: ventricular septal defect (VSD), pulmonary stenosis (PS), overriding aorta, and right ventricular hypertrophy (RVH).

Surgical repair of ToF, typically performed in infancy or early childhood, involves closing the VSD and relieving the RVOT obstruction. This relief of obstruction often requires transannular patching (a patch extending across the pulmonary valve annulus into the RVOT) or extensive resection of the RVOT muscle. While life-saving, these surgical interventions frequently lead to chronic severe pulmonary regurgitation as a long-term sequela.

The pathophysiology of chronic PR in repaired ToF patients is critical. The regurgitant blood flow back into the RV during diastole leads to progressive right ventricular volume overload. Over time, this chronic volume overload causes progressive RV dilation and can eventually lead to RV systolic and diastolic dysfunction. The RV, which is not designed to handle chronic volume overload, dilates and remodels, becoming less efficient. RV dilation and scarring from previous surgery create substrates for ventricular arrhythmias, including sustained ventricular tachycardia, which is a major cause of sudden cardiac death in this population. Patients often experience progressive exercise intolerance, fatigue, dyspnea, and reduced quality of life due to RV dysfunction and decreased forward flow. RV dilation can also lead to functional tricuspid regurgitation, further exacerbating right-sided heart failure symptoms. Significant RV volume overload can cause the interventricular septum to flatten or even bulge into the left ventricle, impacting left ventricular filling and function.

The rationale for transcatheter pulmonary valve intervention (TPVI) in this population is to alleviate chronic PR, prevent or reverse RV remodeling, improve RV function, reduce arrhythmia burden, and enhance exercise capacity. The challenge lies in placing a valve within a highly variable and often severely dilated or previously surgically altered RVOT, making precise device sizing and anchoring paramount. Other congenital heart defects that may require TPVI include truncus arteriosus repair, d-transposition of the great arteries with VSD and PS (Rastelli repair), and pulmonary atresia with intact ventricular septum. However, repaired ToF remains the dominant indication for TPVI worldwide [21].

Understanding the unique anatomical variations and the long-term pathophysiological consequences of surgical repair in CHD patients is foundational for successful patient selection, procedural planning, and the growing application of transcatheter pulmonary valve replacement (TPVR).

Indications and Patient Selection

The decision to proceed with transcatheter pulmonary valve intervention is complex, balancing the burden of pulmonary valve dysfunction against the risks and benefits of the procedure. Patient selection is guided by the type and severity of valve dysfunction, its impact on right ventricular size and function, and the patient's symptoms and exercise capacity.

Indications for Intervention (Stenosis, Regurgitation)

The primary indications for TPVI involve severe pulmonary valve dysfunction, either regurgitation or stenosis, leading to adverse clinical consequences.

Chronic severe PR is by far the most common indication for TPVI, particularly in patients with previously repaired congenital heart disease (CHD), such as tetralogy of Fallot (ToF). The goals of intervening in PR are to alleviate right ventricular volume overload and its sequelae. Indications for intervention in PR generally include: severe pulmonary regurgitation, progressive RV dilation or dysfunction (indexed RVEDV >160 mL/m^2 by CMR), RV systolic dysfunction (RVEF <45–50%), presence of symptoms, arrhythmias, or secondary tricuspid regurgitation [2, 9, 22].

While less common as a sole indication for TPVI, significant pulmonary stenosis can also warrant intervention. This might occur in native PS that was not adequately treated with balloon valvuloplasty, or more commonly, recurrent or residual stenosis within a previously placed RVOT conduit or surgical patch (e.g., in patients with Ross procedure or Rastelli repair). Indications for intervention in PS typically include: significant RVOT obstruction, symptoms (dyspnea, fatigue, or chest pain attributable to RVOT obstruction), progressive RV hypertrophy or dysfunction [22, 23].

It is important to note that many patients presenting for TPVI often have a mixed lesion, with both significant PR and a degree of RVOT obstruction (stenosis) due to the underlying anatomy or previous repairs. In such cases, the overall hemodynamic impact and clinical picture guide the decision.

Timing of Reintervention in Congenital Heart Disease

The optimal timing of reintervention in CHD, particularly for chronic PR after ToF repair, is a subject of ongoing debate and research. The goal is to intervene before irreversible RV damage occurs, but not so early that it necessitates multiple reinterventions over a patient's lifetime. The "sweet spot" often lies in balancing these factors.

Current guidelines and expert consensus emphasize some important considerations for timing. The primary driver for intervention is to prevent long-term, irreversible RV dysfunction and fibrosis. While there is no universally agreed-upon threshold, significant and progressive RV dilation (e.g., indexed RVEDV >160 mL/m^2) and declining RV ejection fraction are strong indicators for intervention. Intervention before RV systolic dysfunction becomes severe (e.g., RVEF <40%) is generally preferred, as post-procedural RV recovery is more likely when intervention occurs before advanced dysfunction. Intervention is generally recommended for symptomatic patients (NYHA class II or higher) with severe PR or PS, as this directly affects their quality of life [21–24].

For asymptomatic patients, objective markers of RV dysfunction or risk for adverse events often guide the decision. These include severe and progressive RV dilation on serial imaging, significant ventricular arrhythmias (NSVT/VT) or other complex arrhythmias, progressive TR, and exercise intolerance that is not fully explained by other factors.

In younger patients, especially those still growing, the timing is more nuanced. TPVI is generally deferred until adolescence or early adulthood (typically >10–12 years old) to allow for sufficient growth, which may reduce the need for multiple reinterventions due to device outgrowing the patient's anatomy. However, if significant symptoms or severe RV dysfunction develop earlier, intervention may be necessary [21, 24].

Patients with previous RVOT conduits (e.g., Rastelli repair, Ross procedure) often require reintervention earlier as conduits are prone to degeneration, calcification, and stenosis/regurgitation over time. The lifespan of a surgical conduit is finite, typically 10–15 years, necessitating reintervention. Patients with transannular patches, while developing PR, may have a more pliable RVOT that can accommodate a transcatheter valve later in life.

While less common, in cases where chronic PR leads to elevated pulmonary artery pressures or RV pressure overload, intervention may be considered to prevent progression to pulmonary hypertension.

In essence, the timing of reintervention for pulmonary valve dysfunction in CHD is a personalized decision made by a multidisciplinary heart team. This team evaluates the patient's overall clinical status, symptom burden, the severity and progression of RV dysfunction and dilation, the specific anatomy of the RVOT, and the potential for device longevity versus the risks of delaying intervention and allowing irreversible RV damage to occur. Serial non-invasive imaging (CMR being particularly valuable) and exercise testing play critical roles in monitoring disease progression and guiding the optimal timing of TPVI [21, 22, 25].

Device Technologies and Techniques

The landscape of transcatheter pulmonary valve intervention has been shaped by the development of specialized devices designed to overcome the unique anatomical challenges of the right ventricular outflow tract (RVOT). These devices broadly fall into two categories: balloon-expandable and self-expandable valves, each with distinct features and optimal applications. Additionally, the concept of valve-in-valve and valve-in-ring procedures has expanded the utility of these technologies.

Balloon-Expandable Valves (Melody, Sapien XT)

Balloon-expandable transcatheter pulmonary valves are characterized by their crimped design onto a balloon, which is then inflated to deploy the valve within the RVOT or a pre-stented conduit. Their deployment offers precise control over valve expansion and positioning. The most commonly used balloon-expandable valves are the Melody and the Sapien XT valves.

The Melody valve was the first transcatheter pulmonary valve to receive CE Mark and FDA approval for clinical use. It consists of a bovine jugular vein valve hand-sutured into a platinum-iridium stent. The stent has an open-cell design that allows for crimping onto a delivery balloon. Delivered via a transfemoral venous approach, the Melody valve is crimped onto a customized balloon catheter. After positioning within the RVOT or conduit, the balloon is inflated, expanding the stent and anchoring the valve. Primarily indicated for use in patients with dysfunctional RVOT conduits (stenotic, regurgitant, or mixed lesions) placed during prior surgical repairs of congenital heart disease (e.g., ToF, truncus arteriosus). The conduit provides a stable platform for valve anchoring. Long-standing clinical experience, established efficacy in conduit populations, and high success rates in treating conduit dysfunction. The balloon-expandable nature allows for precise sizing and deployment. Its open-cell design potentially allows for re-dilation if future growth or restenosis occurs. The limitation of this valve is that it requires a pre-existing surgical conduit or the creation of a stent "landing zone" to ensure stable anchoring. Its profile can be relatively large, sometimes requiring large-bore access. The risk of conduit rupture during balloon dilation is a recognized complication, necessitating careful pre-procedural sizing and preparation [26–28].

Originally designed and approved for aortic valve replacement, the Sapien valves (now commonly Sapien 3 or Ultra) are bovine pericardial valves mounted within a cobalt-chromium frame. Similar to Melody, these valves are balloon-expandable and delivered via a transfemoral venous approach. They are crimped onto a balloon catheter and expanded to deploy the valve. While not specifically designed for the pulmonary position, Sapien valves have been successfully used off-label for TPVR, particularly in challenging anatomies (e.g., heavily calcified conduits, larger RVOTs) or as a bailout strategy. They are increasingly used in valve-in-valve procedures within failing bioprosthetic pulmonary valves or within previously placed Melody valves. Broader range of sizes available (compared to earlier Melody iterations), high radial strength, and a proven track record in aortic applications. Their lower profile delivery systems compared to early Melody systems can be advantageous. The main limitations are that it is not explicitly approved for the pulmonary position and data are derived from off-label use and registries. In addition, it may require higher inflation pressures for deployment in calcified conduits. The frame design might be less forgiving in extremely irregular or very large RVOTs without a stable landing zone [28, 29].

Self-Expandable Valves (Harmony TPV)

Self-expandable transcatheter pulmonary valve (Harmony) utilizes a nitinol frame that expands upon release from a delivery sheath, conforming to the native RVOT or conduit.

The Harmony TPV (formerly called the Harmony Transcatheter Pulmonary Valve System) is specifically designed for implantation in the native RVOT in patients with severe pulmonary regurgitation due to repaired Tetralogy of Fallot or other conditions without a prior surgical conduit. It consists of a porcine pericardial tissue valve integrated into a nitinol frame with a unique "hourglass" shape. The frame has varying radial strength along its length, with greater force at the inflow and outflow aspects to anchor the valve, and a more compliant mid-section to conform to the RVOT [28].

Delivered via a transfemoral venous approach, the Harmony TPV is compressed within a delivery catheter. Upon careful controlled deployment, the nitinol frame self-expands to conform to the RVOT morphology, anchoring the valve.

The Harmony TPV is a groundbreaking innovation, specifically designed for use in the native, non-conduit RVOT in patients with severe PR and significant RV dilation. This addresses a significant unmet need for patients who do not have a surgical conduit suitable for Melody or Sapien valve implantation.

The advantages are the avoidance of the need for a prior surgical conduit since it conforms to the variable native RVOT anatomy. It offers a less invasive option for patients with chronic PR without a defined conduit and it demonstrated significant reduction in PR and RV volume.

The main limitation is that it requires careful patient selection based on RVOT dimensions and morphology to ensure adequate sealing and anchoring, since the hourglass shape might not be suitable for all RVOT anatomies. Another important factor is the risk of left pulmonary artery compression due to the device's bulk, necessitating meticulous pre-procedural CT imaging and careful deployment. Long-term durability data are still accumulating compared to the more established Melody valve [28].

Valve-in-Valve and Valve-in-Ring Procedures

The concept of "valve-in-valve" and "valve-in-ring" (VIR) procedures has significantly expanded the applicability of transcatheter pulmonary valves, offering less invasive options for re-reintervention.

The valve-in-valve procedure involves implanting a transcatheter pulmonary valve (most commonly a Melody or Sapien valve) within a previously implanted, degenerated surgical bioprosthetic valve (e.g., a pulmonary homograft or xenograft) in the RVOT. It's also increasingly used to implant a new transcatheter valve (e.g.,

Sapien) within a failing previously implanted transcatheter valve (e.g., a Melody valve). The degenerated surgical or transcatheter valve provides a stable landing zone for the new transcatheter valve, effectively replacing the failing leaflet function. The main advantages are that it avoids repeat open-heart surgery, which carries increasing risk with each successive operation and provides a less invasive and often safer option for re-reintervention. Careful sizing is critical to avoid paravalvular leak or risk of coronary compression. Pre-stenting of the degenerated valve may be necessary to ensure a uniform cylindrical shape for optimal transcatheter valve seating.

The valve-in-ring procedure involves implanting a transcatheter pulmonary valve within a previously implanted surgical annuloplasty ring that was placed to address tricuspid regurgitation (or less commonly, a non-valved conduit ring). While less common in the primary pulmonary position, this concept extends to other valves (e.g., tricuspid valve). In the pulmonary context, it might involve placing a valve into a non-valved conduit or a surgically placed ring. The rigid annuloplasty ring provides a stable anchor for the transcatheter valve, similar to the VIV principle. It is less frequently used than VIV for pulmonary position, but it is conceptually similar to VIV for creating a landing zone in a less defined anatomical space.

The continuous innovation in device design and refinement of techniques are broadening the indications for TPVI, allowing treatment of more complex anatomies and reducing the need for repeated open-heart surgeries in this vulnerable patient population with congenital heart disease [28].

Procedural Considerations

Transcatheter pulmonary valve intervention requires meticulous planning and execution, leveraging advanced imaging and careful risk mitigation strategies. The unique anatomy of the right ventricular outflow tract (RVOT) and the typically younger patient population necessitate specialized procedural considerations.

Access (Femoral, Jugular, Hybrid Approaches)

The specific device, the patient's anatomy, and the operator's preference primarily determine the choice of vascular access for TPVI.

The most common and preferred access route for the vast majority of TPVI procedures is the transfemoral venous access. The right common femoral vein provides a relatively straight and direct path through the inferior vena cava into the right atrium, right ventricle, and subsequently the pulmonary artery. It is generally safe, familiar to interventionalists, and allows for the use of large-bore sheaths (typically 18–24 Fr, depending on the valve system). Meticulous technique is essential to prevent vascular complications such as hematoma, pseudoaneurysm, or venous thrombosis. Ultrasound guidance for venous puncture is highly recommended to visualize the vessel and avoid inadvertent arterial puncture, especially in younger patients with smaller vessels. In rare cases, severe peripheral venous disease, tortuosity of the IVC, or previous IVC filters may make femoral access challenging or impossible.

Access via the internal jugular vein (typically the right internal jugular vein) can be considered in specific situations. It may be an alternative if femoral access is contraindicated or technically difficult. It can offer a more superior approach, potentially advantageous for certain device delivery systems or complex anatomies. The more acute angulation required to navigate from the superior vena cava into the RVOT can make device delivery and manipulation more challenging. Risks include carotid artery puncture, pneumothorax, and injury to surrounding structures. It is generally reserved for situations where femoral access is not feasible.

In highly complex cases, a hybrid approach combining surgical and percutaneous techniques may be employed. For extremely challenging venous anatomy or in cases where a very large bore sheath is required that cannot be percutaneously inserted, a surgical cutdown to expose the femoral or jugular vein can provide direct, controlled access. In extremely rare and complex scenarios, a direct surgical approach to the RV may be necessary to facilitate valve delivery. This involves a mini-thoracotomy and direct puncture of the RV, offering a straight and controlled path to the pulmonary valve. This approach is reserved for highly specialized centers and specific anatomical challenges where conventional venous access is impossible or unsafe. The advantages of the hybrid approach are that it allows for precise device delivery in otherwise untreatable cases, provides direct visualization for complex maneuvers, and enables immediate surgical repair of any complications. The main limitations are the increased invasiveness compared to purely percutaneous approaches, with associated surgical risks [26].

Imaging Modalities

Comprehensive, real-time imaging is the cornerstone of successful TPVI, guiding every step from pre-procedural planning to post-deployment assessment. A multimodality approach is typically employed.

The fluoroscopy provides real-time X-ray visualization of guidewires, catheters, and the valve delivery system. It is essential for navigating the venous anatomy, crossing the RVOT obstruction or dysfunctional valve, positioning the guidewire in the branch pulmonary arteries, and guiding the overall positioning and deployment of the transcatheter valve. Biplane fluoroscopy or C-arm angulation is crucial to obtain orthogonal views, minimize foreshortening, and accurately assess device position relative to anatomical landmarks. Angiography (contrast injection) in the RVOT and pulmonary artery is performed before and after valve deployment to assess anatomy, measure gradients, and evaluate residual PR or PS. Minimizing radiation exposure, especially in younger patients who may undergo multiple procedures over their lifetime, is paramount. Optimization of fluoroscopy settings and judicious use of angiography are essential.

Echocardiography provides high-resolution, real-time visualization of cardiac structures, complementing fluoroscopy by offering soft tissue detail and hemodynamic information.

Performed under general anesthesia, TEE offers excellent visualization of the pulmonary valve, RVOT, and main pulmonary artery. Pre-procedural assessment of RV size and function, TR severity, and detailed PV/RVOT anatomy.

Intra-procedurally, TEE guides wire crossing, assesses balloon dilation effects, confirms valve positioning, assesses immediate device function (residual PR/PS), and identifies potential complications (e.g., pericardial effusion, device embolization) [4].

Gaining increasing popularity, ICE involves advancing a small ultrasound catheter into the right heart chambers. It provides real-time visualization comparable to TEE, but the operator has direct control over the imaging plane. It allows procedures to be performed under conscious sedation, avoiding general anesthesia. ICE can be particularly useful for guiding wire advancement, assessing leaflet morphology, and evaluating device placement in the RVOT. Its advantage is that it eliminates the need for general anesthesia (reducing procedural risk and recovery time), and provides a unique "from within" perspective. An important limitation is the limited field of view compared to TEE, requiring additional catheter manipulation, with a steeper learning curve for interpretation for some operators [5].

Cardiac CT and CMR are essential for comprehensive pre-procedural planning. CCT provides detailed anatomical information, particularly useful for precisely measuring RVOT dimensions (maximum and minimum diameters), length, calcification, and critical relationships to surrounding structures, especially the coronary arteries. CMR is the gold standard for quantifying RV volumes (RVEDV, RVESV), ejection fraction (RVEF), and pulmonary regurgitation fraction (PRF), crucial for determining the timing of intervention and post-procedural follow-up. Both CCT and CMR data can be used to create 3D anatomical reconstructions, allowing for virtual device implantation and procedural simulation, aiding in device sizing and strategy planning [30].

Management of Coronary Compression Risk

One of the most critical and potentially catastrophic complications of TPVI, particularly when dealing with an unconstrained native RVOT or a rigid conduit, is coronary artery compression. The RVOT and pulmonary artery lie in close anatomical proximity to the left main coronary artery (LMCA) and its branches, as well as the right coronary artery (RCA). Expansion of a transcatheter valve within this space can compress these vessels, leading to myocardial ischemia, infarction, and even death. Meticulous pre-procedural planning is essential to mitigate this risk.

CCT angiography is indispensable. A dedicated CCT acquisition, synchronized with the cardiac cycle, allows for detailed visualization of the coronary arteries, their origins, and their course relative to the RVOT and pulmonary artery. Measurements are taken from the intended valve landing zone to the coronary arteries in various planes.

During the procedure, a balloon dilation test is often performed. This involves placing a large, undeployed balloon (the size of the intended transcatheter valve) in the anticipated landing zone within the RVOT and inflating it while performing a simultaneous coronary artery injection (aortography or selective coronary angiography). If the coronary artery remains widely patent during balloon inflation, the risk of compression is considered low. If any degree of coronary narrowing or compression is observed, it indicates a high risk, and the specific transcatheter valve may be deemed unsuitable for that patient. This is a critical safety step and may lead to a decision to abort the transcatheter procedure in favor of surgical intervention or a different transcatheter strategy.

In some high-risk cases where the balloon inflation test shows borderline compression, a bare-metal stent may be intentionally deployed in the RVOT *prior* to valve implantation to create a more cylindrical and stable landing zone, potentially pushing away structures that could compress the coronary arteries.

While coronary compression is the primary concern, pre-procedural planning also considers the proximity of the intended valve to the tricuspid valve (to avoid leaflet impingement) and the main pulmonary artery bifurcation (to avoid branch pulmonary artery obstruction).

The management of coronary compression risk highlights the complexity and precision required for TPVI. It underscores the importance of a multidisciplinary heart team approach, where interventional cardiologists, cardiac surgeons, advanced imaging specialists, and anesthesiologists collaborate closely to ensure optimal patient selection and procedural safety [31].

Clinical Outcomes and Evidence

The evidence base for transcatheter pulmonary valve intervention has grown substantially since the first Melody valve implantation in 2000. Data from large registries and multicenter studies have established TPVI as a safe and effective treatment option for selected patients with dysfunctional right ventricular outflow tract (RVOT) and pulmonary valve pathology, particularly in the context of congenital heart disease (CHD).

Short- and Long-Term Data

Clinical outcomes for TPVI are predominantly characterized by significant improvements in hemodynamics, right ventricular function, symptoms, and exercise capacity.

Regarding the short-term outcomes, TPVI generally achieves very high technical and procedural success rates, often exceeding 95%. This means successful delivery and deployment of the transcatheter pulmonary valve (TPV) with restoration of adequate RVOT hemodynamics (reduction in pulmonary regurgitation or alleviation of pulmonary stenosis) without major procedural complications. Post-procedure, there is an immediate and dramatic reduction in PR, often to mild or trace levels, and/or a significant decrease in RVOT gradient in stenotic lesions. Within months of TPVI, studies consistently demonstrate a significant reduction in RV end-diastolic volume and RV end-systolic volume, indicating favorable RV reverse remodeling. RV ejection fraction often improves or stabilizes, although the degree of improvement can vary depending on the pre-procedural RV dysfunction. Patients typically experience rapid improvement in symptoms such as dyspnea, fatigue, and exercise intolerance, leading to an enhanced quality of life as measured by validated questionnaires (e.g., Kansas City Cardiomyopathy Questionnaire) and improved functional class (NYHA class) [32].

The reduction in PR and PS is generally sustained over several years. Registry data for the Melody valve, with the longest follow-up, show excellent freedom from reintervention and sustained valve function out to 5–10 years and beyond in a significant proportion of patients. Favorable RV reverse remodeling, initiated acutely, tends to persist or even progress over several years, supporting the notion that earlier intervention can prevent irreversible RV damage. While not always a primary indication, TPVI has been associated with a reduction in the incidence of ventricular arrhythmias, likely due to the decrease in RV volume overload and stress on the myocardial substrate. Long-term survival rates following TPVI are generally excellent, often mirroring those of age-matched healthy populations in the absence of other severe comorbidities. While TPVI is not typically performed to improve overall survival in the immediate term, it aims to prevent the long-term sequelae of chronic RV dysfunction that can ultimately lead to heart failure and premature death. While durable, transcatheter valves are not lifelong solutions. The most common reasons for re-intervention are recurrent PR or PS due to valve degeneration, fracture of the valve stent, or patient growth leading to prosthetic valve stenosis. The expected lifespan of transcatheter pulmonary valves varies, but studies suggest a re-intervention-free survival often around 80–90% at 5 years and 60–70% at 10 years, depending on the device and patient characteristics. The ability to perform a "valve-in-valve" procedure within a failing TPV further extends the patient's surgical freedom [27, 33].

Complications (Endocarditis, Stent Fracture)

While TPVI is generally safe, specific complications associated with the procedure and the implanted devices warrant careful consideration and ongoing monitoring.

TPV endocarditis is a serious, albeit relatively infrequent, complication. Incidence rates vary, but are reported in approximately 2–5% of patients over several years of follow-up, potentially higher than for surgical bioprosthetic valves. Factors associated with increased risk include prior history of endocarditis, infective endocarditis within the first year post-implantation, and the presence of residual PV stenosis or regurgitation. Management typically involves prolonged antibiotic therapy and, in some cases, surgical removal of the infected valve or re-implantation of a new TPV. Due to the difficulty of complete debridement, recurrence is a concern. Lifelong antibiotic prophylaxis for infective endocarditis is recommended for all patients with prosthetic valves, including TPVs [34].

Stent fracture, primarily observed with the Melody valve, can occur in the absence of a stable, rigid landing zone (i.e., when implanted directly into a non-stented RVOT or a poorly supported conduit). Repeated mechanical stress from cardiac motion and blood flow can lead to fatigue fracture of the metal stent frame. Stent fracture can lead to recurrent PS or PR, requiring re-intervention. However, many fractures are asymptomatic and hemodynamically insignificant. Pre-stenting of the RVOT or conduit with a bare-metal stent prior to Melody valve implantation has significantly reduced the incidence of stent fracture by creating a more robust and stable landing zone [35].

As discussed in section "Management of coronary compression risk", coronary compression is a rare but life-threatening complication, mitigated by meticulous pre-procedural imaging and balloon dilation tests.

Access site complications such as hematoma, pseudoaneurysm, or venous thrombosis can occur, though typically managed successfully.

While less common than with aortic or tricuspid valve interventions, new-onset right bundle branch block or complete heart block requiring pacemaker implantation can occur, particularly in patients with pre-existing conduction abnormalities or extensive RVOT scarring.

Device embolization or migration is very rare, but can occur if the valve is improperly sized or inadequately anchored. Often requires immediate retrieval and/or surgical intervention.

Role in Congenital Heart Centers

Transcatheter pulmonary valve intervention has become an indispensable component of the lifelong care strategy for patients with congenital heart disease, particularly those with complex RVOT anatomy and chronic PR/PS.

For suitable candidates, TPVI is now considered the preferred alternative to repeat surgical pulmonary valve replacement due to its less invasive nature, lower procedural morbidity and mortality, and favorable short- and mid-term outcomes.

The complexity of these patients necessitates a dedicated, multidisciplinary Congenital Heart Team. This team typically includes congenital interventional cardiologists, congenital heart surgeons, advanced cardiac imaging specialists (echocardiography, CT, MRI), heart failure specialists, electrophysiologists, and anesthesiologists. The heart team collaboratively evaluates each patient, integrating clinical status, imaging findings, exercise capacity, and electrophysiological data to determine the optimal timing of intervention, device selection, and procedural strategy. This ensures that all therapeutic options (medical management, TPVI, or surgical re-intervention) are considered in a holistic manner.

The role of the congenital heart center extends beyond the procedure itself, encompassing lifelong surveillance, monitoring for device-related complications, and planning for potential future re-interventions. These centers are equipped with the specialized expertise and infrastructure required to manage the unique challenges posed by adults with CHD.

By offering a less invasive option, TPVI helps to defer or potentially avoid repeat open-heart surgeries, thereby reducing the cumulative burden of surgical morbidity and mortality over a patient's lifetime. The increasing volume and complexity of TPVI procedures underscore the need for specialized training and ongoing expertise within dedicated congenital heart centers to ensure optimal patient outcomes and continued innovation in the field.

In conclusion, TPVI represents a transformative therapy in congenital heart disease, providing a highly effective and generally safe alternative to repeat surgery. While long-term vigilance for complications like endocarditis and the need for future re-interventions remain, the overall clinical outcomes, coupled with the ability to manage patients within specialized congenital heart centers, firmly establish TPVI as a cornerstone of modern CHD care [2, 22].

Future Directions

The field of transcatheter pulmonary valve intervention is dynamic, driven by continuous innovation in device technology, expanding clinical indications, and a growing understanding of long-term outcomes in complex congenital heart disease (CHD) patients. The future promises even less invasive, more versatile, and more durable solutions.

Expanding Indications (Native RVOT)

A significant future direction for TPVI lies in expanding its applicability to a broader range of patients, particularly those with native right ventricular outflow tract anatomy.

Historically, TPVI was primarily indicated for patients with failing surgical RVOT conduits due to the need for a rigid landing zone for balloon-expandable valves. However, with the advent of devices like the self-expanding harmony transcatheter pulmonary valve (TPV), intervention in the native, non-conduit RVOT is now feasible for patients with severe PR. Future efforts will focus on developing more precise imaging and clinical criteria to identify which native RVOT anatomies are best suited for current and future self-expanding valves, ensuring optimal anchoring and long-term durability. This includes better characterization of RVOT dilation, muscular hypertrophy, and the extent of annular support. Developing devices and techniques for highly dilated, extremely irregular, or very large native RVOTs, which remain challenging for current technologies.

As data on the benefits of earlier intervention for RV remodeling continue to emerge, there will be a push to identify and treat asymptomatic or mildly symptomatic patients with progressive RV dilation and dysfunction in their native RVOTs before irreversible damage occurs.

While balloon pulmonary valvuloplasty remains the primary treatment for congenital native PS, there may be future roles for TPVI in selected cases of recurrent or severe native PS where balloon dilation is insufficient or where a surgical option is undesirable [28].

Device Innovation

The pipeline for next-generation TPVs is robust, focusing on overcoming current limitations and enhancing device performance and applicability. Future devices will aim for even better conformability to the highly variable and often non-circular RVOTs, ensuring complete sealing to minimize paravalvular leaks, a common challenge in irregular anatomies. This may involve adaptive frames, customizable sizes, or novel sealing skirts. Given the often-dilated and muscular nature of the RVOT, innovative anchoring mechanisms will be crucial to ensure long-term device stability and prevent migration, especially in the native RVOT where there is no rigid conduit for support. Reducing the size of delivery catheters will minimize access site complications, particularly important in younger or smaller patients, and potentially allow for broader patient eligibility. Designing devices with improved radiopacity and echocardiographic visibility will facilitate more accurate intra-procedural guidance and post-implantation assessment [28].

A major focus is on extending the lifespan of transcatheter valves to reduce the need for repeat re-interventions over a patient's long life. This involves material science advancements, improved leaflet design to resist degeneration and calcification, and optimized stress distribution within the stent frame. With a growing number of CHD patients having cardiac implantable electronic devices (CIEDs), future TPV designs may specifically address lead management to avoid impingement, erosion, or interference with the lead's function, potentially by creating dedicated pathways or altering frame designs. The concept of drug-eluting technology, successful in coronary stenting, could potentially be applied to TPVs to reduce tissue ingrowth, inflammation, or calcification, thereby extending device longevity and reducing re-stenosis rates.

Role in Hybrid Procedures

Hybrid procedures, combining surgical and transcatheter techniques, are a rapidly evolving area that promises to offer solutions for highly complex cases that are not amenable to purely percutaneous approaches.

Hybrid approaches can involve a mini-thoracotomy to directly access the RV apex, providing a straight and controlled delivery path for the TPV, particularly useful in patients with challenging venous access or extreme RVOT tortuosity. This direct ventricular access can also allow for surgical pre-stenting or remodeling of the RVOT to create a more suitable landing zone for the transcatheter valve.

Hybrid procedures allow for the simultaneous performance of other necessary surgical interventions (e.g., epicardial arrhythmia ablation, tricuspid valve repair, or closure of residual shunts) during the same procedure as the TPVI, optimizing resource utilization and minimizing multiple procedures for the patient.

The increasing focus on minimally invasive surgical techniques (e.g., robotic-assisted surgery, VATS) may further integrate with transcatheter procedures, offering even less traumatic access or complementary repairs.

For patients with very large, extremely irregular, or highly calcified RVOTs that are beyond the current capabilities of purely transcatheter approaches, hybrid procedures can offer a tailored solution. Surgeons can directly visualize and prepare the RVOT, ensuring optimal conditions for transcatheter valve deployment and anchoring.

Hybrid approaches also serve as crucial salvage strategies in cases of procedural complications during purely percutaneous TPVI or for patients deemed inoperable by conventional surgery but too complex for full transcatheter treatment.

The future of TPVI is characterized by a drive towards greater inclusivity for patients, more sophisticated and durable devices, and a continued emphasis on multidisciplinary collaboration to navigate increasingly complex anatomies and clinical scenarios. These advancements will further solidify TPVI's role as a cornerstone of lifelong care for the growing population of adults with congenital heart disease [36, 37].

Comparative Considerations and Special Populations

The expanding landscape of transcatheter valve interventions now encompasses all four cardiac valves. While each intervention shares fundamental principles of catheter-based delivery, the anatomical, pathological, and demographic nuances of different valve diseases necessitate distinct approaches. This chapter will delve into these comparative considerations, highlighting the unique challenges and opportunities presented by various valve pathologies and patient populations.

Differences in Valve Pathology and Patient Demographics

Transcatheter interventions address a spectrum of valve dysfunctions, primarily stenosis (narrowing) and regurgitation (leakage). However, the underlying causes, valve anatomy, and typical patient profiles vary significantly among the aortic, mitral, tricuspid, and pulmonary valves.

For the tricuspid valve, one main characteristic is the overwhelmingly secondary (functional) tricuspid regurgitation due to right ventricular dilation and annular remodeling from left-sided heart disease or pulmonary hypertension. Primary TR (e.g., rheumatic, Ebstein's anomaly) is rare. Patients often present with advanced right heart failure symptoms, typically elderly, with significant comorbidities and very high surgical risk. The large, highly dynamic, non-planar, and very anterior annulus, that is often severely dilated, with the lack of rigid anatomical constraints makes device anchoring complex. The leaflets are thin and often tethered. Proximity to the conduction system (AV node) and coronary sinus is crucial [2].

On the other hand, the pulmonary valve pathology consists of primarily pulmonary regurgitation or stenosis as long-term sequelae of congenital heart disease (CHD) repair (e.g., Tetralogy of Fallot, truncus arteriosus repair). Native valve disease in adults is rare. The majority of patients are primarily adolescents and young adults who have undergone childhood cardiac surgery. While generally younger and less comorbid than TAVR or TMVR patients, they face the prospect of multiple re-interventions over a lifetime. The most important anatomical feature to keep in mind is the highly variable RVOT morphology, often dilated, muscular, or with surgical patches/conduits. Lack of a true fibrous annulus can make valve anchoring challenging, requiring devices adapted to irregular or "native" RVOTs. Proximity to coronary arteries is a critical consideration [2].

Considerations in Congenital vs Acquired Disease

The distinction between congenital and acquired heart valve disease is fundamental, shaping the indications, procedural challenges, and long-term management strategies for transcatheter interventions.

Most of the interventional procedures address the acquired valve disease (aortic, mitral, tricuspid in adults), which can be degenerative (calcification, myxomatous degeneration), ischemic, rheumatic (less common in developed countries for new cases) or secondary to LV disease. Patients are typically older adults with comorbidities, reflecting a lifetime of wear-and-tear or systemic diseases impacting the heart. The goals of intervention are symptom relief, improvement in quality of life, prevention of progressive ventricular dysfunction, and potentially improved survival. Intervention often occurs when symptoms are significant or ventricular function is compromised. While dynamic, acquired valve annuli often provide more stable and predictable landing zones for devices compared to the highly variable post-surgical anatomy in CHD. For these patients, often there is need for a single definitive intervention, with re-intervention considered if the prosthetic valve degenerates after many years, or if the initial intervention for regurgitation proves incomplete [2, 9].

For patients with congenital valve disease (pulmonary, and some tricuspid/mitral/aortic in younger patients), developmental anomalies present at birth often require multiple surgical interventions throughout life. The valve pathology is frequently a long-term consequence of these repairs (e.g., chronic PR after ToF repair). These are younger patients, often adolescents or young adults, with a history of complex cardiac surgeries. While generally healthier than elderly acquired disease patients, they carry the burden of lifelong CHD. The goal of intervention is to prevent or reverse ventricular remodeling, improve exercise capacity, reduce arrhythmia burden, and *delay* the need for repeat open-heart surgery, thereby extending "surgical freedom." The anatomy is highly variable and often severely distorted by previous surgeries (patches, conduits, resections). This makes device sizing, anchoring, and avoidance of critical structures (e.g., coronary arteries in pulmonary interventions) particularly challenging. A staged approach is common. Transcatheter interventions are often part of a sequence of procedures over a patient's lifetime. The understanding is that a transcatheter valve, like a surgical bioprosthesis, has a finite lifespan, and future re-interventions (surgical or transcatheter valve-in-valve) will likely be necessary. The goal is to maximize the intervals between interventions [22, 23].

Pediatric vs Adult Patients

The patient's age significantly impacts every aspect of transcatheter valve intervention, from device selection and procedural considerations to post-procedural care and long-term follow-up. While adult congenital heart disease (ACHD) specialists increasingly manage younger adults with CHD, the truly pediatric population presents unique challenges.

Smaller body size and ongoing somatic growth are major considerations. Device sizes need to be appropriate for smaller anatomies, and the potential for the valve to be "outgrown" by the patient is a significant concern. This often necessitates larger future devices or repeat interventions as the child grows.

Smaller vessel caliber increases the risk of vascular complications (e.g., bleeding, thrombosis, vessel damage) with large-bore catheters. This often requires meticulous technique, sometimes necessitating surgical cutdown for access, or a longer hospital stay for monitoring. In adults, larger vessels generally allow for easier and safer percutaneous access, although tortuosity or peripheral vascular disease can be issues.

In pediatric patients, general anesthesia is almost universally required due to the need for patient immobility, airway control, and complex imaging during long procedures. In adults, many procedures (e.g., TAVR, some TTVR) can be performed under conscious sedation, reducing risks and recovery time.

The conduction system in smaller hearts can be in closer proximity to the valve annulus, potentially increasing the risk of new-onset heart block during valve implantation, particularly in the tricuspid and aortic positions.

Fewer devices are specifically designed and approved for pediatric anatomies. Off-label use of adult devices (e.g., smaller TAVR valves for pulmonary position) is common. There is a greater need for customized or highly conformable devices for complex CHD anatomies.

Lifelong follow-up is critical in pediatric patients, as these patients will require multiple interventions (surgical or transcatheter) over decades. The strategy involves careful timing to defer surgery, maximize intervals between procedures, and utilize valve-in-valve techniques where possible. Counseling families about this lifelong journey is paramount.

In summary, while transcatheter technologies offer profound benefits across all four heart valves, a nuanced understanding of the distinct pathological, anatomical, and demographic profiles of each patient group is essential for successful patient selection, procedural planning, and the delivery of optimal, individualized care. The future of transcatheter interventions will undoubtedly see further specialization and refinement to address these unique comparative considerations [22, 23].

Summary and Conclusions

The landscape of structural heart disease intervention has been profoundly reshaped by the advent and rapid evolution of transcatheter therapies for the right-sided heart valves. Once considered "forgotten" in comparison to their left-sided counterparts, the tricuspid and pulmonary valves now benefit from an expanding arsenal of innovative devices and refined techniques, offering new hope for patients previously deemed unsuitable for conventional surgery.

Key Takeaways from Current Practice

Current practice highlights several critical advancements and established principles in transcatheter right-sided valve therapies.

Transcatheter tricuspid valve and pulmonary valve interventions have emerged as crucial treatment options for high-risk patients with severe, symptomatic tricuspid regurgitation or significant pulmonary regurgitation/stenosis due to congenital heart disease (CHD). These therapies offer less invasive alternatives to repeat open-heart surgery, which carries significant morbidity and mortality in these often-fragile populations.

Data from pivotal clinical trials (e.g., TRILUMINATE Pivotal for tricuspid repair, TRISCEND II for tricuspid replacement) and large registries consistently demonstrate the safety and efficacy of these procedures. Patients experience significant improvements in symptoms, quality of life, functional capacity, and favorable ventricular remodeling.

Device innovation has been paramount. For the tricuspid valve, edge-to-edge repair (e.g., TriClip, PASCAL) is well-established, with various transcatheter tricuspid valve replacement (TTVR) systems (e.g., EVOQUE, Intrepid) rapidly gaining traction. For the pulmonary valve, balloon-expandable valves (Melody, Sapien) remain the standard for conduit dysfunction, while self-expanding valves (Harmony TPV) have revolutionized treatment for the native right ventricular outflow tract (RVOT).

Success hinges on meticulous procedural planning and execution. This includes strategic access route selection (predominantly transfemoral venous), comprehensive multi-modality imaging guidance (fluoroscopy, TEE, ICE, pre-procedural CT/MRI), and diligent management of specific risks such as coronary compression (for PV interventions) and vascular complications.

Unlike the largely homogenous elderly population for TAVR, right-sided valve interventions serve diverse groups. Tricuspid patients are typically older adults with acquired functional TR and advanced heart failure. Pulmonary valve patients are often younger, with complex congenital heart disease, facing the challenge of lifelong disease management and potential serial re-interventions.

Role of the Multidisciplinary Team

The complexity inherent in transcatheter right-sided valve interventions underscores the non-negotiable role of the multidisciplinary heart team. This collaborative model is fundamental to optimizing patient outcomes.

The Heart Team, comprising interventional cardiologists, cardiac surgeons, advanced imaging specialists, heart failure specialists, electrophysiologists, and anesthesiologists, collectively assesses the patient's overall clinical status, comorbidities, anatomical suitability, and life expectancy. This holistic approach ensures all therapeutic avenues are considered.

For complex conditions like TR and the myriad anatomies in CHD, the team determines the optimal timing of intervention, selects the most appropriate device, and devises the safest and most effective procedural strategy. This includes deciding between repair vs. replacement, or transcatheter vs. surgical options.

The team proactively identifies potential complications and develops contingency plans. For instance, in TPVI, the risk of coronary compression is rigorously assessed and managed through team-based discussion and specialized imaging protocols.

For congenital heart disease patients, the congenital heart team is crucial for lifelong surveillance, monitoring valve and RV function, anticipating future re-interventions (e.g., valve-in-valve procedures), and counseling patients and families on the long-term journey.

Outlook for Transcatheter Right-Sided Valve Therapies

The future of transcatheter right-sided valve therapies is incredibly promising, marked by continuous innovation and expanding clinical utility.

Next-generation devices with enhanced conformability, improved sealing mechanisms, lower delivery profiles, and increased durability are expected. Innovations in anchoring mechanisms will address highly dilated or irregular native annuli, particularly for the tricuspid and pulmonary valves. Devices specifically designed to navigate and mitigate issues with pre-existing CIED leads will also emerge.

As devices become more versatile and data on long-term outcomes mature, indications will likely broaden. For TR, this could mean intervening earlier in symptomatic patients before irreversible RV damage. For PR, further expansion into native RVOTs will continue, potentially even for asymptomatic patients with objective markers of RV dysfunction.

Advanced imaging techniques (e.g., 3D CT/MRI, strain imaging) combined with clinical data and novel biomarkers will allow for even more precise patient phenotyping and risk stratification. This will help identify ideal candidates for specific devices and optimize the timing of intervention for maximum long-term benefit.

Hybrid approaches, combining minimally invasive surgical techniques with transcatheter interventions, will offer solutions for the most complex cases, enabling access to challenging anatomies and facilitating concomitant procedures.

Future research will focus on head-to-head comparisons between different devices and strategies (e.g., repair vs. replacement for TR, different TPV types) to guide optimal patient pathways. The integration of transcatheter therapies with optimal guideline-directed medical therapy for heart failure will also be a key area of study.

In conclusion, transcatheter interventions for the tricuspid and pulmonary valves represent a paradigm shift in cardiovascular medicine. By offering safe, effective, and less invasive alternatives, they are transforming the lives of patients previously facing limited options. The continued evolution of technology, combined with the unwavering commitment to a multidisciplinary heart team approach, ensures a bright future for this vital and rapidly advancing field.

References

1. Hahn RT, et al. Intraprocedural imaging of transcatheter tricuspid valve interventions. JACC Cardiovasc Imaging. 2019;12(3):532–53.
2. Baumgartner H, et al. 2017 ESC/EACTS guidelines for the management of valvular heart disease. Eur Heart J. 2017;38(36):2739–91.
3. Sorajja P, et al. Transcatheter repair for patients with tricuspid regurgitation. N Engl J Med. 2023;388(20):1833–42.
4. Nguyen CT, et al. Echocardiographic guidance for diagnostic and therapeutic percutaneous procedures. Cardiovasc Diagn Ther. 2011;1(1):11–36.
5. Basman C, Parmar YJ, Kronzon I. Intracardiac echocardiography for structural heart and electrophysiological interventions. Curr Cardiol Rep. 2017;19(10):102.
6. Monaco GD, et al. Transcatheter tricuspid valve replacement: current options and future perspectives. Rev Cardiovasc Med. 2025;26(1):25712.
7. Andreas M, et al. Tricuspid valve disease and cardiac implantable electronic devices. Eur Heart J. 2024;45(5):346–65.
8. Tang GHL, et al. Tricuspid transcatheter edge-to-edge repair for severe tricuspid regurgitation: 1-year outcomes from the TRILUMINATE randomized cohort. J Am Coll Cardiol. 2025;85(3):235–46.
9. Nishimura RA, et al. 2017 AHA/ACC focused update of the 2014 AHA/ACC guideline for the management of patients with valvular heart disease: a report of the American College of Cardiology/American Heart Association Task Force on Clinical Practice Guidelines. Circulation. 2017;135(25):e1159–95.
10. Elkasaby MH, et al. Transcatheter tricuspid valve intervention compared to isolated tricuspid valve surgery in tricuspid regurgitation patients: a systematic review and meta-analysis. JACC. 2024;83(13_Supplement):1137–47.
11. Fam NP, et al. Intracardiac echocardiography for guidance of transcatheter tricuspid edge-to-edge repair. EuroIntervention. 2018;14(9):e1004–5.
12. Baldus S, et al. Transcatheter valve repair of tricuspid regurgitation with the PASCAL system: TriCLASP study 30-day results. Catheter Cardiovasc Interv. 2022;100(7):1291–9.
13. Kodali SK, et al. 1-year outcomes of transcatheter tricuspid valve repair. J Am Coll Cardiol. 2023;81(18):1766–76.
14. Gray WA, et al. 1-year outcomes of cardioband tricuspid valve reconstruction system early feasibility study. JACC Cardiovasc Interv. 2022;15(19):1921–32.
15. Besler C, Meduri CU, Lurz P. Transcatheter treatment of functional tricuspid regurgitation using the trialign device. Interv Cardiol. 2018;13(1):8–13.
16. Blasco-Turrión S, et al. Bicaval TricValve implantation in patients with severe symptomatic tricuspid regurgitation: 1-year follow-up outcomes. JACC Cardiovasc Interv. 2024;17(1):60–72.
17. Arnold Suzanne V, et al. Quality of life after transcatheter tricuspid valve replacement. JACC. 2025;85(3):206–16.
18. Lederman RJ, et al. Transcaval access and closure best practices, vol. 16(4). JACC: Cardiovasc Interven; 2023. p. 371–95.
19. Hahn RT, et al. Transcatheter valve replacement in severe tricuspid regurgitation. N Engl J Med. 2025;392(2):115–26.
20. Suradi HS, Hijazi ZM. Percutaneous pulmonary valve implantation. Glob Cardiol Sci Pract. 2015;2015(2):23.
21. Meca Aguirrezabalaga JA, et al. Pulmonary regurgitation after repaired tetralogy of Fallot: surgical versus percutaneous treatment. Ann Transl Med. 2020;8(15):967.

22. Baumgartner H, et al. 2020 ESC guidelines for the management of adult congenital heart disease. Eur Heart J. 2021;42(6):563–645.
23. Stout KK, et al. 2018 AHA/ACC guideline for the management of adults with congenital heart disease: executive summary: a report of the American College of Cardiology/American Heart Association Task Force on Clinical Practice Guidelines. J Am Coll Cardiol. 2019;73(12):1494–563.
24. Therrien J, et al. Optimal timing for pulmonary valve replacement in adults after tetralogy of Fallot repair. Am J Cardiol. 2005;95(6):779–82.
25. Brancaccio G, et al. The impact of tricuspid regurgitation on timing pulmonary valve replacement in ACHD patients after tetralogy of Fallot repair. Int J Cardiol Congen Heart Dis. 2025;20:100577.
26. Driesen BW, et al. Percutaneous pulmonary valve implantation: current status and future perspectives. Curr Cardiol Rev. 2019;15(4):262–73.
27. Jones TK, et al. Long-term outcomes after melody transcatheter pulmonary valve replacement in the US investigational device exemption trial. Circ Cardiovasc Interv. 2022;15(1):e010852.
28. Patel ND, et al. Transcatheter pulmonary valve replacement: a review of current valve technologies. J Soc Cardiovasc Angiograph Interven. 2022;1(6)
29. Plessis J, et al. Edwards SAPIEN Transcatheter pulmonary valve implantation: results from a French registry, vol. 11(19). JACC: Cardiovascular Interventions; 2018. p. 1909–16.
30. Boutsikou M, Tzifa A. Noninvasive imaging prior to percutaneous pulmonary valve implantation. Hell J Cardiol. 2022;67:59–65.
31. Velázquez Martín M, et al. Coronary compression following percutaneous pulmonary valve implantation despite a negative balloon sizing test: lessons learnt from this unusual complication. Cardiovasc Revasc Med. 2022;40:135–8.
32. Pagourelias ED, et al. Right ventricular remodelling after transcatheter pulmonary valve implantation. Catheter Cardiovasc Interv. 2017;90(3):407–17.
33. McElhinney DB, et al. Short- and medium-term outcomes after transcatheter pulmonary valve placement in the expanded multicenter US melody valve trial. Circulation. 2010;122(5):507–16.
34. Lourtet-Hascoët J, et al. Infective endocarditis after transcatheter pulmonary valve implantation in patients with congenital heart disease: distinctive features. Arch Cardiovasc Dis. 2023;116(3):159–66.
35. McElhinney DB, et al. Stent fracture, valve dysfunction, and right ventricular outflow tract reintervention after transcatheter pulmonary valve implantation, vol. 4(6). Circulation: Cardiovasc Interven; 2011. p. 602–14.
36. Li Q, Ling Y, Gan C, Feng Y, Zhao Z. Hybrid approach to transcatheter pulmonary valve replacement in patients with excessively large anatomy. Cardiology in the Young. 2025;35(6):1292–7. https://doi.org/10.1017/S1047951125001842.
37. Zhang S, Meng Q, Qi H, Sun J, Li Y, Qian X. Quadricuspid pulmonic valve with pulmonary artery aneurysm. Quant Imaging Med Surg. 2024;14(1):1272–5. https://doi.org/10.21037/qims-23-898. Epub 2024 Jan 2. PMID: 38223076; PMCID: PMC10784045.

Advanced Aortic Valve Repair Strategies

11

Aureliu Batrinac and Malakh Shrestha

Introduction

The aortic root and aortic valve form a complex functional unit essential for optimal cardiac hemodynamics. Pathologies affecting this structure—such as aneurysms, dissections, or primary aortic insufficiency—can severely compromise cardiac function and pose life-threatening risks. While aortic valve replacement with mechanical or biological prostheses has historically been the standard solution, the development and refinement of native valve repair and preservation techniques have revolutionized the management of these conditions. These techniques, though technically demanding and requiring a deep understanding of 3D anatomy and physiology, offer patients significant long-term benefits, including lower thrombosis and hemorrhage rates, avoidance of long-term anticoagulation (especially for mechanical prostheses), more physiological valve function, and potentially longer durability of the repaired valve compared to bioprostheses. This article targets cardiac surgeons, interventional cardiologists, cardiology residents, and researchers, providing an in-depth analysis of the field.

A. Batrinac (✉)
Cardiovascular Surgery, Department of Cardiovascular Surgery, Medpark International Hospital, Chisinau, Moldova

M. Shrestha
Aortic Surgery at the Mayo Clinic Rochester Minnesota, Rochester, MN, USA

Mayo Clinic Aortic Center, Rochester, MN, USA

G. Tinică, A. Burlacu (eds.), *Surgical, Hybrid and Minimally Invasive Structural Cardiac Interventions*, https://doi.org/10.1007/978-3-032-16676-0_11

Anatomy of the Aortic Root and Aortic Valve

The aortic root represents the proximal outflow segment of the left ventricle, located between the ventriculo-aortic junction and the sinotubular junction (STJ). It is a dynamic, three-dimensional structure composed of (see Table 11.1):

- *Sinuses of Valsalva*: Three funnel-shaped dilatations (right coronary, left coronary, and non-coronary sinuses). Their walls are thin and elastic.
- *Commissures and Coronary Attachment Points*: The three commissures of the aortic valve attach at the STJ level. Coronary ostia typically open into the coronary sinuses (left in the left sinus, right in the right sinus), usually below the upper edge of the commissures, but position may vary.
- *Aortic Valve (Aortic Semilunar Valve)*: Composed of three triangular cusps (or leaflets), highly resistant, with a layered structure:
  - *Ventricularis (fibrillar layer)*: Ventricular surface exposed to blood flow.
  - *Spongiosum*: Middle layer rich in proteoglycans, providing elasticity.
  - *Fibrosus*: Arterial layer, thick and resistant, composed of densely packed collagen fibers ensuring structural integrity. The free edge (*margo liber*) is thickened (Arantius nodule centrally and lunulae laterally), ensuring tight closure.
- *Ventriculo-Aortic Junction (VAJ)*: A complex annular structure comprising:

Table 11.1 Key anatomical elements of the aortic root and critical relationships

Anatomical element	Description	Functional/surgical significance
Sinuses of valsalva	3 dilatations (right, left, non-coronary)	Facilitate valve closure via vortices; contain coronary ostia; thin wall prone to dilation
Aortic cusps	3 cusps (right, left, non-coronary); layered (ventricularis, spongiosum, fibrosus)	Ensure closure tightness; integrity of the fibrosus layer is critical. *Margo liber* with Arantius nodule
Ventriculo-aortic junction (VAJ)	"True" annulus—discontinuous fibrous crown-like ring at the lowest cusp attachment points	Defines the valvular orifice; reference for measurement and suturing in repair
Commissures	Superior attachment points of cusps at the STJ	Support cusp tension; their geometry determines coaptation
Sinotubular junction (STJ)	Upper boundary of the root where sinuses merge	Critical diameter; dilation causes aortic insufficiency via commissural traction ("STJ Oversizing")
Coronary ostia	Openings in coronary sinuses (left in left sinus, right in right sinus)	Must be correctly reimplanted during root surgery; variable position
Membranous septum	Below the right-noncoronary commissure	Proximity to the His bundle; risk of AV block with deep suturing
Mitro-aortic/ aorto-mitral fibrous continuity	Connective tissue between aortic (non-coronary) and mitral valves	Critical for structural stability; excessive dissection may destabilize the mitral valve

  - *True Aortic Annulus*: A discontinuous fibrous "crown-like" ring at the lowest attachment points of the cusps. Not a complete circular ring. Defines the valvular orifice.
  - *Intercuspal Commissures*: Superior support zones attached at the STJ.
- *Sinotubular Junction (STJ)*: The upper boundary of the aortic root where the sinuses merge to form the tubular ascending aorta. STJ diameter is critical for valve function.
- *Ventriculo-Aortic Functional Complex (Aortico-Ventricular Unit)*: Includes:
  - *Membranous Septum*: Located below the commissure between the non-coronary and right cusps.
  - *Mitro-Aortic Fibrous Continuity*: Connective tissue between the aortic and mitral valves (at the level of the non-coronary cusp).
  - *Aorto-Mitral Fibrous Continuity (Aorto-Mitral Interval)*: Direct connection between the aortic and anterior mitral annuli.
- *Suspension of the Aortic Valve*: Cusps are supported by tension between their inferior (VAJ) and superior (commissures at STJ) attachment points. The geometry of the sinuses of Valsalva facilitates valve closure by creating vortices that reduce mechanical stress on the cusps [1–3].

Physiology of the Aortic Root and Valve

The function of the aortic root and valve is inextricably linked, ensuring:

1. *Efficient Systolic Opening*: Allows blood ejection from the left ventricle with minimal resistance. The conical geometry of the outflow tract and root minimizes turbulence.
2. *Tight Diastolic Closure*: Prevents blood regurgitation into the left ventricle.
   - *Key Mechanisms*:
     - Cusp elasticity and recoil.
     - Sinus of Valsalva geometry: Creates diastolic blood vortices that "push" cusps centrally, enabling rapid/sealed closure with minimal mechanical stress.
     - Optimal STJ diameter (~90% of annular diameter): Prevents cusp prolapse. Dilated STJ reduces commissural tension, causing insufficiency.
     - *Height-to-Opening Ratio (HOO)*: For optimal coaptation, cusp height (H) must be sufficient relative to orifice diameter (O). HOO <0.8 (especially <0.75) indicates high risk of post-repair insufficiency.
     - Cusp symmetry: Essential for uniform coaptation.
3. *Dynamic Suspension*: Cusps are passively tensioned between attachment points. Disruption of root geometry (annular/STJ dilation, asymmetric sinus dilation) compromises coaptation.
4. *Coronary Reservoir*: Sinuses enable diastolic coronary perfusion by allowing blood flow back toward coronary ostia.

Pathologies of the Aortic Valve and Root

Pathologies requiring complex repair/preservation fall into two overlapping categories (Table 11.2) [4, 5]:

A. *Primary Aortic Valve Pathologies (with Normal/Near-Normal Root)*:
   - *Degenerative Aortic Insufficiency*: Isolated prolapse due to elongated/ruptured marginal chordae (*frenula*) or excess cusp tissue. Cusps are typically thin/mobile. May be idiopathic or associated with Barlow syndrome (thick, redundant, myxomatous cusps) or Marfan syndrome.
   - *Rheumatic Aortic Insufficiency*: Commissural fusion, cusp retraction, and fibrosis. Repair is more challenging and less frequent than in degenerative pathology.
   - *Aortic Endocarditis*: Cusp destruction (perforations, abscesses), large vegetations. Repair is possible if destruction is limited and infection controlled.
   - *Congenital Aortic Stenosis (Bicuspid/Unicuspid)*: Bicuspid valve repair (AVr) is an option in selected cases with predominant insufficiency and favorable anatomy.

Table 11.2 Classification of aortic root pathologies and repair implications

Pathology	Key features	Implications for valve repair/preservation
Idiopathic degenerative aneurysm	Initially normal cusps; symmetric/asymmetric root dilation.	Repair often feasible (David/Yacoub). Monitor closely for late annular dilation.
Marfan syndrome	Symmetric progressive dilation; normal cusps prone to elongation/prolapse; high dissection/rupture risk.	*David I reimplantation* preferred (stabilizes annulus). Yacoub contraindicated.
Loeys-Dietz syndrome	Aggressive dilation; rupture risk at smaller sizes; normal/near-normal cusps.	*David I reimplantation* recommended due to high risk. Yacoub offers no annular support.
Bicuspid aortic valve (BAV)	Variable anatomy (Sievers type 0,1,2); asymmetric dilation (less affected non-coronary sinus); high valvulopathy risk.	Complex repair: cusp correction (plication, pericardial patch) + root correction (modified David/Yacoub).
Type A aortic dissection	Emergency; acute insufficiency; normal cusps may prolapse; detached commissures; dissected root.	Repair possible in select cases: commissure refixation, cusp resuspension, David on dissected tissue. High risk.
Isolated STJ dilation	Normal sinuses/annulus; enlarged STJ → commissural traction → insufficiency.	Simplified technique: STJ reduction (banding or reimplantation/remodeling with small graft).

B. *Aortic Root Pathologies (Causing Secondary Aortic Insufficiency)*:

- *Aortic Root Aneurysm (Type A Ascending Aorta)*: Idiopathic/degenerative dilation (most common). Associated with:
  - *Marfan syndrome* (FBN1 mutations; progressive root dilation, secondary cusp elongation/prolapse).
  - *Loeys-Dietz syndrome* (TGFBR1/2/SMAD3 mutations; aggressive arterial dilation, high rupture/dissection risk).
  - *Vascular Ehlers-Danlos syndrome* (COL3A1 mutations; tissue fragility).
  - *Bicuspid aortic valve (BAV)* (1–2% prevalence; asymmetric root dilation/aneurysm; Sievers classification).
  - *Aortitis* (e.g., Takayasu, giant cell arteritis, radiation-induced).
- *Type A Aortic Dissection Involving the Root*: Acute severe insufficiency due to cusp prolapses, annular dilation, or commissural detachment. Valve preservation may be feasible in experienced centers.
- *Isolated STJ Dilation*: Causes insufficiency via "STJ oversizing." Repair may require STJ reduction alone.

Diagnostics of Aortic Valve and Root Pathologies

Accurate diagnosis and detailed morphological evaluation are critical for patient selection [6, 7].

A. *Non-Invasive Imaging*:

- *Transthoracic Echocardiography (TTE)*: Initial investigation. Assesses valve function, ventricular dimensions, ejection fraction, and root/ascending aorta dimensions. Limited for detailed root/cusp morphology.
- *Transesophageal Echocardiography (TEE)*: *Gold standard* for pre-operative valve/root morphology:
  - Precise measurements (VAJ, sinuses, STJ, ascending aorta).
  - Cusp assessment (number, thickness, mobility, prolapse, retraction).
  - Mechanism of insufficiency (annular/STJ dilation, cusp prolapse).
  - Coaptation height, vena contracta width (VCW).
  - Height-to-opening ratio (HOO).
  - Dissection detection.
- *CT Angiography (3D Reconstruction)*: *Essential for surgical planning*:
  - 3D measurements of all segments (VAJ, sinuses, STJ, ascending aorta, arch, descending aorta).
  - Geometric root assessment (symmetry, shape).
  - Anatomical relationships (coronaries, supra-aortic vessels).
  - Calcification detection.
  - Full thoracic/abdominal evaluation.

- *Cardiac MRI*: Alternative to CT; excellent functional assessment (regurgitant volume/fraction, ventricular mass). Tissue characterization (edema, hemorrhage in dissection).

B. *Invasive Diagnostics*:

- *Cardiac Catheterization (Coronary Angiography)*: Indicated for patients with coronary risk factors to identify lesions requiring concurrent revascularization. Not needed for root/insufficiency evaluation if non-invasive imaging is conclusive.

Advanced Repair Techniques for Aortic Valve and Root Preservation in Root Aneurysm

The core principle is *restoring normal root geometry and correcting structural cusp pathology* to ensure stable coaptation. Two main strategies:

A. *Aortic Valve Repair (AVr) for Primary Cusp Pathology (Normal Root)* [8, 9]:

- *Indications*: Isolated cusp prolapse (usually right/non-coronary), degenerative insufficiency, or BAV with favorable anatomy.
- *Key Techniques*:
  - *Free Margin Plication*: Shortening prolapsed cusps via suturing (central or at lunulae).
  - *Resection of Redundant Tissue*: Rare (e.g., Barlow syndrome).
  - *Pericardial Patch Plasty*: For perforations or retracted cusps (glutaraldehyde-treated autologous pericardium).
  - *Geometric Rebalancing*: Adjustments for symmetry and coaptation height (HOO >0.8). Intraoperative saline test under pressure is essential.
  - *Annuloplasty*: For moderate annular dilation (>25–28 mm):
    - *Subcommissural Annuloplasty*: Sutures below commissures to reduce annular circumference. Limited efficacy.
    - *External Aortic Ring Annuloplasty*: Synthetic/pericardial ring placed *externally* around VAJ (Lansac technique). Superior stability.
    - *External Suture annuloplasty with Gor* -Tex 0 suture (Schäfers technique).

B. *Valve-Sparing Aortic Root Replacement (VSARR) for Root Aneurysm* [10–13]:

- *Indications*: Root aneurysm (>50 mm; >45 mm in Marfan/BAV/Loeys-Dietz/symptomatic) with repairable native valve (thin/mobile cusps, no severe calcification/retraction). Final intraoperative assessment (inspection/saline test) is decisive.
- *Key Techniques*:

1. *Reimplantation (David Procedure)*:
   - Native valve implanted inside a Dacron graft. Entire root resected; only commissural "buttons" preserved.
   - *Critical Steps*:
     – Root mobilization (extensive dissection below VAJ).
     – Subannular suture placement (secures VAJ diameter; prevents dilation).
     – Commissural reimplantation at neo-STJ.
     – Saline test for coaptation.
     – Coronary button reimplantation.
   - *Variants*: David I (straight graft), David IV/V (neo-sinus creation).
   - *Advantages*: Complete annular support. *Preferred for connective tissue disorders (Marfan, Loeys-Dietz) and significant annular dilation.*
   - *Risks*: Heart block (deep subannular sutures), geometric distortion.
2. *Remodeling (Yacoub Procedure)*:
   - Dacron graft tailored into three "tongues" sutured to the native VAJ. Commissures fixed at neo-STJ. *No subannular support.*
   - *Advantages*: Preserves native 3D geometry; technically simpler.
   - *Disadvantages*: *Contraindicated in connective tissue disorders due to late annular dilation risk.*
   - *Stabilization*: Add external ring ("Yacoub + Ring"), or Yacoub and Gor-Tex suture annuloplasty.
3. *Combined Techniques*:
   - *Valsalva Grafts*: Preformed sinuses for more physiological flow.
   - *BAV Repair + VSARR*: Cusp correction (plication/patch) + root stabilization (usually David).

C. *Intraoperative Decision-Making and Saline Test* [14–16]:

- Valve preservation decided after direct inspection.
- *Saline test under pressure assesses*:
  - Coaptation height (>8–10 mm).
  - Symmetry.
  - Residual insufficiency.
  - Estimated HOO.
- Convert to AVR if coaptation is inadequate or insufficiency > grade I–II.

Complications of Surgery

Early Complications

- Bleeding/re-transfusion, stroke, myocardial dysfunction, coronary injury (during reimplantation), complete AV block (David procedure), residual insufficiency, infection, operative mortality (1–5%) [17, 18].

Late Complications

- Recurrent aortic insufficiency (main cause of reoperation; due to cusp degeneration, annular dilation, or residual aortic dilation) [19–21].
- Aortic stenosis (rare).
- Endocarditis (risk similar to bioprostheses).
- Progressive aortic dilation/dissection/rupture (connective tissue disorders).
- *10-year freedom from reintervention:* >85–90% in experienced centers (David for Marfan) [22–24].

Conclusions and Perspectives

Advanced aortic valve repair/preservation represents the pinnacle of modern cardiac surgery. The *David procedure* is optimal for connective tissue disorders; *Yacoub* may suit degenerative aneurysms with stable annuli (add external ring). Rigorous patient selection, 3D imaging, and intraoperative saline testing are paramount. Lifelong imaging surveillance is mandatory. Future directions include refined prostheses, computational modeling, and hybrid approaches [25, 26].

References

I. Anatomy and Physiology

1. Anderson RH, et al. The anatomy of the aortic root. Anat Rec. 2008;291(3):288–98.
2. Sutton JP, et al. The forgotten interleaflet triangles: a review of the surgical anatomy of the aortic valve. Ann Thorac Surg. 1995;59(2):419–27.
3. Kunzelman KS, et al. Aortic root and valve relationships: impact on surgical repair. J Thorac Cardiovasc Surg. 1993;106(3):435–42.

II. Pathologies and Diagnostics

4. Hiratzka LF, et al. 2010 ACCF/AHA/AATS/ACR/ASA/SCA/SCAI/SIR/STS/SVM Guidelines for thoracic aortic disease. J Am Coll Cardiol. 2010;55(14):e27–e129.
5. Erbel R, et al. 2014 ESC Guidelines on aortic diseases. Eur Heart J. 2014;35(41):2873–926.
6. Michelena HI, et al. Natural history of asymptomatic bicuspid aortic valve. Circulation. 2011;123(18):1993–2000.
7. Bonow RO, et al. 2020 ACC/AHA Guideline for valvular heart disease. J Am Coll Cardiol. 2020;77(4):e25–e197.

III. Surgical Techniques and Outcomes

A. Valve Repair (AVr)

8. Schäfers HJ, et al. Preservation of the bicuspid aortic valve. J Thorac Cardiovasc Surg. 2013;145(3 Suppl):S46–51.

9. Aicher D, et al. Aortic valve repair leads to low valve-related complications. Eur J Cardio-Thorac Surg. 2010;37(1):127–32.

B. Valve-Sparing Root Replacement (VSARR)

10. David TE, et al. Aortic valve-sparing operation. J Thorac Cardiovasc Surg. 1992;103(4):617–22.
11. Yacoub MH, et al. Remodeling of the aortic valve annulus. J Thorac Cardiovasc Surg. 1998;115(5):1081–90.
12. Lansac E, et al. Aortic ring standardization. Eur J Cardio-Thorac Surg. 2005;28(3):391–6.
13. de Kerchove L, et al. Valsalva graft in David procedure. J Thorac Cardiovasc Surg. 2015;149(2 Suppl):S30–5.

C. Bicuspid Aortic Valve and Connective Tissue Disorders

14. Fazel SS, et al. Aortic root performance in VSARR. J Thorac Cardiovasc Surg. 2008;136(3):657–63.
15. Patel ND, et al. VSARR for bicuspid valves. Ann Cardiothorac Surg. 2016;5(4):324–31.
16. Cameron DE, et al. David procedure in Marfan syndrome. J Thorac Cardiovasc Surg. 2016;151(1):179–88.

IV. Imaging Diagnostics

17. Lang RM, et al. Echocardiography chamber quantification. J Am Soc Echocardiogr. 2015;28(1):1–39.
18. Blanke P, et al. CT imaging in aortic valvular disease. J Cardiovasc Comput Tomogr. 2019;13(6):309–15.

V. Complications and Long-Term Outcomes

19. Boodhwani M, et al. Long-term outcomes after VSARR. Circulation. 2014;130(11 Suppl 1):S53–8.
20. Matalanis G, et al. Aortic valve repair in Australia. Heart Lung Circ. 2011;20(9):555–62.
21. Jassar AS, et al. VSARR in Loeys-Dietz syndrome. Ann Thoracic Surg. 2012;94(5):1466–9.

VI. Comprehensive Reviews

22. El Khoury G, et al. Aortic valve repair: current status. Eur J Cardio-Thoracic Surg. 2018;55(1):1–11.
23. Bissell MM, et al. Aortic dilation in BAV disease. Circulation. 2013;127(8):886–8.
24. David TE. Surgical treatment of aortic valve endocarditis. J Thorac Cardiovasc Surg. 2018;155(1):95–100.

VII. Guidelines and Consensus

25. Writing Committee Members. 2023 ACC/AHA/SCAI Statement on Interventional Cardiology. J Am Coll Cardiol. 2023;81(24):2373–407.
26. Vahanian A, et al. 2022 ESC/EACTS Guidelines for valvular heart disease. Eur Heart J. 2022;43(7):561–632.

Tailored Interventions for Adults with Congenital Heart Defects: A Modern Perspective

12

Alessandro Varrica, Alessandro Frigiola, Andrei Țăruș, and Alessandro Giamberti

Introduction

Brief Epidemiology

Advances in pediatric cardiology have transformed congenital heart disease (CHD) from a predominantly fatal condition in infancy to a chronic disease across the lifespan. In high-income countries, survival to adulthood now exceeds 97% among children born with CHD [1]. Consequently, the population of adults with CHD (ACHD) now surpasses the pediatric population [2, 3]. For example, data from the United States in 2010 reported approximately 2.4 million CHD survivors, of whom 1.4 million (~60%) were adults (~6.16 per 1000 adults) [3]. Globally, the estimated number of adults living with CHD is around 13 million [4]. This population is also aging: by 2010, two-thirds of CHD patients were adults, and projections suggest that 11% of ACHD patients will be aged 60 years or older by 2030 [3]. Although ACHD patients exhibit increased mortality compared to age-matched controls, more than 75% of those surviving to age 18 reach their sixties [5].

Today, ACHD patients are predominantly managed in specialized congenital heart centers. Both European and North American guidelines emphasize life-long structured care. The 2020 European Society of Cardiology (ESC) guidelines stress individualized decision-making, encompassing timing, risk stratification, and intervention selection [6, 7]. The 2018 American College of Cardiology (ACC)/American Heart Association (AHA) guidelines provide Class I recommendations for structured transition programs and sustained care throughout adulthood [7].

A. Varrica · A. Frigiola · A. Giamberti
IRCCS Policlinico San Donato, San Donato Milanese, Italy

A. Țăruș (✉)
Faculty of Medicine, University of Medicine and Pharmacy "Grigore T Popa", Iasi, Romania

Institute of Cardiovascular Diseases "Prof. Dr. George I.M. Georgescu", Iasi, Romania

G. Tinică, A. Burlacu (eds.), *Surgical, Hybrid and Minimally Invasive Structural Cardiac Interventions*, https://doi.org/10.1007/978-3-032-16676-0_12

Challenges in Transitioning to Adult CHD Care

Transitioning from pediatric to adult congenital care presents persistent clinical and psychosocial challenges. A significant proportion of CHD patients become lost to follow-up during adolescence, with only a minority successfully transferring to ACHD-specific services. In some cohorts, the transfer rate to ACHD centers is as low as 15% [2]. Barriers include reluctance to leave familiar pediatric providers, insufficient awareness of long-term care needs, geographic limitations, psychosocial stressors, and insurance-related issues. Structured transition programs, reinforced patient education, and interdisciplinary collaboration are essential to ensure safe and effective progression to adult care [2, 7].

Key Differences Between Pediatric and Adult CHD Patients

As CHD patients age, their clinical profile and healthcare needs evolve substantially. Pediatric CHD management predominantly focuses on anatomical correction, early survival, and prevention of developmental delays. In contrast, adult CHD care is defined by the need for long-term surveillance, management of acquired comorbidities, and prevention of late complications such as arrhythmias, progressive heart failure, and endocarditis.

Adults often present with surgically altered anatomy and may require re-intervention decades after initial repair. Furthermore, adults with CHD face unique life-stage challenges, including pregnancy, employment, and psychosocial adaptation, necessitating a broader and more nuanced care model. These distinctions require not only a different clinical skill set but also a shift in care philosophy toward multidisciplinary, individualized management. Differences in care models, clinical priorities, and complication profiles between pediatric and adult CHD populations are summarized in Table 12.1.

Tailored Interventions in Adult CHD Patients

The management of ACHD is inherently heterogeneous. A universal therapeutic approach is not feasible due to variation in anatomical complexity, prior interventions, hemodynamic status, comorbidities, and patient-specific goals [7, 8]. Contemporary guidelines emphasize personalized treatment strategies based on these variables [6].

Important factors influencing tailored intervention include:

- *Anatomical substrate:* Lesion-specific approaches are necessary, such as pulmonary valve replacement in repaired tetralogy of Fallot [7].
- *Surgical history:* Prior sternotomies increase reoperation risk, often favoring transcatheter or hybrid interventions [9].

Table 12.1 Key differences between pediatric and adult CHD patients

Parameter	Pediatric CHD	Adult CHD
Primary focus	Defect repair and survival	Long-term management and quality of life
Anatomy	Typically native anatomy	Post-surgical or post-interventional anatomy
Complications	Heart failure (acute), cyanosis	Arrhythmias, heart failure (chronic), endocarditis
Comorbidities	Usually absent	Often present (hypertension, diabetes, etc.)
Intervention goals	Definitive correction	Symptom control, re-intervention, prevention
Imaging	Echocardiography primary	Multimodality (echo, MRI, CT, 3D modeling)
Treatment approach	Protocol-driven	Highly individualized (tailored)
Care model	Pediatric cardiology-led	Multidisciplinary ACHD team

- *Physiological status:* Parameters such as ventricular function, pulmonary vascular resistance, and arrhythmia burden inform procedural planning [8, 10].
- *Comorbidities:* Conditions such as coronary artery disease or diabetes impact both procedural risk and post-intervention recovery [5, 7].
- *Patient-centered goals:* Considerations such as pregnancy planning, employment, and quality of life are critical to shared decision-making [8].

Advanced imaging modalities and interdisciplinary ACHD teams facilitate individualized treatment planning. Select patients may benefit from hybrid surgical-percutaneous procedures or pre-procedural 3D modeling. A proposed clinical pathway to guide these tailored interventions is illustrated in Fig. 12.1.

Comparison of Intervention Types in Adult CHD

The expanding population of adult CHD patients has led to a diversification of treatment approaches, including conventional surgery, catheter-based interventions, and hybrid strategies that combine both. Selection of the optimal intervention is highly patient-specific and depends on anatomical complexity, surgical history, comorbid burden, and patient preferences.

Surgical approaches remain the gold standard for complex repairs and situations where long-term durability is paramount. However, advancements in percutaneous technologies have enabled effective, less invasive alternatives for many conditions, such as transcatheter valve replacement and device closures. Hybrid procedures, which integrate surgical exposure with catheter-based therapy, are particularly useful for high-risk reoperations or anatomically challenging lesions.

The spectrum of interventions applied in ACHD care is outlined in Table 12.2, providing a comparative overview of indications, benefits, and limitations associated with each modality.

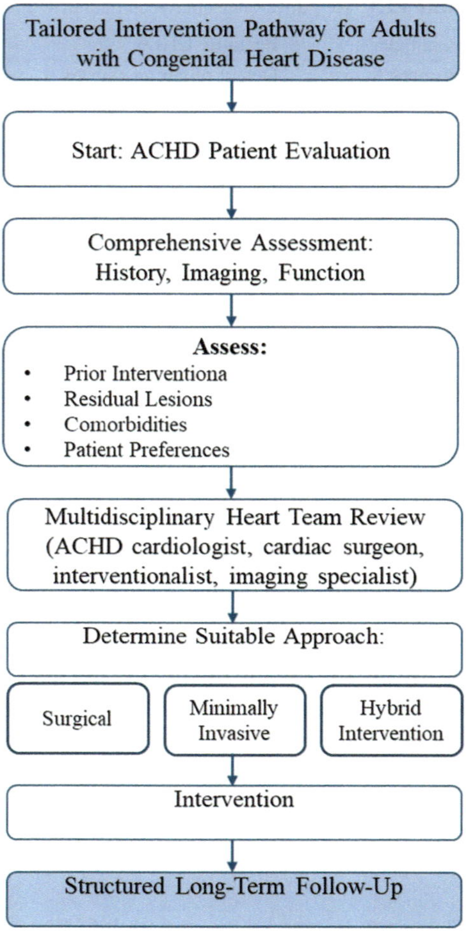

Fig. 12.1 Decision pathway for tailored interventions in adults with congenital heart disease

Table 12.2 Comparison of intervention types in adult CHD

Intervention type	Typical indications	Advantages	Limitations
Surgical	Complex re-operations, valve replacements, conduit revisions	Definitive repair, direct visualization, durability	Higher morbidity, longer recovery, adhesions from prior surgery
Minimally invasive	ASD/VSD closure, pulmonary valve implantation, coarctation stenting	Reduced trauma, faster recovery, often under conscious sedation	Limited by anatomy, device availability, vascular access
Hybrid	Multiple lesions, complex anatomy, re-intervention after surgery	Combines benefits of surgery and percutaneous methods	Requires specialized center, multidisciplinary team

Classification of Adult Congenital Heart Defects

ACHD is commonly classified by two key dimensions: the anatomical complexity of the defect (simple, moderate, or complex) and the surgical history (repaired vs. unrepaired lesions). This dual framework aids risk stratification, guides follow-up intensity, and informs long-term management.

Complexity of Defects: Simple vs. Complex

Simple lesions include defects such as small atrial septal defects (ASD), ventricular septal defects (VSD), and mild valvular lesions, which typically have minimal hemodynamic impact and low re-intervention rates [11]. In contrast, *complex defects* comprise more severe anomalies like tetralogy of Fallot (TOF), transposition of the great arteries (TGA), truncus arteriosus, and single-ventricle physiology, which usually require staged surgical palliation during infancy and necessitate lifelong specialized care [6, 12, 13]. Many adults with complex CHD are postoperative survivors with residual hemodynamic issues or prosthetic material that predispose them to late complications, including arrhythmias and heart failure [14, 15].

Repaired vs. Unrepaired Lesions

The surgical history of a CHD patient significantly influences their current physiological status and clinical risk. *Repaired lesions*—whether fully corrected or palliated—can still be associated with residual defects, valve dysfunction, and late sequelae, particularly if the repair was complex or performed late in childhood [16, 17]. In contrast, *unrepaired lesions* may either represent mild anomalies not requiring intervention or defects that progressed to inoperability (e.g., Eisenmenger physiology in large shunts). These patients are at heightened risk for complications such as pulmonary hypertension, cyanosis, and end-organ dysfunction [18].

Diagnostic Work-Up and Patient Stratification

Accurate diagnosis and effective stratification are essential components in the lifelong management of ACHD [19]. Likewise, tailored risk stratification tools have been developed to predict outcomes and aid clinical decision-making. Current international guidelines [6, 7] emphasize a multidisciplinary team approach to interpret these diagnostic findings and formulate individualized management plans.

Non-invasive Imaging Modalities

Transthoracic Echocardiography (TTE) remains the initial and most widely used modality due to its availability and capacity to evaluate ventricular function, valve hemodynamics, and residual shunts. However, echocardiography alone may be insufficient in postoperative or complex cases with poor acoustic windows [19]. For example, imaging the branch pulmonary arteries or venous connections by TTE can be suboptimal in certain anatomies (e.g., after an arterial switch or in anomalous pulmonary venous return), in which case advanced imaging is required.

Cardiac Magnetic Resonance Imaging (CMR) offers high-resolution, radiation-free evaluation of anatomy and function, and is particularly valuable for assessing right ventricular volume and function in repaired TOF and Fontan physiology [7]. It enables serial quantification of ventricular dimensions, myocardial fibrosis via late gadolinium enhancement, and flow measurements essential for procedural timing. When CMR is contraindicated, cardiac computed tomography (CT) provides excellent spatial resolution, particularly for assessing extracardiac structures, coronary anomalies, and calcified conduits.

Computer Tomography (CT) when CMR is contraindicated, cardiac CT provides excellent spatial resolution, particularly for assessing extracardiac structures, coronary anomalies, and calcified conduits, allows for rapid acquisition, and has been optimized to minimize radiation exposure [7, 20]. Three-dimensional modeling (Fig. 12.2), derived from CT or CMR datasets, has gained increasing application in pre-interventional planning for patients with complex anatomies [21].

Invasive Imaging and Hemodynamic Assessment

Cardiac catheterization remains a cornerstone diagnostic modality in selected ACHD patients. It provides direct hemodynamic measurements, allowing for the assessment of pulmonary artery pressures, pulmonary vascular resistance, shunt quantification (Qp:Qs), and ventricular end-diastolic pressures. This is particularly essential in patients with suspected pulmonary hypertension, complex shunt physiology, or unclear gradients not fully resolved by non-invasive imaging.

Additionally, catheterization enables coronary angiography in patients with a history of arterial switch, anomalous coronary arteries, or those over 40 years of age undergoing reintervention. Coronary angiography is crucial for identifying acquired coronary artery disease and evaluating coronary anatomy in complex congenital substrates prior to surgery or transcatheter procedures.

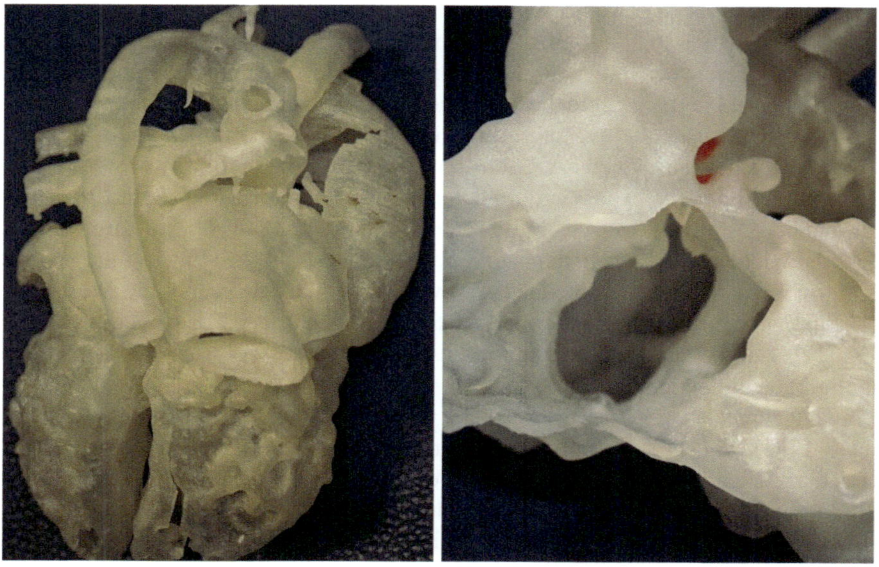

Fig. 12.2 3D reconstructed heart model in patients with double outlet right ventricle (DORV), evaluation for the creation of intra-cardiac baffle between VSD and aorta

Tailored Interventions for ASD and VSD in Adults

Introduction

ASDs and VSDs are common congenital heart lesions that often present or persist into adulthood. Timely closure of significant septal defects is indicated in adults to prevent complications such as right heart failure, arrhythmias, and pulmonary hypertension. Even in patients over 40 years old, repairing an ASD can improve long-term survival and functional status compared to leaving it untreated [22]. Multiple therapeutic approaches are available—including percutaneous transcatheter device closure, conventional surgical repair, and hybrid techniques—and the choice of intervention must be tailored to the patient's anatomy and clinical scenario. Key factors influencing the decision include defect size and location, the presence of adequate rims or support for device placement, coexistent cardiac issues (e.g., valve disease or arrhythmias), and the patient's surgical risk or preference.

Atrial Septal Defect in Adults

Transcatheter Closure Transcatheter device closure has become the preferred first-line treatment for secundum ASDs in adults due to its minimally invasive nature and excellent outcomes. Multiple studies and meta-analyses have shown that transcatheter ASD closure is as effective as surgery in achieving defect closure, with the added benefits of lower complication rates, shorter hospital stays, and faster recovery [23]. In a 2022 systematic review (33 studies), transcatheter closure had significantly fewer peri-procedural complications and a hospital stay about 4 days shorter on average than surgical repair. There was no significant difference in overall mortality between the two approaches in adults, underscoring that both are generally safe [24]. Transcatheter ASD closure also avoids the morbidity of sternotomy and cardiopulmonary bypass required for surgery. Notably, long-term data from adult cohorts show that survival after device closure is equivalent to surgical closure, though device-treated patients may have a small risk of needing re-intervention (e.g., for a residual shunt or device issue) within the first few years [25]. Most reinterventions occurred early and were related to residual leaks or device problems (Fig. 12.3), and overall findings support using transcatheter closure in the majority of eligible adult patients [25].

From a technical standpoint, transcatheter closure is suitable for persistent foramen ovale (PFO) (Fig. 12.4a) and ostium secundum ASDs with adequate rim tissue for device anchoring (Fig. 12.4b). Generally, defects up to ~35 mm in diameter can be closed with currently available occluder devices, provided there is at least a 5 mm rim of septal tissue around the hole (especially at the posterior-inferior and superior rims). Complex or atypical ASDs can present challenges: large secundum defects

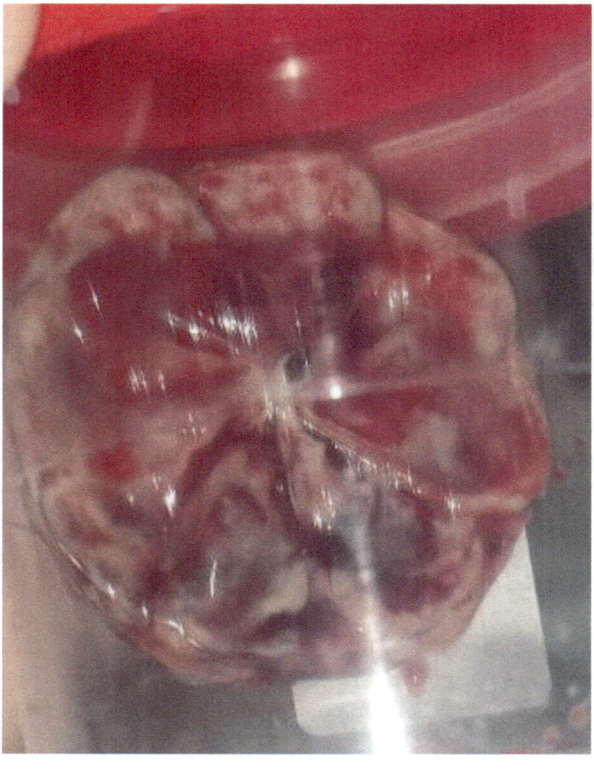

Fig. 12.3 ASD closure device extracted after thrombus formation

(>38–40 mm), multifenestrated septums, or those with deficient rims (e.g., near the vena cava or coronary sinus) may not securely hold a device. If an ASD is too large or lacks sufficient surrounding tissue, or if it is a different type (such as ostium primum or sinus venosus ASD), transcatheter closure is often not feasible and surgical repair is indicated [26]. Additionally, the presence of significant *pulmonary arterial hypertension* (PAH) can influence the strategy. Device closure can be performed in adults with moderately elevated pulmonary pressures as long as there is net left-to-right shunt, but if irreversible pulmonary vascular disease (Eisenmenger physiology) has developed, closure is contraindicated regardless of technique. Careful hemodynamic assessment (including shunt fraction Qp:Qs and pulmonary vascular resistance) is done in adults with long-standing ASDs to ensure it is safe to close the defect.

Surgical Repair Surgical closure of ASDs has been performed for decades and remains a very important option—especially for cases not amenable to devices. Surgically, a patch (often pericardium or synthetic material) is sewn over the septal opening via open-heart surgery. One major advantage of surgery is that virtually no defect is too large or complex to be closed; the surgeon can directly repair multi-hole or very large ASDs and address associated anomalies (such as anomalous pulmonary venous return in sinus venosus ASD, or valve clefts in primum ASD) during the same operation. In contrast to device closure, surgical closure is not limited by defect size or rim anatomy. Modern surgical outcomes for isolated ASD in adults are excellent. Operative mortality is extremely low in experienced centers, and long-term results are durable. For instance, a series of adult ASD surgical patients reported no early or late deaths and 25-year survival over 90% after suture or patch closure [27]. Goris et al. followed 28 adults who underwent surgical VSD/ASD closure and found no deaths and only one reoperation over an average 13-year follow-up. Surgical closure reliably eliminates the shunt and relieves right heart vol-

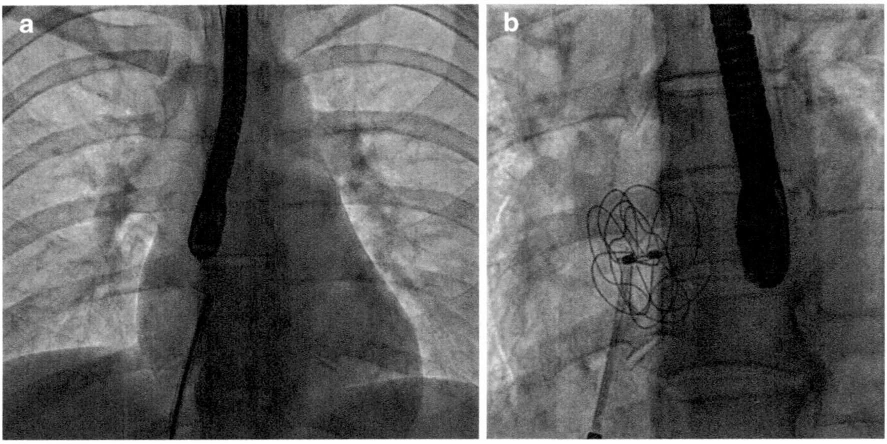

Fig. 12.4 (**a**) Delivery of PFO closure device. (**b**) ASD closed with septal occluder device

ume overload, leading to improvements in symptoms and cardiac remodeling. One consideration in older ASD patients is that longstanding atrial enlargement may have led to atrial arrhythmias (e.g., atrial fibrillation or flutter); closure of the defect may not reverse these arrhythmias, and indeed adults post-ASD repair should be monitored for arrhythmia onset. Some centers will perform a concomitant maze procedure or pulmonary vein isolation during ASD surgery if atrial fibrillation is present. Another consideration is tricuspid regurgitation (TR) secondary to right heart dilation—this often improves once the ASD is closed and RV volume overload is resolved. Notably, studies have shown that even without surgical tricuspid annuloplasty, significant functional TR can regress after percutaneous ASD closure due to normalization of right heart size and pressures [28]. If TR is severe, however, a surgical approach allows the opportunity to perform a tricuspid valve repair (annuloplasty) at the time of ASD patching for optimal results. Overall, surgery "still has a place" for ASD treatment in adults [24], especially for defects unsuitable for device closure or when concomitant surgical procedures are needed. With minimally invasive techniques (such as mini-thoracotomy or robotic-assisted ASD closure), the surgical impact can be reduced, though these are specialized approaches. The choice between device vs surgery should be individualized: transcatheter closure is favored for eligible secundum ASDs given its lower morbidity, while surgery is reserved for non-secundum defects, very large or unfavorably located secundum ASDs, or patients requiring additional repairs.

Ventricular Septal Defect in Adults

Indications and Challenges Ventricular septal defects in adults are less common than ASDs because large VSDs usually present in infancy and are repaired early, or else may lead to severe pulmonary hypertension if unrepaired. Nonetheless, some adults have unrepaired moderate congenital VSDs, residual post-surgical VSDs, or (less commonly) acquired defects (e.g., post-myocardial infarction VSD, which is a distinct scenario). Indications for closing a congenital VSD in adulthood include evidence of significant left-to-right shunt (typically Qp:Qs >1.5) with left heart volume overload, significant chamber enlargement, or clinical symptoms such as exercise intolerance. Even asymptomatic moderate VSDs are often closed in adults to prevent long-term complications like heart failure, arrhythmias, or infective endocarditis. Another common indication is aortic regurgitation (AR) due to VSD prolapse—VSDs in the membranous or outlet septum can lead to aortic cusp prolapse and AR over time; repairing the VSD can stabilize or improve the valve function if done early. On the other hand, if a VSD has led to severe pulmonary vascular disease, closure is contraindicated. Thus, similar to ASD, a careful hemodynamic assessment is done; adults with VSD and elevated pulmonary artery pressures may undergo vasodilator testing to determine if closure is possible without causing hemodynamic collapse.

Transcatheter Device Closure Less invasive transcatheter closure of VSDs has been developed over the past two decades, but its application in adults is more limited and technically complex than ASD closure. Still, for certain VSD types, percutaneous closure offers a valuable alternative to surgery. The best candidates are muscular VSDs—these are often accessible via catheter from the venous or arterial side and have an ample rim of muscle for device seating (Fig. 12.5). Many muscular VSDs in adults are small and may not require intervention unless symptomatic; however, sizable muscular defects causing volume overload can be successfully closed with devices. Perimembranous VSDs (located in the membranous septum near the aortic valve) represent the most common type of VSD and are more challenging for transcatheter closure due to proximity to the cardiac conduction system and adjacent valves. There are occluder devices designed for perimembranous VSDs (e.g., the Amplatzer perimembranous VSD Occluder), but in some regions these have been restricted or withdrawn over concerns of heart block. Nonetheless, experienced centers (particularly in Asia and Europe) have reported success with device closure of perimembranous VSDs in carefully selected patients. A meta-analysis of 7 studies (3134 patients, including children and some adults) found that percutaneous closure of perimembranous VSDs achieved similar procedural success as surgical repair (≈99% in both) when patients were appropriately selected, without a higher risk of major complications like complete heart block or significant valvular regurgitation [29]. Notably, there was no statistical difference in the rate of complete heart block between device vs surgical closure in these studies (pooled risk ~1% in each group) [29]. This suggests that with current techniques, transcatheter closure can be done safely in the short term, though careful patient selection is critical. The same meta-analysis showed that device closure was associated with significantly shorter hospital stays and virtually eliminated the need for blood trans-

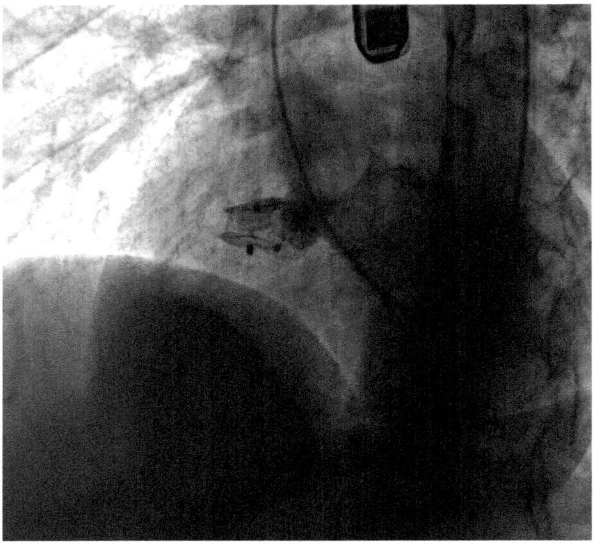

Fig. 12.5 Implantation of 2 septal occluders for muscular VSD closure

fusions compared to surgery [29], underscoring the less invasive nature of the percutaneous approach.
Technical advances have improved the safety of VSD device closure. One major concern historically was complete atrioventricular block (cAVB) due to device pressure on the delicate atrioventricular conduction bundle (especially in perimembranous VSDs). More recent long-term data are encouraging: in a large single-center experience with 149 transcatheter VSD closures (pediatric and adult patients, 104 perimembranous), the incidence of complete heart block was only 0.7% (1 out of 149) during a median 6-year follow-up [30]. Other studies similarly report high success with muscular VSD devices—Chessa et al. treated 40 adult VSD patients (both muscular and perimembranous) with devices and had no device embolizations or procedural deaths; about 15% had minor complications (most commonly transient arrhythmias) [31]. In that series, one complex case with a residual post-surgical VSD did ultimately require surgery after device implantation due to persistent leak, highlighting that some device closures may need a backup surgical solution.

In summary, transcatheter VSD closure is an effective treatment in adults when anatomy is favorable. It is most often employed for muscular VSDs or small-to-moderate perimembranous VSDs with sufficient rims and distance from valves. Advantages include avoidance of open-heart surgery and quicker recovery; however, meticulous attention is required to minimize conduction injury (e.g., sizing the device not too oversized, and monitoring the ECG closely during and after the procedure). Long-term surveillance after device closure is important, as latent heart block can (rarely) develop days to weeks post-procedure—patients are often kept on telemetry for a few days and followed with regular ECGs [30]. Also, any residual shunt or new valve regurgitation would need follow-up, though significant persisting defects are uncommon when the device is well-seated.

Surgical VSD Closure Surgery remains the gold-standard therapy for VSDs, especially for large perimembranous or doubly-committed VSDs in adults. Surgical repair typically involves a patch closure via a ventriculotomy or through the right atrium (for membranous defects near the tricuspid valve). The strengths of surgery are its reliability and completeness: a surgeon can directly close virtually any VSD and simultaneously address associated issues (such as repairing an aortic valve cusp if prolapse/AR is present, or closing multiple VSDs if more than one defect exists). In an adult patient, if there is significant AR resulting from the VSD, surgery allows for correction of both the VSD and the aortic valve (either repair or replacement) in one setting. Surgical outcomes in adult VSD patients are generally very good, although data are from relatively small series since it's uncommon to operate on VSDs de novo in adulthood. In one study of adults (mean age ~40) undergoing surgical VSD closure, there was no operative mortality and long-term follow-up showed excellent quality of life [27]. The most frequent long-term issue was mild residual aortic regurgitation in some patients (especially those who already had valve prolapse), but no patient progressed to severe heart failure . Surgical closure, of course, carries the general risks of open-heart surgery, including a small but non-zero risk of complications like bleeding, infection, or stroke, and a recovery period due to the sternotomy. However, with modern techniques, most adult VSD surgical patients recover uneventfully and enjoy improvement in symptoms. Notably, surgery virtually eliminates the VSD shunt immediately, which can be critical in cases of large shunts or endocarditis. In the context of endocarditis on a VSD, surgery allows debridement of infected tissue and patch closure in a controlled manner, which is often lifesaving. Also, unlike device closure, surgical closure is not constrained by weight or vascular access, so it is the only option in cases where a device can't be delivered—though this is less relevant in adults who usually have adequate access.

When weighing device vs. surgery for a VSD in an adult, the defect's anatomy is paramount. For a moderate-size perimembranous VSD with good margins and no severe valve prolapse, a transcatheter approach *may* be possible in an experienced center, potentially sparing the patient a sternotomy. On the other hand, for a large perimembranous VSD (especially if >8–10 mm or with anterior extension), or if there is important associated AR, surgery is the safer and more definitive choice. The 2018 American guidelines on adult congenital heart disease also suggest that closure (by any method) should be undertaken if the shunt is significant and pulmonary pressures are not prohibitive, to prevent deterioration [7]. Importantly, if a transcatheter attempt is made and fails (e.g., device cannot be safely positioned or a complication occurs), prompt conversion to surgical repair is indicated—hence such procedures are done with a surgical backup team available. Fortunately, the need for urgent surgical bailout in elective device closures is rare.

Hybrid Perventricular Approach A specialized hybrid technique has been developed that blurs the line between surgery and percutaneous intervention. In a hybrid VSD closure, a surgeon provides a small access (often a mini thoracotomy or subxiphoid incision) to the beating heart, and an occluder device is delivered through the myocardium into the VSD under echocardiographic guidance—all without cardiopulmonary bypass. This approach is especially useful for muscular VSDs that are not easily reached via traditional transcatheter routes (for example, an apical muscular VSD in a small child), and it avoids the need for a full open-heart procedure. In pediatric patients and some adults, hybrid closure has been shown to be safe and effective in experienced centers. A recent comparative study in children demonstrated that the hybrid method can achieve outcomes similar to open surgery, with the added benefits of shorter operation times, shorter hospital stays, and improved cosmetic results [32]. In that study, hybrid VSD closure was performed in a select group and had high success, highlighting it as a viable alternative [32]. For adults, hybrid approaches are less commonly needed (since transcatheter from the groin is usually feasible given larger patient size), but they might be considered in scenarios such as: an adult with multiple VSDs where some can be patched surgically and others closed with a device in the same session, or in a high-risk surgical patient where avoiding cardiopulmonary bypass is desired. Hybrid ASD closures are rarely reported (ASDs are readily accessible by transcatheter in most cases), but conceptually a minimally invasive surgical assist could be used if needed (for instance, to place a device directly through an atrial wall puncture in challenging anatomy).

Overall, the hybrid technique exemplifies a tailored approach—combining the strengths of surgery and catheterization—and can be reserved for patients who fall in the gray zone between one method and the other.

Management of Aortic Coarctation in Adults: Tailored Procedural Selection and Techniques

Introduction

Coarctation of the aorta (CoA) is a congenital narrowing of the aortic arch, comprising about 5–10% of congenital heart defects [33, 34]. While often diagnosed and repaired in infancy, some patients reach adulthood with untreated or residual CoA. Adult presentations include native coarctation (Fig. 12.6), re-coarctation after childhood repair, and post-repair complications such as aneurysms at the repair site. Untreated CoA leads to severe hypertension and early cardiovascular mortality (mean survival ~35 years) [34]. Thus, intervention is indicated in adults with significant CoA (generally a peak gradient >20 mmHg or >50% luminal narrowing with hypertension) [35]. Multiple treatment modalities are available—catheter-based interventions, open surgical repair, and hybrid approaches—and the optimal strategy must be individualized. Historically, open surgery (resection and end-to-end anastomosis) was the standard from the first repair in 1944 through the late twentieth century [36]. Transcatheter techniques emerged in the 1980s (balloon angioplasty) and 1990s (stent implantation) to avoid thoracotomy in older patients [37]. Today, most adult CoA patients are managed with endovascular stenting, although surgical or hybrid repair is selected in certain anatomical or patient scenarios.

Catheter-Based Interventions

Balloon Angioplasty Stand-alone balloon dilatation was one of the first transcatheter therapies for CoA. It can acutely relieve obstruction but has a high incidence of elastic recoil and intimal injury in adults, often leading to residual gradients or aneurysm formation [38]. As a result, balloon angioplasty alone is now seldom used in adults except in specific scenarios (e.g., as a palliative measure or when stenting is contraindicated).

Endovascular Stenting Endovascular stent implantation is the cornerstone of adult CoA treatment (Fig. 12.7). Large observational studies have shown that stenting achieves excellent immediate gradient reduction comparable to surgery, with lower acute complication rates and shorter hospital stay [38]. Stents provide radial support to prevent recoil and protect against vessel wall tears better than ballooning alone. Both bare-metal and covered stents are available. Bare-metal stents (e.g., balloon-expandable stainless steel stents) were common in early practice but are increasingly replaced by covered stent grafts in adults. Covered stents can seal inti-

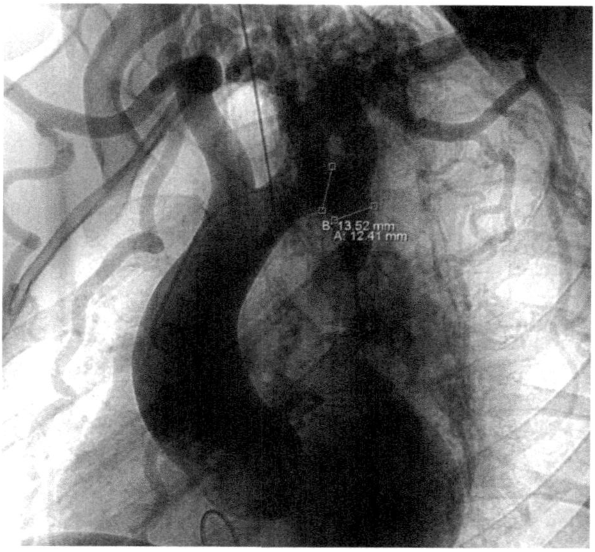

Fig. 12.6 Natural history of coarctation of aorta in a 23-year-old patient

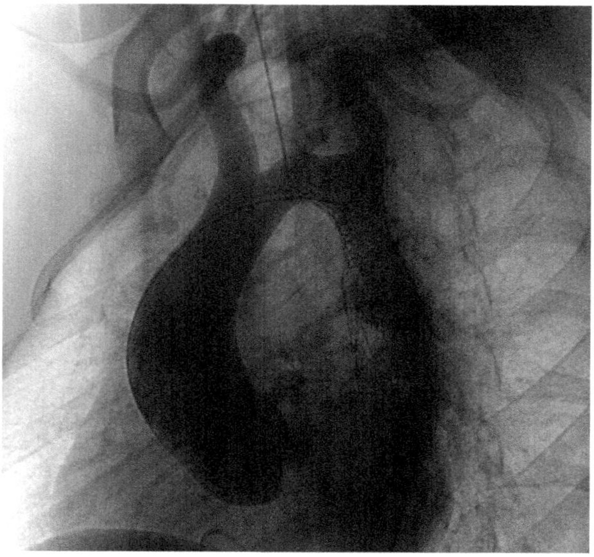

Fig. 12.7 Final result after endovascular treatment of aortic coarctation

mal tears and exclude aneurysms, reducing the risk of catastrophic rupture [39]. Modern series report primary use of covered stents for native adult CoA, reserving bare stents for select cases (such as very tortuous anatomy or when covering a branch is undesirable) [39]. For example, in a multicenter study of 93 adults (mean age 44) treated endovascularly, over 90% received either a balloon-expandable covered stent or a longer stent-graft, whereas only ~10% received an uncovered stent [39]. This shift reflects the priority to minimize aortic wall injury in older patients.

The immediate outcomes of stenting in adults are excellent. Stent placement typically reduces the peak systolic pressure gradient to near-zero (from ~20–30 mmHg down to <5–10 mmHg), with a high procedural success rate [39].
Unlike surgery, stenting avoids thoracotomy and has no risk of spinal cord ischemia in the short segment typically treated; hospital stays are significantly shorter (often 1–3 days) than with open repair [38]. On the other hand, stented patients require lifelong imaging surveillance for stent integrity and may need planned re-interventions. Particularly, young adults treated with a relatively small stent may undergo staged redilatation as they grow or if residual gradient appears [34]. Even in fully grown adults, approximately 10–15% of cases require a re-intervention within 5 years, often for minor restenosis or to extend the stent in a long-segment lesion [39].

Open Surgical Repair

Open surgery via left thoracotomy remains an important option, especially for anatomically complex coarctations and in young, low-risk patients. Several surgical techniques are available, chosen according to CoA anatomy:

Resection with End-to-End Anastomosis The classic operation involves excising the coarcted segment and directly suturing the ends of the aorta together. In adults, this is feasible for discrete coarctations with adequately mobile aortic ends. However, adults often have a rigid aorta and extensive collateral vessels, limiting mobility. Thus, simple end-to-end repair is less often possible in older patients. When achievable, it eliminates the diseased segment entirely and reconstructs a normal aortic continuity. Historically, in infants this approach had high re-coarctation rates due to a small anastomosis, but in adults re-stenosis is less common if a tension-free repair is attained [35].

Patch Aortoplasty This technique (opening the coarctation longitudinally and sewing in a patch to enlarge the lumen) was once used to reduce recurrence rates. However, patch repairs in early series led to aneurysm formation in 20–40% of cases, as the native wall opposite the patch dilated over time [40]. Even with improved materials (PTFE patches), aneurysm risk remained appreciable. Consequently, patch aortoplasty is now generally avoided in adults. Leaving the abnormal aortic tissue in situ with a patch is considered suboptimal due to the risk of pseudoaneurysm at the repair site.

Interposition Graft Replacement In contemporary adult practice, a common surgical approach is resection of the coarctation followed by insertion of a prosthetic Dacron graft to bridge the gap (Fig. 12.8). This is performed via a left posterolateral thoracotomy. Many centers favor graft interposition in adults because it ensures a wide, turbulence-free repair and maintains native aortic continuity without tension [41]. Meticulous surgical technique is required to avoid injury to adjacent structures

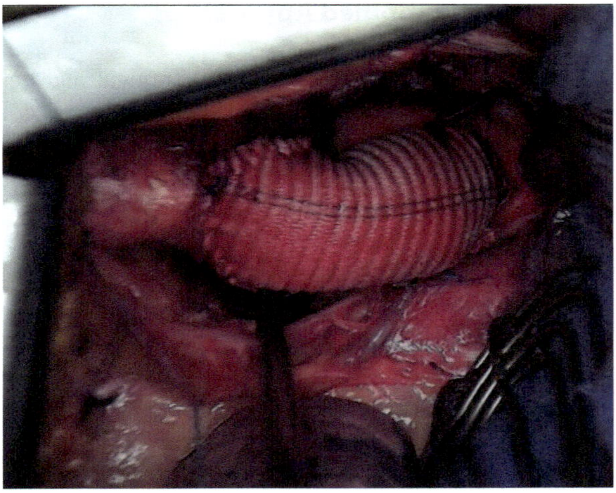

Fig. 12.8 Dacron tube that bridges the coarctation gap

(recurrent laryngeal nerve, vagus nerve, esophagus) and to control extensive intercostal collaterals that may cause bleeding. Use of partial cardiopulmonary bypass (left heart bypass) during the repair can maintain distal perfusion and reduce ischemia to the spinal cord and abdominal organs, especially in longer repairs [34]. With graft repairs, results are excellent: operative mortality in experienced centers is near 0%, and strokes or paraplegia are exceedingly rare [41].

Extra-Anatomic Bypass In complex or re-do scenarios, an extra-anatomic bypass can be employed—typically an ascending-to-descending aortic bypass graft placed via a median sternotomy (tunneling the graft through the posterior pericardium). This approach is especially useful if the coarctation is long or involves the arch, or if the patient simultaneously requires open heart surgery (e.g., aortic valve replacement) [42]. A large single-center series of 80 adult patients with "complex" CoA demonstrated that ascending-to-descending bypass can be performed with low morbidity and 0% early mortality [42]. In that study, many patients had extensive arch hypoplasia or previous failed repairs; concomitant cardiac procedures (e.g., valve replacement, CABG) were often done in the same operation. The 5- and 10-year outcomes showed excellent relief of upperbody hypertension and a 94% survival at 10 years [42]. This underscores that extra-anatomic bypass is a safe, effective one-stage solution for adults with CoA and other cardiac lesions, avoiding the need for two separate surgeries. Some experts, however, reserve this method for cases where a lateral thoracotomy repair is not feasible. Others argue that a well-done aortic graft replacement via the left chest is preferable to an extra-anatomic route for long-term flow dynamics [34]. In practice, the choice may depend on the surgeon's exposure: for instance, a patient with severe arch hypoplasia plus aortic valve disease might best be served by a median sternotomy to address both, whereas an isolated but long coarctation might be handled by an ascending-to-descending bypass or a staged hybrid.

Hybrid and Combined Approaches

Hybrid approaches—combining open surgical and endovascular techniques—are employed for adults with coarctation in the setting of complex anatomy or concomitant pathology. The goal of a hybrid strategy is to minimize the invasiveness of repair while still addressing issues that a single modality cannot optimally treat alone. Common scenarios include:

- *CoA with Arch Vessel Involvement:* If the coarctation or an associated aneurysm invades on the aortic arch (near or involving the left subclavian or left common carotid artery), a purely endovascular stent might require covering major branches. In such cases, a hybrid approach can preserve branch perfusion. For example, surgeons may perform a carotid-subclavian bypass or ascending-to-subclavian bypass to revascularize the left arm, then an endovascular stent-graft is deployed across the coarctation extending into the arch without causing arm ischemia [43]. This strategy is used for proximal thoracic aortic stent grafting when the left subclavian artery needs to be sacrificed for an adequate landing zone.
- *CoA with Large Aneurysm (Post-Repair or Native):* Patients who developed a sizable aneurysm at a prior coarctation repair site (e.g., a Dacron patch aneurysm) or a concomitant aneurysm just distal to a coarctation represent high-risk cases. Open redo surgery for a pseudoaneurysm can be challenging and hazardous. A hybrid operation can be performed: for instance, an "elephant trunk" procedure (open surgical graft placed in the arch with a free distal end) followed by a second-stage endovascular completion into the descending aorta. Modern variations include the frozen elephant trunk, where a stent-graft is sewn onto the end of an arch graft and deployed downstream in the same operation. In a Cleveland Clinic series of 14 adults with prior coarctation repairs who developed large post-coarctation aneurysms, hybrid repairs (open arch surgery combined with endograft insertion) were executed with 0% perioperative mortality and no strokes or paralysis [43]. As an example, one hybrid strategy is a two-stage approach: first, a surgical graft is placed from the ascending aorta to just beyond the left subclavian (fixing arch pathology), and second, an endovascular stent-graft is placed to bridge the distal arch/ upper descending aorta (covering the coarctation and aneurysm) [43].
- *CoA with Concomitant Cardiac Lesions:* Adults with coarctation often have other cardiac abnormalities, notably bicuspid aortic valve (with stenosis or root dilation) or coronary artery disease. A hybrid approach allows simultaneous treatment. For example, a patient with severe aortic valve disease and coarctation might undergo surgical aortic valve replacement and ascending aorta replacement via sternotomy, and in the same setting or staged, have a stent placed in the descending aorta to relieve the coarctation. This avoids the need for a second large open procedure via thoracotomy. Similarly, if cardiopulmonary bypass is initiated for an intracardiac repair, the team can also elect to repair the coarctation under the same anesthesia by placing a stent via a trans-femoral route or via

the open aorta (an antegrade stent delivery through the opened ascending aorta). Hybrid open/endovascular methods thus offer a tailored solution for patients with "multi-level" disease. In all these approaches, careful heart team planning is essential. Decisions on hybrid strategies consider the exact location of disease, urgency (e.g., impending aneurysm rupture may prompt an endovascular-first approach), and patient condition. Notably, the presence of an aneurysm or arch hypoplasia may force a hybrid or open solution when endovascular alone would be suboptimal (for instance, if there is no safe landing zone for a stent graft due to proximity of the left carotid artery).

Decision Criteria for Modality Selection

Choosing the optimal treatment for an adult with coarctation involves evaluating multiple patient-specific and anatomical factors.

Lesion Anatomy and Location The morphology of the coarctation is a primary determinant. A short, discrete coarctation in the typical juxtaductal location is ideal for stenting, as endovascular outcomes are superb in this setting [40]. Conversely, long-segment narrowing or arch hypoplasia may favor a surgical or hybrid approach. If the transverse arch is significantly small or the coarctation extends over a lengthy aorta, placing multiple stents or a very long stent graft can be less effective or risk covering great vessels. In such cases, an extended end-to-end surgical repair or an ascending-to-descending bypass with or without stent assistance may yield a more complete relief. Lesions very close to the left subclavian artery origin also raise concern: a stent might occlude the subclavian artery. If coverage of the subclavian is anticipated and the patient has robust collaterals, a covered stent may be placed deliberately across it (accepting sacrifice of that artery), but often surgeons will revascularize or transpose the subclavian first (hybrid strategy). Thus, coarctations involving the arch or proximal descending aorta require a tailored plan balancing open vs endo.

Presence of Aneurysm or Fragile Aorta An associated aortic aneurysm or a history of prior patch repair that has dilated is a strong indication for using covered stent technology or a hybrid approach. Endovascular repair is generally preferred for post-surgical pseudoaneurysms because it avoids re-dissection of scarred tissue and can exclude the aneurysm with a graft. For example, in adults with prior coarctation patch repairs who develop aneurysmal degeneration, covered stentgrafts have become the treatment of choice, showing high success in excluding aneurysms with low complication rates. If the aneurysm is large or involves the arch, a combined open plus TEVAR approach may be needed as discussed. In contrast, if no aneurysm is present and the aortic wall appears healthy, a bare-metal stent might suffice for a simple narrowing. Overall, a "fragile" aorta (older age, extensive calcification, or cystic medial changes) pushes the decision toward covered stents or surgical replacement to mitigate rupture risk.

Patient Age and Comorbidities Patient characteristics heavily influence modality. Younger adult patients (e.g., in their 20s–30s), especially those who are otherwise healthy and active, may be candidates for surgery if the anatomy is not amenable to an easy stent. Surgical repair in a young, low-risk adult offers a one-and-done solution with possibly lower re-intervention rates. On the other hand, older patients or those with significant comorbidities (e.g., COPD, prior thoracotomy, frailty) are often better served by endovascular treatment due to the higher risk of open surgery. In practice, many adults over 50 years or with significant medical issues will be steered toward stenting unless contraindicated.

History of Prior Coarctation Repair Whether the patient has had a previous repair (and what type) is crucial. Re-coarctation after childhood surgery frequently occurs in a scarred segment that might be complex to reoperate. Transcatheter stenting has shown excellent results for recurrent coarctation and avoids the high risk of redo thoracotomy. Indeed, current guidelines and experiences recommend catheter-based intervention as first-line for adults with prior coarctation repair who present with a re-narrowing [6, 7]. The heart team should review the prior operative reports, imaging, and current anatomy to decide if a different modality now is advantageous.

Concurrent Cardiac Pathologies Coarctation in adults is frequently accompanied by other issues like bicuspid aortic valve disease (aortic stenosis or regurgitation) and ascending aortic aneurysm, or less commonly, ventricular septal defect and others. The need to address these conditions can dictate the approach. If an adult requires open heart surgery for valve or ascending aorta, it may be prudent to handle the coarctation in the same hospitalization via a one-stage or staged hybrid strategy. For example, an adult with a large ascending aneurysm and coarctation might undergo ascending aortic replacement (open) plus stenting of the coarctation in a planned hybrid sequence. Alternatively, some surgeons perform an ascending-to-descending bypass during the valve/aorta surgery to simultaneously relieve the coarctation without needing a stent. On the other hand, if the coarctation is the only issue or accompanied only by systemic hypertension, an endovascular-first approach spares the patient an open operation. The presence of significant aortic valve disease or coronary disease pushes the decision toward involving open surgical components.

Technical Considerations Finally, certain technical factors can influence strategy. Vascular access is one; most adult CoA stents are delivered via femoral arteries. If an adult has severely diseased or small femoral/iliac arteries that cannot accommodate a large sheath, alternative routes (transsubclavian or surgical conduit on the aorta) are options, but these add complexity and might tilt toward open repair in some cases. The risk of spinal cord ischemia is low for localized coarctation repairs, but if a very long stent graft is needed (extending far down the descending aorta), the team might stage the procedure or use spinal drains as precautions—considerations more relevant in extensive stent-grafting than in focal coarctation stenting. If such extensive coverage is anticipated, a hybrid or open surgical approach with lower spinal risk may be favored. Another factor is the urgency of intervention: in hypertensive emergencies or heart failure due to CoA, a quicker endovascular solution may be chosen for prompt relief.

Conclusions

Adult aortic coarctation is a complex condition that requires individualized management. A variety of interventional, surgical, and hybrid techniques are available, each with distinct advantages depending on patient and anatomical factors. Endovascular stenting has become first-line therapy for most adult coarctations due to its high efficacy and low invasiveness, particularly in native or recurrent narrowings that are discrete and in patients for whom surgery poses higher risk. Open surgical repair (via graft interposition or bypass) remains crucial for cases with long-segment disease, arch hypoplasia, or in young healthy patients where a one-time durable fix is desired. Hybrid approaches combining surgery and catheter techniques exemplify the heart-team strategy in managing associated pathologies—for instance, addressing an arch aneurysm or valvular lesion surgically while relieving the coarctation with a stent in the same setting. Optimal results are achieved by tailoring the treatment modality to the patient's anatomy, prior intervention history, and overall clinical condition.

Tailored Interventions in Adult TOF Patients Post-surgical Repair

Introduction

TOF is a congenital cardiac anomaly that has seen dramatically improved survival due to early surgical repair [44]. In the modern era, over 90% of TOF patients reach adulthood after primary repair in infancy. However, "repaired" TOF is not cured—most adults have residual hemodynamic lesions and progressive sequelae that require ongoing surveillance and intervention [45]. The most frequent issues in adults with repaired TOF include chronic pulmonary regurgitation (due to transannular patch or valvotomy in the initial repair), residual VSD or right ventricular outflow tract (RVOT) obstruction, and progressive aortic root dilatation with aortic valve regurgitation. These can lead to right ventricular (RV) volume overload, arrhythmias (notably ventricular tachycardia associated with QRS prolongation >180 ms), left ventricular (LV) dysfunction, and risk of sudden cardiac death.

Pulmonary Valve Replacement (PVR) in Adult TOF

Chronic pulmonary regurgitation (PR) is the most prevalent residual lesion after TOF repair. Surgical relief of RVOT obstruction often involves disrupting the pulmonary valve, leading to free PR in ~80% of cases. PR is initially well-tolerated, but over years it causes progressive RV volume overload, dilation, and systolic dysfunction [46]. PR has been shown to be a key determinant of RV contractile dysfunction in repaired TOF, and chronic PR contributes to ventricular arrhythmias and exercise intolerance. Approximately 35–40% of TOF patients undergo PVR within 30 years of initial repair [9], underscoring how commonly this intervention is needed in adulthood.

Surgical PVR—Technique and Outcomes Surgical pulmonary valve replacement remains the standard for most adult TOF patients, especially those with large RVOTs or concomitant lesions. It is typically performed via median resternotomy with cardiopulmonary bypass. If significant RVOT aneurysm or scar tissue is present, that tissue is resected and a viable outflow tract is reconstructed. Bioprosthetic valves (e.g., bovine jugular vein grafts or porcine valves mounted in a conduit) are most commonly used for the pulmonary position, as mechanical valves carry high risk of thrombosis in the low-pressure RVOT and would mandate lifelong anticoagulation (Fig. 12.9). A homograft is another option, especially if the RVOT requires replacement of a large conduit. At surgery, any residual subpulmonary muscle bundles can be resected and branch pulmonary artery stenoses addressed with patch angioplasty if needed. The tricuspid valve is often evaluated; if significant TR is present, an annuloplasty may be performed concurrently to improve RV function post-PVR. In addition, many centers perform intraoperative cryoablation or arrhythmia lesion set (e.g., right atrial isthmus ablation or ventricular scar incision) in patients with documented arrhythmias, aiming to reduce post-PVR tachyarrhythmia recurrence. These concomitant procedures contribute to a comprehensive "tailored" surgical approach. Surgical PVR in experienced hands has low operative risk. Contemporary series report perioperative mortality <1% [47]. In a meta-analysis of 3118 patients, pooled 30-day mortality was 0.87% and 5-year survival ~97.8%, highlighting the excellent early and mid-term outcomes [47].

The main drawback of surgical PVR is the limited lifespan of bioprosthetic valves. All bioprostheses will eventually degenerate or calcify, typically within 10–15 years, necessitating redo PVR (Fig. 12.10). In fact, the meta-analysis noted that about 4.9% of patients required a redo PVR by 5 years, and 15–20% by 10 years is common [47]. Therefore, a young adult TOF patient may expect two to three PVRs in their lifetime if done surgically. This has driven interest in less invasive options and in optimizing the timing (to delay initial PVR until absolutely indicated but not waiting so long as to incur irreversible harm). Nonetheless, surgical PVR remains extremely effective at alleviating PR and improving hemodynamics in the near term. Long-term survival after PVR is high, with studies showing >90% 10-year survival and low incidence of sudden death or heart failure [48]. Most patients feel symptomatic relief and increased exercise tolerance within months after the procedure.

Transcatheter PVR—Technique and Outcomes In the last 15 years, transcatheter pulmonary valve implantation (TPVI) has emerged as an important alternative to

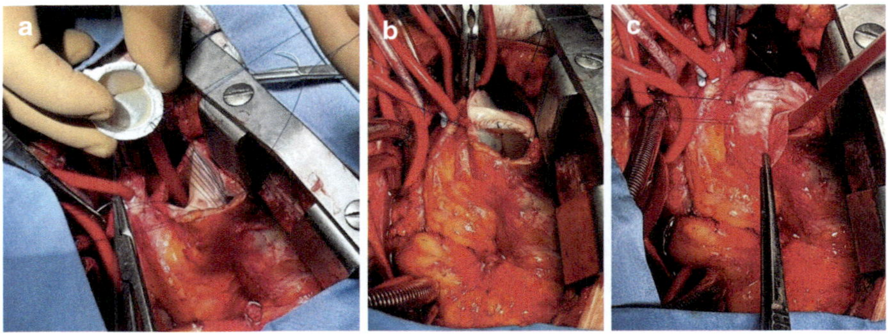

Fig. 12.9 (**a**) Suture of the bioprosthesis in pulmonary position. (**b**) Bioprosthesis fixed in pulmonary position with sutured pericardial patch for anterior wall reconstruction. (**c**) Trimming of the pericardial patch for proper pulmonary artery and right ventricular closure

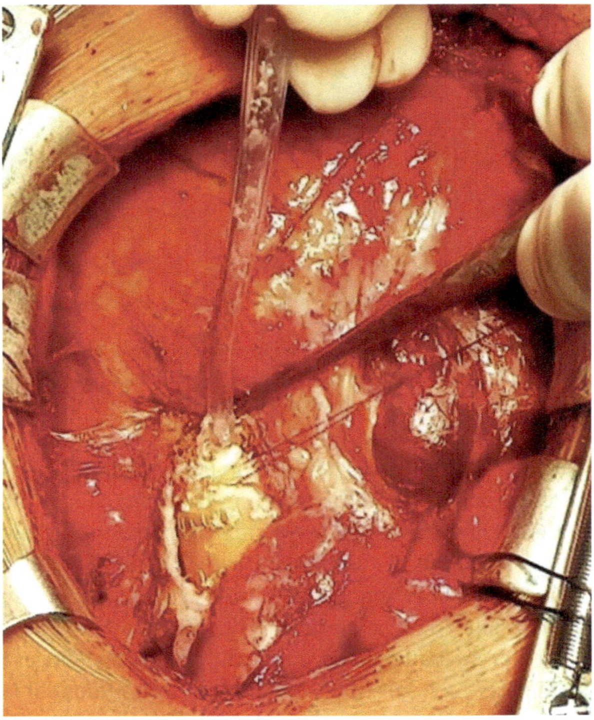

Fig. 12.10 Calcified biointegral bioconduit in pulmonary position after previous ToF repair

open PVR in selected TOF patients. TPVI is less invasive and is particularly attractive for patients with a pre-existing RV-PA conduit or bioprosthetic valve that has become regurgitant or stenotic. The two most commonly used devices are the Melody valve (Medtronic)—a bovine jugular vein valve mounted in a stent and the Edwards Sapien 3 valve (a balloon-expandable bovine pericardial valve, originally

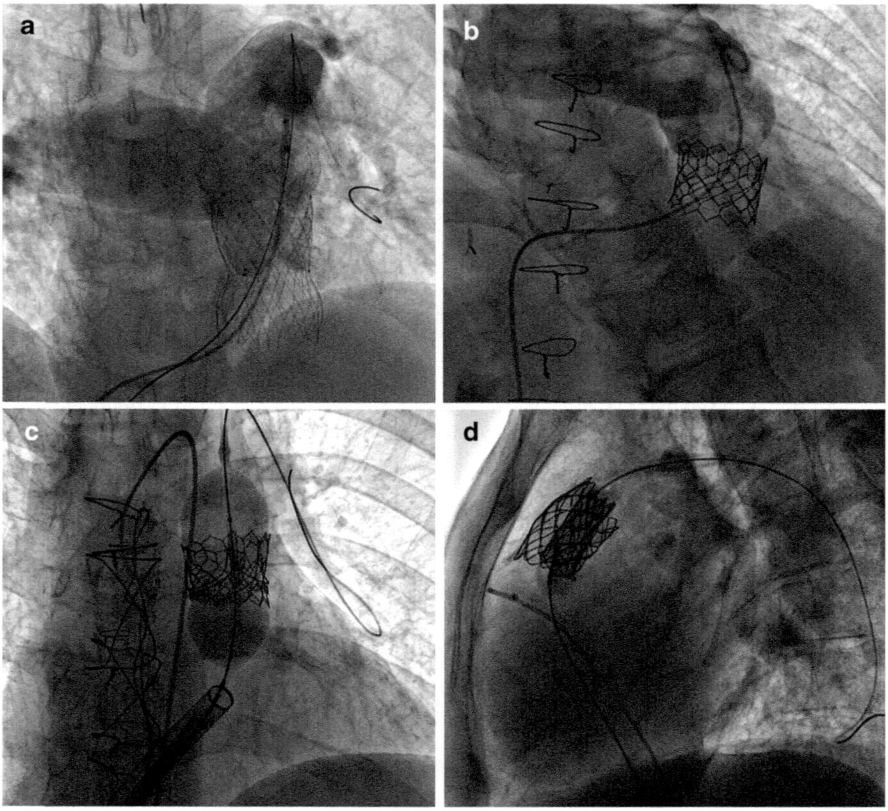

Fig. 12.11 (**a**) TPVI with self-expandable prosthesis. (**b**) TPVI with balloon-expandable prosthesis. (**c**) TPVI valve-in-valve procedure with balloon-expandable prosthesis. (**d**) TPVI with balloon-expandable prosthesis on previously implanted stent for support

for aortic position, used off-label in pulmonary position). More recently, newer TPV systems such as the self-expanding Harmony valve (for large native outflow tracts) and the Alterra adaptive pre-stent + Sapien system have been approved to expand TPVI to patients with enlarged native RVOTs not suitable for Melody or Sapien alone [49]. These innovations have extended catheter-based therapy to a broader range of adult TOF anatomies (Fig. 12.11).

Not every patient is a candidate for TPVI. Generally, TPVI is favored if the anatomy is "conduit-like", meaning a circumferential landing zone—either a calcified homograft or surgical conduit—of appropriate diameter (typically 16–28 mm for current devices) [49]. If the native RVOT was repaired with a large patch and is very dilated (Fig. 12.12), surgical PVR or a hybrid approach may be required to first downsize the outflow tract. An important pre-procedure step is *coronary artery compression testing*: because the RVOT lies adjacent to coronary branches, a balloon is inflated at the intended valve site under angiographic observation to ensure

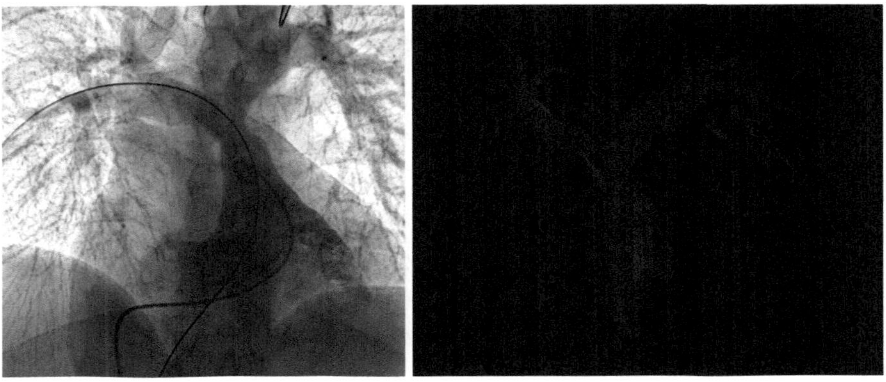

Fig. 12.12 Angiography with 3D reconstruction of the trapeze shape RVOT in TOF, contraindication for TPVI

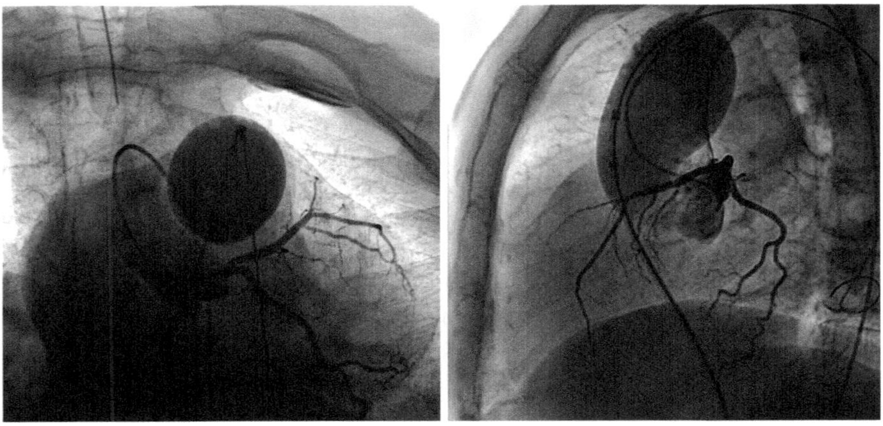

Fig. 12.13 Negative ballon coronary compression test in two incidences prior to TPVI

no coronary is impinged before deploying a TPV (Fig. 12.13) [7]. This safeguards against catastrophic coronary compression by the TPV stent (Fig. 12.14). If risk is present, surgical PVR is indicated instead. The TPVI procedure itself involves balloon-prestenting of the RVOT or conduit (to create a stable scaffold) followed by deployment of the valve-on-stent. The procedure is usually well tolerated with short hospital stay.

Outcomes of TPVI have continually improved and now approach surgical outcomes for the appropriate subset. Acute success rates are >95%, with dramatic reduction in PR and RVOT gradient. The Melody valve IDE trial reported no procedural mortality and excellent hemodynamic results; at discharge, >98% had no more than mild PR and significantly reduced RV pressures [50]. Over the long term, TPV durability is reasonable though slightly inferior to surgical valves. In the

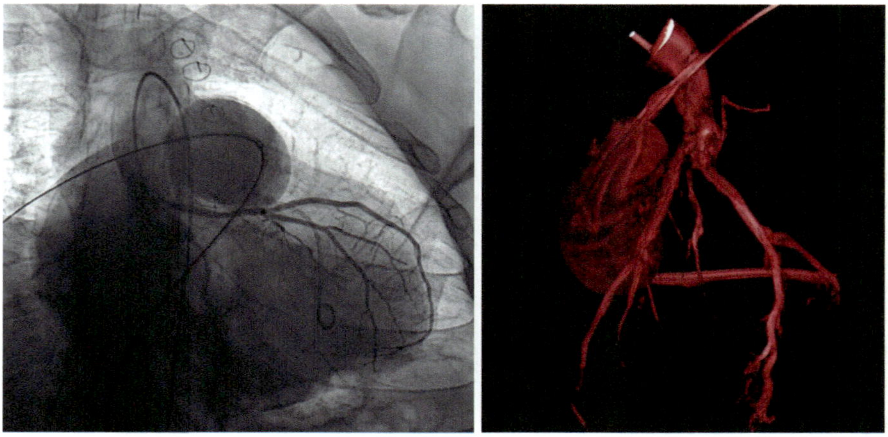

Fig. 12.14 Positive balloon coronary compression test prior to TPVI

U.S. Melody valve 10-year report, estimated freedom from TPV reoperation was 79% at 10 years and freedom from any TPV re-intervention (including catheter dilations or valve-in-valve) was 60% [50].

Hybrid Strategies A hybrid approach may be employed in select situations to combine surgical and transcatheter advantages. One example is a large native RVOT where a full surgical PVR would be very invasive: instead, a surgeon can place a surgical band or reducer to create a smaller landing zone [51], then a TPV is implanted either intraoperatively or in a staged catheterization. Another hybrid scenario is simultaneous surgical and cath interventions—e.g., intraoperative stenting of branch pulmonary arteries under direct vision, or using cardiopulmonary bypass to facilitate a difficult catheter placement. Overall, hybrid approaches are individualized and used in specialized centers for anatomically complex cases [52].

In summary, *PVR in adult TOF is a safe and effective intervention* that should be performed at the appropriate time—neither too late (to avoid permanent RV damage) nor too early (to avoid unnecessary early reoperations). Individualized care, considering anatomy, symptoms, and imaging findings, is critical in the decision for surgical vs transcatheter PVR.

Residual Ventricular Septal Defect (VSD) and RVOT Obstruction

Residual defects after TOF repair can include a small VSD leak or residual RVOT/pulmonary stenosis. While less common than PR, these issues can significantly impact hemodynamics if substantial. In one series from the early era, 28 of 41 reoperations were for residual VSD and 11 for residual RVOT obstruction [53], highlighting their historical importance. Modern surgical techniques have reduced their incidence, but adult cardiology guidelines still address these lesions.

Residual VSD

Many repaired TOF patients have tiny residual "shunts" with negligible hemodynamic effect. However, a significant residual VSD can cause left-to-right shunting, leading to LV volume overload, increased pulmonary blood flow, and risk of heart failure or pulmonary hypertension over time. Indications for closure of a residual VSD are similar to native VSDs: any VSD with a substantial shunt (Qp:Qs ≥1.5–2.0) or that causes RV/LV volume overload should be closed, regardless of symptoms. The 2020 ESC guidelines agree that VSD closure is recommended if there is evidence of significant LV overload (unless contraindicated by severe pulmonary vascular disease) [6]. Even a smaller VSD may merit intervention if it coexists with other lesions (like PR or TR) and contributes to overall hemodynamic stress. Conversely, if the residual VSD is trivial (Qp:Qs <1.3) and not causing enlargement of the heart, it can be managed conservatively with periodic monitoring. Importantly, any residual VSD (even small) poses an endocarditis risk due to turbulent flow, so patients require endocarditis prophylaxis and surveillance.

Surgical Closure The traditional approach for a significant residual VSD is surgical reoperation. This is performed via sternotomy and cardiopulmonary bypass, often approaching through the right atrium (for perimembranous defects) or directly through the RVOT if the VSD is proximal. The defect is patched (or occasionally sutured if very small) to achieve complete closure. Surgical outcomes for isolated VSD reoperation are excellent—mortality is low (in one early series 93% survival was reported, and in modern series operative mortality is <1–2%) and long-term results are good, with substantial symptomatic improvement [54]. Surgical closure is preferred if the VSD is large, in a difficult location for devices (e.g., adjacent to the valves), or if the patient is already undergoing surgery for another reason (such as concomitant PVR or RVOT revision). Many residual VSDs in TOF are located near the patch margin close to the right ventricle outflow—these can often be accessed and closed during a PVR surgery without much added risk. One must take care to avoid injury to the conduction system when closing septal defects; this risk is low but present, similar to primary VSD surgery.

Transcatheter Closure In the past two decades, percutaneous device closure has become an option for certain postoperative VSDs, avoiding reoperation. This strategy is typically reserved for moderate-size residual VSDs (say 4–10 mm) in suitable locations, such as muscular VSDs or gaps between patch and septum, where a device can be safely positioned [55]. Device closure can be challenging in post-surgical anatomy due to irregularly shaped defects and patch material, but improvements in occluder devices have increased success rates. A recent series of 12 patients who underwent percutaneous closure of postoperative VSDs (median defect ~6–7 mm) reported an 83% success rate, with 10 of 12 closed successfully and 2 cases requiring surgical backup due to device embolization [55]. No long-term complications were seen in the successful cases aside from one trivial residual leak and one mild RVOT obstruction on follow-up. These results demonstrate that transcatheter closure is feasible yet technically demanding, often requiring advanced imaging and careful sizing to avoid complications. The risk of device embolization is the main acute concern. Other potential complications include heart block valve interference or residual shunts. Thus, patient selection is critical. Generally, a percutaneous approach is favored for moderate defects in older children or adults where anatomy is amenable and surgical risk is higher or the patient strongly desires to avoid re-sternotomy. If the defect is large (>10–12 mm), has multiple fenestrations, or is very close to the AV valves, surgical closure remains the safer option.

Hybrid Approaches Occasionally, a hybrid technique is used for residual VSDs that are difficult to close by catheter alone. In such cases, a surgeon can provide direct access (e.g., via a small ventriculotomy or through a transatrial approach), and then a catheter device is deployed under direct visualization. This can secure device positioning and minimize bypass time. Hybrid VSD closures are not common but can be valuable in complex anatomies—they combine the precision of surgery with the avoidance of a full cardiopulmonary bypass run (in some instances).

Residual Right Ventricular Outflow Tract (RVOT) Obstruction

Residual RVOT obstruction can take several forms: a narrowing at the pulmonary valve annulus (Fig. 12.15), hypertrophic muscle bands in the RV infundibulum, distal stenosis in a pulmonary artery branch, or obstruction in a prosthetic RV-PA conduit. In the context of repaired TOF, causes include an intentionally small transannular patch (to avoid PR, at the expense of a gradient), incomplete resection of subvalvular muscle, or later acquired stenosis (e.g., calcification of a conduit or conduit-valve stenosis). Significant RVOT obstruction imposes pressure overload on the RV, which can lead to RV hypertrophy, fibrosis, and dysfunction if untreated. It may also contribute to exercise intolerance and arrhythmias. Thus, identifying and relieving significant RVOT obstruction is important in adult TOF follow-up.

Catheter Interventions For discrete valvular pulmonary stenosis, balloon pulmonary valvuloplasty is the first-line treatment in adults, as it can fracture the fused commissures and enlarge the orifice without surgery [7]. Balloon dilation can also be used for isolated distal obstructions like branch pulmonary artery stenoses; often, stents are implanted in branch PAs to maintain patency if the vessels are large enough to accommodate stents (Fig. 12.16). In patients with an RV-PA conduit, transcatheter stenting of the conduit can relieve stenosis (Fig. 12.17), and if regurgitation is also present, placing a transcatheter valve will treat both issues. In fact, guidelines consider it reasonable to perform conduit interventions (stent or TPVI) in adults with moderate or greater conduit stenosis if there is reduced exercise capacity or arrhythmia related to the RV pressure load. Percutaneous techniques thus play a major role in managing residual RVOT obstruction, especially when it is distal or related to prior conduit. Many adult congenital centers will attempt a transcatheter relief of RVOT or branch PA obstruction before resorting to surgery, given the lower

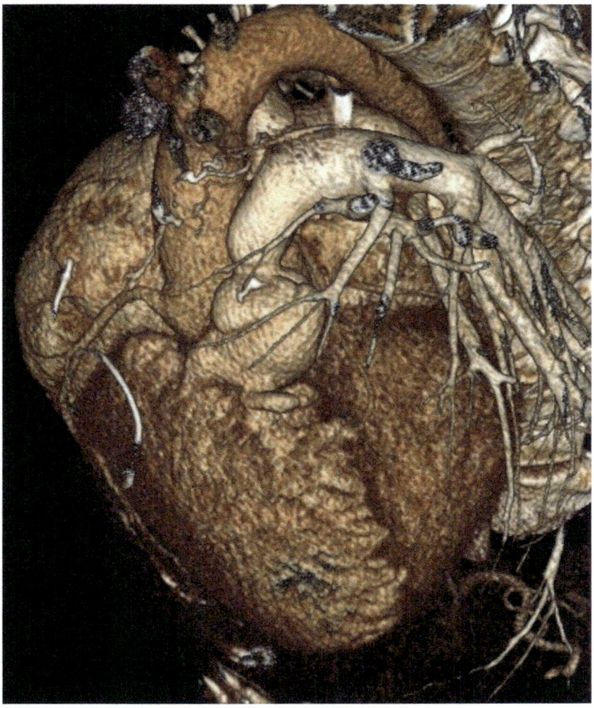

Fig. 12.15 Pulmonary valve severe stenosis in a 24 24-year-old patient after infant TOF repair

acute risk. Success rates of balloon valvuloplasty for isolated valvular PS in adults are high, often achieving >50% reduction in gradient, though mild residual stenosis may remain. Stenting of conduits or branches also yields significant gradient relief; however, if multiple stenotic areas or very diffuse narrowing exists, surgery might be preferable for a more complete result.

Surgical Relief Surgery is indicated when anatomy is not amenable to catheter therapy or when concomitant issues require open surgery. Surgical options depend on the level of obstruction: subvalvular muscle bundles are resected (a transventricular or transatrial approach can be used to cut away hypertrophic muscle in the RVOT). If the pulmonary annulus is small and obstructive, the surgeon can perform a transannular patch enlargement (accepting the creation of free PR, which may then necessitate placing a valve; often a valved conduit or a pericardial patch plus bioprosthetic valve will be used in that scenario to avoid leaving the patient with severe PR). For conduit stenosis, a full conduit replacement may be done (surgically inserting a new homograft or valved tube) (Fig. 12.18). Branch PA stenoses can be addressed with patch angioplasty of the branch, sometimes approached through the pulmonary arteriotomy. The risks of surgical RVOT revision are similar to primary TOF surgery but generally quite low in experienced centers, especially if not accompanied by multiple other procedures. One must be mindful of scarring and collateral vessels from prior surgery (e.g., close to the aorta or coronary arteries). Reports

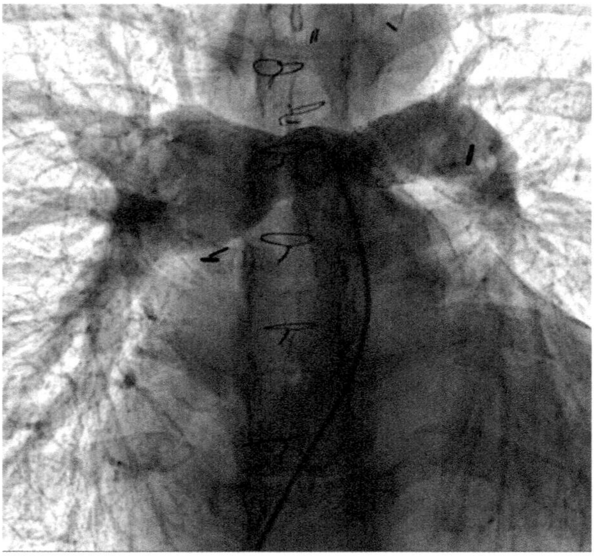

Fig. 12.16 Left pulmonary artery stent

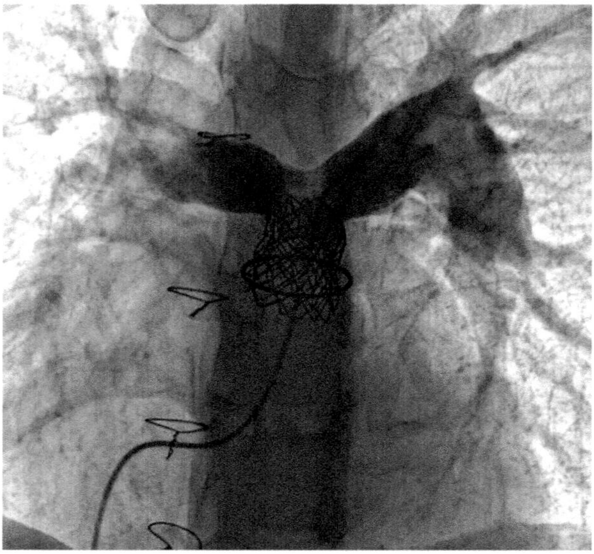

Fig. 12.17 Stent placement for PA-RV conduit stenosis

from reoperative TOF surgeries show that relief of RVOT obstruction carries low mortality and markedly improves RV pressure. Modern results are even better, with surgical reintervention for RVOT obstruction typically having excellent relief and rare major complications.

Hybrid Approaches A combined approach may occasionally be used, such as intraoperative balloon dilation of a distal PA that the surgeon cannot effectively

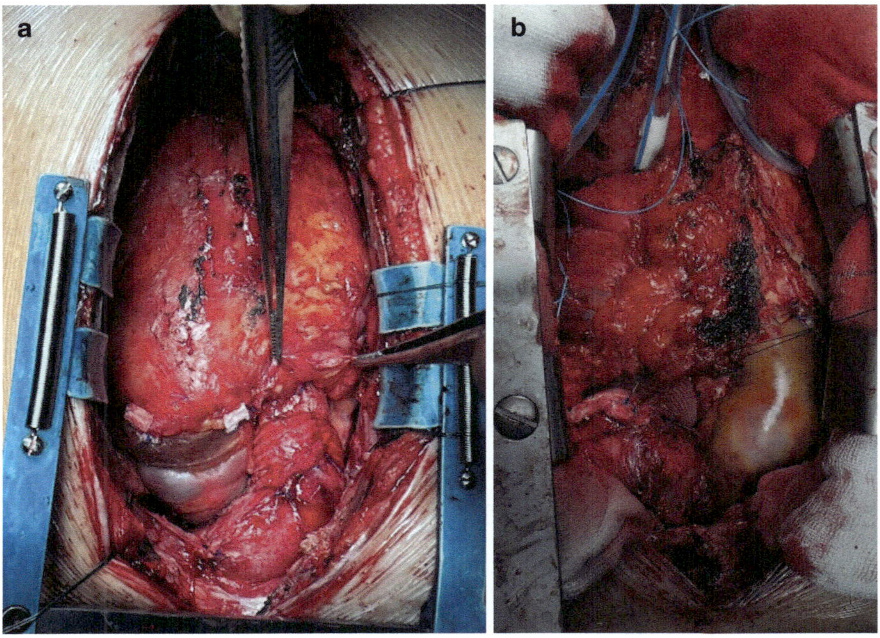

Fig. 12.18 Reconstruction of PA with homograft and ascending aorta replacement. (**a**) Levocardia, (**b**) Dextrocardia

patch (with the surgeon providing access via a pulmonary arteriotomy). Another example is the placement of a stent in a conduit during surgery under direct vision—this might be done if a Melody valve is planned to be placed later inside the stent, allowing the patient to avoid a conduit replacement. These specialized techniques are individualized to the patient needs.

Tailored Interventions in Adult TGA Patients Post-surgical Repair

Introduction

Dextro-transposition of the great arteries (D-TGA) is a complex congenital defect that historically required inventive surgical solutions for survival. Throughout the 1960s–70s, the atrial switch procedures (Mustard and Senning operations) were the standard correction, creating intra-atrial baffles to reroute blood at the atrial level [56]. This achieved physiological (but not anatomical) repair, leaving the morphologic RV as the systemic ventricle. In the mid-1980s, the arterial switch operation (ASO) developed by Jatene supplanted atrial switches for D-TGA, restoring anatomically correct ventriculo-arterial connections [56]. For the subset of D-TGA with VSD and pulmonary stenosis, the Rastelli procedure (introduced 1969) became the preferred repair, using a VSD patch to direct the LV to the aorta and a conduit to connect the RV to the pulmonary arteries. Each of these operations results in a unique physiology that, as patients reach adulthood, can give rise to specific long-term complications. Indeed, late problems are common—one center reported that atrial switch patients frequently required reoperation for baffle complications (stenosis or leaks) decades after the initial surgery [57]. Meanwhile, arterial switch survivors face issues of the "neo-aorta," coronaries, and pulmonary arteries in the long term, and Rastelli patients often need multiple conduit replacements over their lifetime. These complications often require tailored re-interventions, ranging from transcatheter procedures to surgical or hybrid approaches, depending on the anatomy and the issue at hand.

Atrial Switch (Mustard/Senning)—Late Complications and Interventions

Adults who had a Mustard or Senning procedure in childhood commonly present with one or more long-term sequelae of the atrial switch anatomy. The chief issues are baffle stenoses, baffle leaks,

Baffle Obstruction (Stenosis) Obstruction of the synthetic or autologous atrial baffle is a frequent late complication. Narrowing can occur at the SVC limb or IVC limb of the systemic venous baffle, leading to venous. In Mustard/Senning cohorts, baffle stenosis has been reported in a significant fraction of patients and can occur decades postoperatively as the baffle materials shrink or scar. The preferred treatment is percutaneous transluminal balloon angioplasty and stenting of the baffle if anatomy allows. Reports have demonstrated that stenting of SVC/IVC baffle obstructions is highly effective at relieving venous pressure and improving symptoms, avoiding the morbidity of redo open-heart surgery [57, 58]. In a large single-center experience, transcatheter intervention successfully relieved Mustard/Senning baffle stenosis in the majority of cases (45 of 50 attempts), with only 5 patients (10%) referred to surgery for complex anatomies not amenable to stenting [57]. If percutaneous stent placement is not possible (e.g., if the baffle is very tortuous or completely obstructed), a surgical baffle revision or replacement can be performed, although reoperation carries higher risk in these re-do patients [57]. Notably, some centers have even adopted hybrid approaches—for instance, deploying a stent intra-operatively under direct visualization in the OR when transcatheter access to the baffle is challenging [59]. Such innovative combined techniques underscore the goal of minimizing risk while relieving obstructions.

Baffle Leaks Atrial baffle leaks are another long-term problem, often resulting from suture line dehiscence or patch degeneration. Clinically, a significant baffle leak creates a shunt that can cause arterial desaturation due to systemic venous blood leaking into the pulmonary venous side (right-to-left shunt)—essentially an "atrial level" right-to-left shunt similar to an ASD. There is also risk of paradoxical

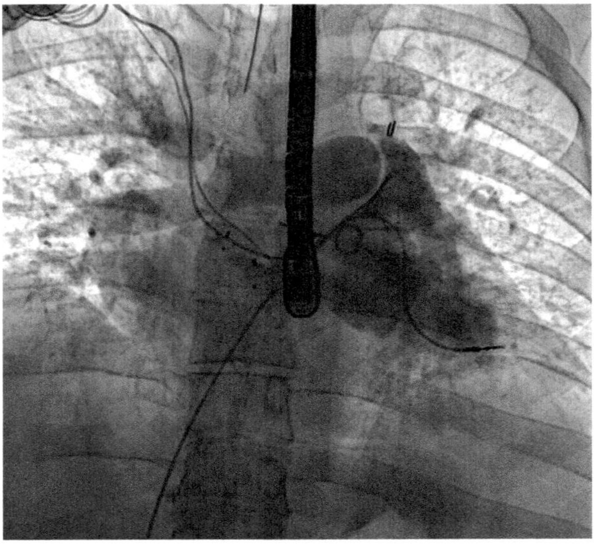

Fig. 12.19 Intra-arterial baffle leak after Senning operation was closed with percutaneous occluders

embolism if clots traverse the leak. Small leaks may be well-tolerated, but larger leaks usually warrant closure. Transcatheter device closure is the first-line therapy for baffle leaks in most cases [57]. Covered stents or occluder devices (e.g., Amplatzer septal or duct occluders) can be deployed within the baffle to seal the defect, often at the same time as addressing any stenosis (Fig. 12.19). In the previously mentioned series, 16 occlusion devices and 18 covered stents were used to successfully close baffle leaks in dozens of patients [57]. Only if percutaneous closure fails or is contraindicated would surgical patch repair of a baffle leak be pursued.

Arterial Switch Operation (ASO)—Late Complications and Interventions

This anatomic repair spares the RV from systemic work and avoids the baffles of an atrial switch. As a result, the long-term outcomes after ASO have been excellent: most patients survive into adulthood with preserved exercise capacity and good quality of life [56, 60]. Surgical mortality in experienced centers is under 5%, and 20-year survival exceeds 90% in most series [61]. The major late complications seen in adult ASO patients tend to fall into three categories: coronary artery complications, neoaortic (root/valve) complications, and issues with the pulmonary outflow (supravalvular pulmonary stenosis).

Coronary Artery Complications During the arterial switch, the coronary arteries are detached from the native aorta and reimplanted into the neo-aorta. Early postoperative coronary insufficiency (due to kinking or stenosis at the reimplantation site)

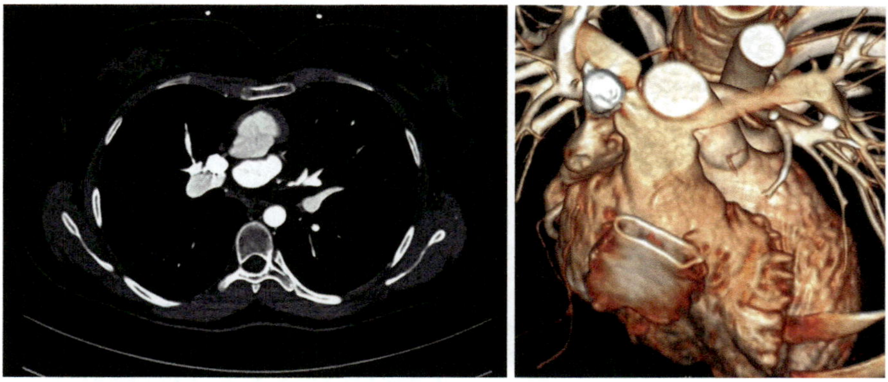

Fig. 12.20 Left coronary artery occlusion in a patient after neonatal ASO

is a known hazard in the first days/weeks after ASO. Those that survive to adulthood typically do not have an obvious early coronary issue. However, there remains a long-term risk of late coronary ostial stenosis or insufficiency—fibrotic narrowing at the coronary reattachment site or ostial stretching that can progress silently (Fig. 12.20). Adults with prior ASO may rarely present with myocardial ischemia, and in some cases sudden cardiac death in ASO survivors has been attributed to occult coronary obstructions. Routine follow-up includes screening for ischemia (e.g., stress testing, coronary CT angiography) in this population. If a significant coronary lesion is confirmed, the preferred intervention is percutaneous coronary intervention (PCI) with stenting, performed by an experienced adult congenital interventionalist [60]. PCI in ASO patients has shown good mid-term results, with one review noting ~95% average stenosis relief and sustained patency in most cases [60]. In contrast, coronary artery bypass grafting is rarely utilized—because the coronaries originate from the neo-aortic root (often without sizable side branches to graft onto) and the young age of patients, CABG is only reported in ~2–9% of cases. Overall, freedom from any coronary re-intervention 20 years after ASO is very high (≈75–99% in various series) [60]. In summary, adult ASO patients should be evaluated for ischemic symptoms periodically, and if coronary narrowing is found, PCI is usually effective; surgical or hybrid approaches are rarely needed for the coronaries in this era [4].

Neopulmonary Artery Stenosis The LeCompte maneuver, integral to the ASO, involves bringing the branch pulmonary arteries forward in front of the aorta. This can sometimes create an angulation or mild compression of one or both pulmonary artery branches (Fig. 12.21). Additionally, the surgical anastomosis between the native pulmonary root (now attached to RV) and the pulmonary artery confluence can become a site of narrowing as the patient grows. Consequently, supravalvular and branch pulmonary artery stenosis is one of the most common late issues after arterial switch. In fact, pulmonary artery stenosis is reported as the most frequent indication for re-intervention in ASO survivors, more common than neoaortic valve

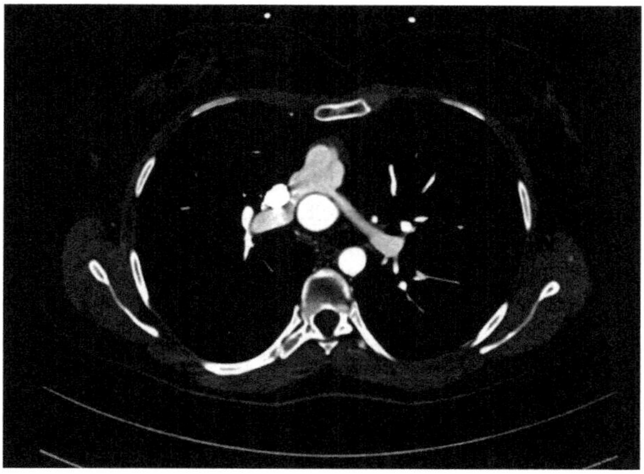

Fig. 12.21 Pulmonary branch stenosis in patient after ASO and LeCompte maneuver

problems in the second and third decades [62]. Patients may be asymptomatic or have reduced exercise tolerance; imaging will show narrowing (often of the left pulmonary artery) with elevated right ventricular pressures on echocardiogram. For moderate or severe stenoses, transcatheter relief is usually the first step. Balloon angioplasty can be attempted, but often stenting of the branch PA is needed to achieve a lasting increase in vessel diameter [62]. Stenting has high acute success in relieving the gradient, but it is not without risks in ASO patients. Notably, the proximity of the branch PAs to the ascending aorta and coronary buttons means that an expanding PA stent can compress the coronary arteries or even erode into the aorta if not carefully sized. There are reports of PA stenting in ASO leading to life-threatening complications such as left main coronary compression and creation of an aorto-pulmonary fistula. To mitigate these risks, interventionalists now routinely perform advanced imaging (e.g., cardiac CT or selective angiography) to delineate the course of coronaries relative to the PA, and they may use covered stents to prevent a fistula if the anatomy is tenuous [62]. If a branch PA stenosis is very long segment or involves the bifurcation severely, surgical repair is indicated—this can entail patch angioplasty of the branch PAs or the main PA. In some cases, especially if both branches are small, surgeons may reconstruct the bifurcation with pericardial patches or use a short conduit. Surgical outcomes for PA augmentation are generally good, though re-stenosis can occur. In one series, criteria for surgery included failure of catheter intervention or complex multi-level stenoses, and surgical reconstruction achieved relief with low mortality [62].

Neo-aortic Root Dilation and Valve Regurgitation Perhaps the most emblematic late complication of the arterial switch is the issue of the neo-aorta. In the ASO, the pulmonary valve and root become the new aortic valve and root (facing systemic pressure). The pulmonary root tissues are thinner and more distensible, which makes progressive aortic root dilation a real concern over time. Along with root enlargement, the neoaortic valve (originally a trileaflet pulmonary valve) may develop regurgitation due to stretching of the sinotubular junction and valve annulus. Studies have documented that mild neo-aortic regurgitation is very common by adolescence—for instance, a meta-analysis found only ~48% of ASO patients were free from at least mild aortic regurgitation at 20 years [63, 64]. Fortunately, moderate or severe aortic regurgitation is much less frequent: freedom from ≥moderate regurgitation was ~88% at 20 years (meaning about 12% had moderate AR by 20 years, rising to ~21% by 30 years) [64]. Neo-aortic root dilation has a similar prevalence, affecting over half of patients by 20+ years post-switch (often mild dilation of the root or ascending aorta) [64]. The etiology is likely multifactorial—original pulmonary root size mismatch, growth, and long-term pressure load all contribute. Surgical options include aortic valve repair (if cusps are salvageable and the issue is mainly annular dilatation; a David procedure or similar root remodeling may be attempted) versus valve replacement with root replacement (Bentall procedure) if the valve is not easily repairable. Neo-aortic root surgery in ASO patients has been reported in only a small minority so far—on the order of 3–5% by the 20–30 years mark [64]. When such surgery is needed, it is a complex reoperation often involving reimplantation of coronaries into the new graft; however, outcomes have generally been favorable if performed before severe LV dysfunction occurs.

Rastelli Procedure—Late Complications and Interventions

The Rastelli operation is employed for patients with TGA who have a large VSD and RV outflow tract obstruction (e.g., pulmonary stenosis), a subset sometimes termed "TGA-VSD-PS." In the Rastelli procedure, the surgeon closes the VSD in such a way as to route the LV blood through the VSD to the aorta, and inserts a prosthetic RV-to-PA conduit to establish flow from the RV to the pulmonary arteries. This achieves anatomical correction (the LV becomes the systemic pump into the aorta), but at the expense of introducing a prosthetic conduit and an intraventricular baffle. Adults who underwent Rastelli repairs in childhood almost universally face the need for multiple re-interventions during their lifetime. The two main problem areas are: (1) conduit degeneration, (2) subaortic obstruction (related to the VSD baffle).

RV-PA Conduit Degeneration By design, the Rastelli includes a prosthetic or homograft conduit connecting the right ventricle to the pulmonary artery. These conduits have a limited lifespan—they do not grow with the patient and tend to develop progressive stenosis and/or regurgitation due to calcification and tissue degeneration. Studies have shown that *essentially all* Rastelli conduits will require replacement in time. For example, in a large series of 101 Rastelli patients, 44 patients needed reoperation for conduit stenosis during a median 8.5-year follow-up [65]. The median longevity of a conduit is on the order of 10–15 years (shorter in childhood, often slightly longer once an adult-sized conduit is placed). Thus, adult Rastelli patients are frequently those who have already had one or two conduit replacements in adoles-

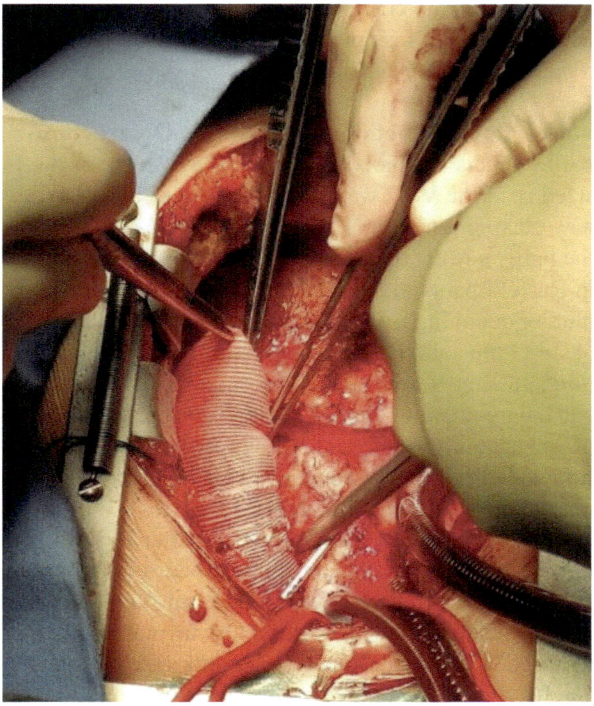

Fig. 12.22 PA-RV conduit replacement after Rastelli operation

cence and present with a worn-out conduit in their 20s or 30s (Fig. 12.22). Intervention is indicated when conduit obstruction causes RV hypertension or when severe conduit valve regurgitation causes RV volume overload. The traditional treatment has been surgical conduit replacement, reoperating to implant a new homograft or valved tube between the RV and PA. Surgical risk for isolated conduit replacement in a young adult is acceptable (often <3% mortality in experienced centers), but many of these patients will need repeat operations over their lifetime. In the last 10–15 years, a game-changing therapy has been the development of TPVI. If the old conduit is of sufficient diameter and has a suitable landing zone, a bovine jugular vein valve mounted in a stent (Melody valve) or a newer self-expanding valve can be delivered via catheter and expanded inside the old conduit, restoring valve function and relieving stenosis without open-heart surgery. TPVI has transformed the care of RV-PA conduits. Outcomes have been very good: the Melody valve U.S. trial reported >90% freedom from any re-intervention at 5 years and excellent hemodynamic results [66]. In other words, transcatheter valves can nearly halve the frequency of surgeries. Of course, TPVI is not always feasible—the conduit may be too small or heavily calcified to safely dilate. In such cases, a hybrid approach can be used: the surgeon may place a fresh conduit or enlarging patch, and then a transcatheter valve can be implanted in a subsequent step when the patient is more stable. In some instances, bare-metal stents are first placed to crack calcium and enlarge a narrowed conduit, and then a valve is delivered. If TPVI is not possible or the anatomy is unfavorable, surgical replacement remains the gold standard.

Subaortic Obstruction (LVOT/Baffle Obstruction) The Rastelli intraventricular baffle directs LV blood across the VSD to the aorta. If this tunnel is not perfectly sized or if the VSD was small and had to be enlarged, there is a risk of creating a new obstruction in the LVOT. Moreover, as the heart grows and geometry changes, the baffle can encroach on the LV outflow or the aortic valve. Subaortic obstruction in Rastelli patients often manifests as a rising LVOT gradient, a new systolic murmur, or declining LV function due to afterload. In the earlier-cited series, 11 patients (11% of the cohort) required surgical reoperation specifically for subaortic obstruction late after Rastelli [65]. This often necessitated takedown of the RV-PA conduit and enlargement of the VSD or revision of the baffle. The surgical solution depends on the anatomy: some patients simply need the VSD re-patched with a larger baffle (to widen the tunnel), whereas others might have muscle bundles or tissue obstructing the outflow that can be resected.

In summary, subaortic obstruction after Rastelli is managed by reoperation, tailored to how the baffle can be modified; it's important to relieve it before the LV suffers irreversible damage. Long-term data suggest that a need for VSD/baffle enlargement is associated with a less favorable prognosis—in one study, those who required VSD enlargement had higher risk of late death or transplant [67]. Thus, careful surgical technique at initial repair and vigilant follow-up are key.

Tailored Management of Tricuspid Valve Regurgitation in Adult ccTGA

Overview of ccTGA and Its Challenges

Congenitally corrected transposition of the great arteries (ccTGA) is a rare cardiac anomaly characterized by both atrioventricular and ventriculoarterial discordance. This "double discordance" results in physiologically normal circulation, but the morphologic RV supports systemic circulation and the systemic AV valve is the morphologic TV [7]. Many ccTGA patients reach adulthood without early intervention, but over time the systemic RV faces progressive pressure/volume overload, leading to RV dysfunction, severe systemic TV regurgitation, arrhythmias, and heart failure [6, 7]. In fact, natural history data show high rates of deterioration by mid-adulthood—up to 50% of unoperated ccTGA patients experience heart failure, significant TR, arrhythmias or sudden death by age 40 [7].

Systemic Tricuspid Valve Regurgitation in ccTGA

Systemic AV valve regurgitation is a critical prognostic factor in ccTGA [68]. The morphologic TV, situated in the systemic AV position, often has structural abnormalities and becomes incompetent over time under systemic pressures [69]. Progressive severe TR exacerbates systemic RV volume overload and dysfunction. Thus, managing the systemic TV is central to ccTGA care.

Indications and Timing for Tricuspid Valve Surgery

Surgical intervention is indicated for symptomatic ccTGA adults with severe TR as long as systemic RV systolic function is preserved or only mildly depressed (ejection fraction >40%) [7]. For asymptomatic patients, surgery is considered reasonable if there is progressive RV dilation or early dysfunction [70]. If systemic RV is severely depressed, isolated valve surgery carries prohibitive risk and alternatives like heart transplantation or double-switch repair are considered [71].

Tricuspid Valve Repair vs. Replacement

Tricuspid valve replacement has been the preferred approach in ccTGA adults because valve repair has a high failure rate [68]. In a series of 57 ccTGA patients undergoing TV surgery, those who received valvuloplasty had a 60% recurrence of significant TR in long-term follow-up [68]. In contrast, prosthetic replacement reliably eliminates regurgitation and is associated with improved functional outcomes [68, 72].

Surgical intervention can reverse some functional deterioration: patients after TV replacement experienced improved exercise capacity and RV metrics [72]. Subjective symptom status in ccTGA can be unreliable; objective measures should guide the timing rather than symptoms alone [72]. Valve surgery should be performed in experienced adult congenital heart centers.

Tailored Interventions in Adults with Univentricular Heart Physiology—Fontan Circulation

Patients with univentricular heart physiology, particularly those palliated with the Fontan operation, represent a growing cohort within ACHD. The unique circulatory dynamics of the Fontan circuit create long-term challenges that frequently necessitate surgical, interventional, or hybrid interventions.

Fontan Circuit Obstruction

Fontan pathway obstructions may occur at surgical anastomoses or in conduits due to somatic outgrowth, thrombosis, or calcification. These obstructions lead to elevated venous pressures and diminished cardiac output. Intervention is indicated in symptomatic patients or when hemodynamically significant gradients are present (Fig. 12.23).

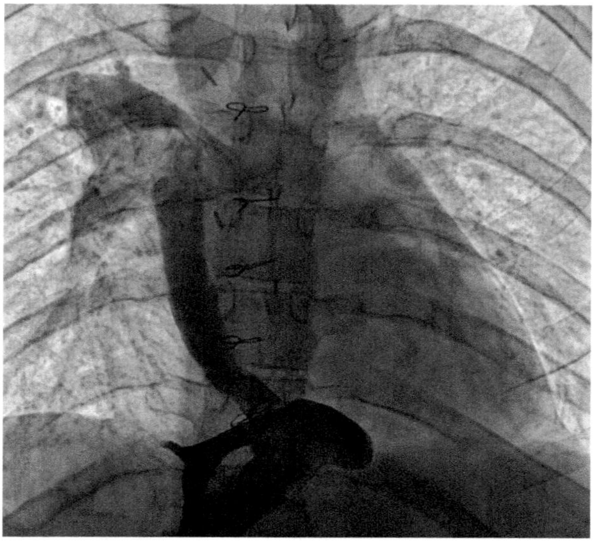

Fig. 12.23 Extra-cardiac Fontan conduit stenosis

Interventional Approach Stenting of narrowed segments is the preferred first-line therapy. Bare-metal or covered stents are selected based on anatomy, and intravascular lithotripsy may be used in calcified conduits (Fig. 12.24) [73, 74]. Relief of gradients improves symptoms and may also benefit liver congestion and exercise capacity [75].

Surgical/Hybrid Approach In cases of extensive obstruction or failed catheter-based therapy, surgical revision or Fontan conversion may be necessary [76]. However, operative risk is considerable in re-operations.

Systemic Atrioventricular Valve Regurgitation

Significant systemic AV valve regurgitation, especially in patients with morphologic right ventricles, contributes to Fontan failure and volume overload.

Surgical Approach Valve repair is preferred when feasible, using techniques such as annuloplasty or leaflet augmentation. Valve replacement (typically bioprosthetic) is indicated when repair is not durable [77, 78]. Surgery is often performed alongside Fontan revision or conversion. Timing is crucial. Patients with preserved ventricular function and moderate regurgitation may benefit most. Severe regurgitation with poor ventricular function carries higher operative risk and lower postoperative benefit [79].

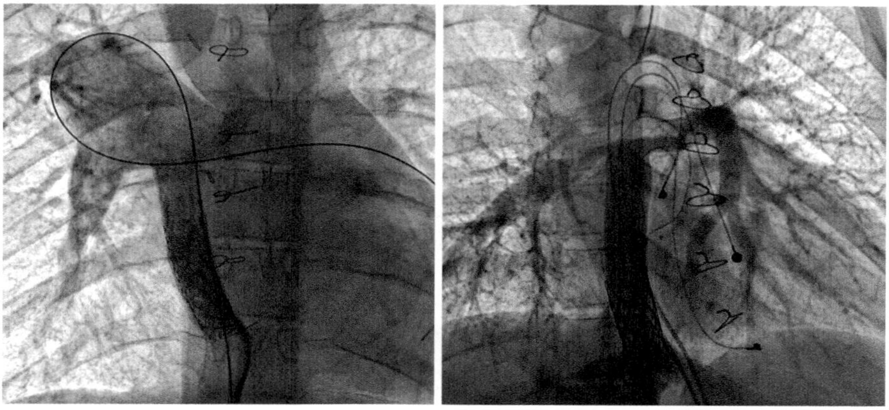

Fig. 12.24 Stenting of extra-cardiac Fontan conduit

Atrial Arrhythmias

Arrhythmias, especially intra-atrial reentrant tachycardia, are prevalent in older Fontan patients and may lead to hemodynamic instability.

Interventional Approach Catheter ablation, with 3D electroanatomic mapping, is effective in terminating reentry circuits [80]. Trans-baffle puncture is often required for access in extracardiac Fontans.

Surgical Approach In refractory cases, conversion from atriopulmonary Fontan (Fig. 12.25) to extracardiac conduit, combined with biatrial Maze procedure and pacemaker implantation, is performed [81].

Plastic Bronchitis

Plastic bronchitis is a severe lymphatic complication involving bronchial cast formation. Interventional Approach: Dynamic contrast lymphangiography identifies aberrant lymphatic flow to the airways. Targeted embolization of leaking lymphatics using coils or glue can resolve symptoms [82, 83].

Protein-Losing Enteropathy (PLE)

PLE manifests as hypoalbuminemia and edema due to protein leakage into the gastrointestinal tract.

Interventional Approach Stenting of narrowed Fontan pathways and transcatheter fenestration may relieve elevated venous pressures [84].

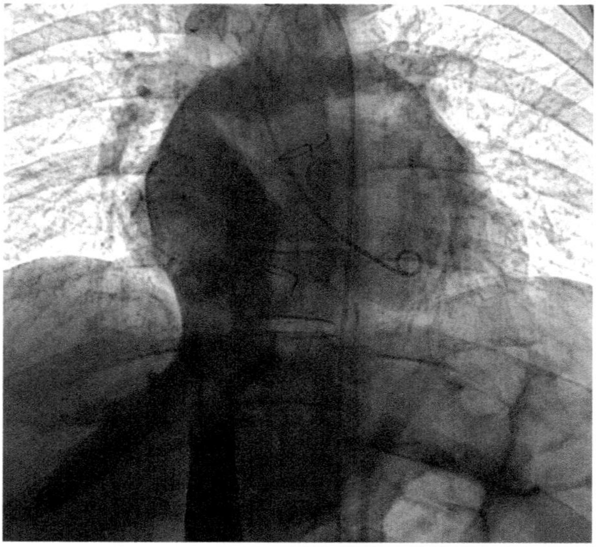

Fig. 12.25 Atriopulmonary Fontan

Table 12.3 Common interventions in adult Fontan complications

Complication	Intervention	Selection criteria	Outcome
Fontan pathway obstruction	Stent, surgical revision	Hemodynamic gradient, symptoms	High success with stenting
AV valve regurgitation	Repair or replacement	Severe regurgitation, preserved function	Improved symptoms, variable survival
Atrial arrhythmias	Ablation, Fontan conversion	Refractory arrhythmia, sinus node dysfunction	Rhythm control in ~50% at 5 years
Plastic bronchitis	Lymphatic embolization	Recurrent casts, abnormal lymphatics	Resolution in ~80% cases
Protein-losing enteropathy	Fenestration, lymphatic embolism	Hypoalbuminemia, failed medical therapy	Palliation or cure in select cases
Fontan liver disease	Surveillance, combined transplant	Cirrhosis, HCC risk	Improved survival with combined transplant

Lymphatic Interventions Novel transhepatic lymphatic embolization of gut-draining lymphatics is an emerging therapy [85].

Surgical Options In refractory cases, surgical creation of fenestration or Fontan revision may be attempted. Transplantation is often required in end-stage disease [86] (Table 12.3).

Conclusion

The management of adults with congenital heart defects requires a nuanced, multidisciplinary, and patient-specific approach that accounts for the complexity of prior repairs, comorbidities, and evolving anatomical substrates. This chapter has illustrated how interventions must be individually tailored rather than generalized, guided by lesion type, physiological burden, imaging findings, and patient-centered goals. The growing ACHD population benefits from the convergence of advanced diagnostic modalities, emerging transcatheter technologies, and refined surgical techniques—often in hybrid configurations—to optimize outcomes and minimize morbidity. Transitions from pediatric to adult care must be well-structured to avoid loss to follow-up, while lifelong surveillance is essential to prevent late complications such as arrhythmias, heart failure, and valve deterioration. Across the spectrum of defects—from ASDs and VSDs to complex post-repair TOF and TGA—therapeutic decisions should be evidence-based but flexible, accommodating the patient's age, anatomy, preferences, and long-term prognosis. As these patients increasingly reach advanced age, new challenges will emerge that further test the adaptability of congenital heart programs. Ultimately, the future of ACHD care lies in raising specialized centers, maintaining long-term registries, and continually integrating innovation with individualized care philosophy to improve both survival and quality of life.

References

1. Moons P, Bratt EL, De Backer J, Goossens E, Hornung T, Tutarel O, et al. Transition to adulthood and transfer to adult care of adolescents with congenital heart disease: a global consensus statement of the ESC Association of cardiovascular nursing and allied professions (ACNAP), the ESC working group on adult congenital heart disease (WG ACHD), the Association for European Paediatric and Congenital Cardiology (AEPC), the pan-African Society of Cardiology (PASCAR), the Asia-Pacific pediatric cardiac society (APPCS), the inter-American Society of Cardiology (IASC), the Cardiac Society of Australia and New Zealand (CSANZ), the International Society for Adult Congenital Heart Disease (ISACHD), the world heart federation (WHF), the European congenital heart disease organisation (ECHDO), and the global Alliance for rheumatic and congenital hearts (global ARCH). Eur Heart J. 2021;42(41):4213–23.
2. Gurvitz M, Valente AM, Broberg C, Cook S, Stout K, Kay J, et al. Prevalence and predictors of gaps in care among adult congenital heart disease patients: HEART-ACHD (the health, education, and access research trial). J Am Coll Cardiol. 2013;61(21):2180–4.
3. Gilboa SM, Devine OJ, Kucik JE, Oster ME, Riehle-Colarusso T, Nembhard WN, et al. Congenital heart defects in the United States: estimating the magnitude of the affected population in 2010. Circulation. 2016;134(2):101–9.
4. van der Linde D, Konings EE, Slager MA, Witsenburg M, Helbing WA, Takkenberg JJ, et al. Birth prevalence of congenital heart disease worldwide: a systematic review and meta-analysis. J Am Coll Cardiol. 2011;58(21):2241–7.
5. Tutarel O, Kempny A, Alonso-Gonzalez R, Jabbour R, Li W, Uebing A, et al. Congenital heart disease beyond the age of 60: emergence of a new population with high resource utilization, high morbidity, and high mortality. Eur Heart J. 2014;35(11):725–32.

6. Baumgartner H, De Backer J, Babu-Narayan SV, Budts W, Chessa M, Diller GP, et al. 2020 ESC guidelines for the management of adult congenital heart disease. Eur Heart J. 2021;42(6):563–645.
7. Stout KK, Daniels CJ, Aboulhosn JA, Bozkurt B, Broberg CS, Colman JM, et al. 2018 AHA/ACC guideline for the Management of Adults with Congenital Heart Disease: a report of the American College of Cardiology/American Heart Association task force on clinical practice guidelines. Circulation. 2019;139(14):e698–800.
8. Egbe AC, Miranda WR, Lopez-Jimenez F, Connolly HM. Atherosclerotic cardiovascular disease in adults with congenital heart disease. JACC Adv. 2022;1(2):100026.
9. Hickey EJ, Veldtman G, Bradley TJ, Gengsakul A, Manlhiot C, Williams WG, et al. Late risk of outcomes for adults with repaired tetralogy of Fallot from an inception cohort spanning four decades. Eur J Cardiothorac Surg. 2009;35(1):156–64; discussion 64
10. Kempny A, Hjortshoj CS, Gu H, Li W, Opotowsky AR, Landzberg MJ, et al. Predictors of death in contemporary adult patients with Eisenmenger syndrome: a multicenter study. Circulation. 2017;135(15):1432–40.
11. Marelli AJ, Ionescu-Ittu R, Mackie AS, Guo L, Dendukuri N, Kaouache M. Lifetime prevalence of congenital heart disease in the general population from 2000 to 2010. Circulation. 2014;130(9):749–56.
12. Khairy P, Ionescu-Ittu R, Mackie AS, Abrahamowicz M, Pilote L, Marelli AJ. Changing mortality in congenital heart disease. J Am Coll Cardiol. 2010;56(14):1149–57.
13. Tutarel O. Acquired heart conditions in adults with congenital heart disease: a growing problem. Heart. 2014;100(17):1317–21.
14. Mandalenakis Z, Rosengren A, Skoglund K, Lappas G, Eriksson P, Dellborg M. Survivorship in children and young adults with congenital heart disease in Sweden. JAMA Intern Med. 2017;177(2):224–30.
15. Verheugt CL, Uiterwaal CS, van der Velde ET, Meijboom FJ, Pieper PG, van Dijk AP, et al. Mortality in adult congenital heart disease. Eur Heart J. 2010;31(10):1220–9.
16. Moons P, Bovijn L, Budts W, Belmans A, Gewillig M. Temporal trends in survival to adulthood among patients born with congenital heart disease from 1970 to 1992 in Belgium. Circulation. 2010;122(22):2264–72.
17. Kempny A, Dimopoulos K, Uebing A, Diller GP, Rosendahl U, Belitsis G, et al. Outcome of cardiac surgery in patients with congenital heart disease in England between 1997 and 2015. PLoS One. 2017;12(6):e0178963.
18. Diller GP, Kempny A, Alonso-Gonzalez R, Swan L, Uebing A, Li W, et al. Survival prospects and circumstances of death in contemporary adult congenital heart disease patients under follow-up at a large tertiary centre. Circulation. 2015;132(22):2118–25.
19. Szugye N. Greater than the sum of its parts: multimodality imaging in adults with congenital heart disease. Cardiovasc Diagn Ther. 2024;14(6):1176–85.
20. Spanaki A, Kabir S, Stephenson N, van Poppel MPM, Benetti V, Simpson J. 3D approaches in complex CHD: where are we? Funny printing and beautiful images, or a useful tool? J Cardiovasc Dev Dis. 2022;9(8)
21. Mylotte D, Pilote L, Ionescu-Ittu R, Abrahamowicz M, Khairy P, Therrien J, et al. Specialized adult congenital heart disease care: the impact of policy on mortality. Circulation. 2014;129(18):1804–12.
22. Konstantinides S, Geibel A, Olschewski M, Görnandt L, Roskamm H, Spillner G, Just H, Kasper W. A comparison of surgical and medical therapy for atrial septal defect in adults. N Engl J Med. 1995;333(8):5.
23. Ooi YK, Kelleman M, Ehrlich A, Glanville M, Porter A, Kim D, et al. Transcatheter versus surgical closure of atrial septal defects in children: a value comparison. JACC Cardiovasc Interv. 2016;9(1):79–86.
24. Chambault ALOK, Brown LJ, Mellor SL, Sorathia N, Thomas AE, Kothari N, Harky A. Transcatheter versus surgical closure of atrial septal defects: a systematic review and meta-analysis of clinical outcomes. Cardiol Young. 2022;1(32):9.

25. Kotowycz MA, Therrien J, Ionescu-Ittu R, Owens CG, Pilote L, Martucci G, et al. Long-term outcomes after surgical versus transcatheter closure of atrial septal defects in adults. JACC Cardiovasc Interv. 2013;6(5):497–503.
26. Wood KP, Fleming GA, Chamberlain RC. Update on Transcatheter device closure of congenital septal defects. Curr Cardiol Rep. 2023;25(9):1083–93.
27. Bol Raap G, Meijboom FJ, Kappetein AP, Galema TW, Yap SC, Bogers AJ. Long-term follow-up and quality of life after closure of ventricular septal defect in adults. Eur J Cardiothorac Surg. 2007;32(2):215–9.
28. Kim M, Lee PH, Kim DH, Jung SH, Lee SA, Lee S, et al. Transcatheter versus surgical closure of atrial septal defect in adult patients with tricuspid regurgitation. Heart. 2022;108(24):1957–63.
29. Saurav A, Kaushik M, Mahesh Alla V, White MD, Satpathy R, Lanspa T, et al. Comparison of percutaneous device closure versus surgical closure of peri-membranous ventricular septal defects: a systematic review and meta-analysis. Catheter Cardiovasc Interv. 2015;86(6):1048–56.
30. Bergmann M, Germann CP, Nordmeyer J, Peters B, Berger F, Schubert S. Short- and long-term outcome after interventional VSD closure: a single-center experience in pediatric and adult patients. Pediatr Cardiol. 2021;42(1):78–88.
31. Chessa M, Butera G, Negura D, Bussadori C, Giamberti A, Fesslova V, et al. Transcatheter closure of congenital ventricular septal defects in adult: mid-term results and complications. Int J Cardiol. 2009;133(1):70–3.
32. Adilbekova A, Marassulov S, Baigenzhin A, Kozhakhmetov S, Nurkeyev B, Kerimkulov A, et al. Hybrid versus traditional method closure of ventricular septal defects in children. JTCVS Tech. 2024;24:137–44.
33. Dikmen N, Ozcinar E, Eyileten Z, Hasde AI, Yazicioglu L, Kaya B, et al. Comparative analysis of surgical and endovascular approaches for isolated aortic coarctation repair across age groups: outcomes and long-term efficacy. J Clin Med. 2024;13(19)
34. Hafen L, Shutze WP, Potluri S, Squiers JJ, DiMaio JM, Brinkman WT. Heart team approach for comprehensive management of aortic coarctation in the adult. Ann Cardiothorac Surg. 2022;11(1):37–45.
35. Alkashkari W, Albugami S, Hijazi ZM. Management of Coarctation of the aorta in adult patients: state of the art. Korean Circ J. 2019;49(4):298–313.
36. Kvitting JP, Olin CL. Clarence Crafoord: a giant in cardiothoracic surgery, the first to repair aortic coarctation. Ann Thorac Surg. 2009;87(1):342–6.
37. Vriend JW, Mulder BJ. Late complications in patients after repair of aortic coarctation: implications for management. Int J Cardiol. 2005;101(3):399–406.
38. Forbes TJ, Kim DW, Du W, Turner DR, Holzer R, Amin Z, et al. Comparison of surgical, stent, and balloon angioplasty treatment of native coarctation of the aorta: an observational study by the CCISC (congenital cardiovascular interventional study consortium). J Am Coll Cardiol. 2011;58(25):2664–74.
39. Erben Y, Oderich GS, Verhagen HJM, Witsenburg M, van den Hoven AT, Debus ES, et al. Multicenter experience with endovascular treatment of aortic coarctation in adults. J Vasc Surg. 2019;69(3):671–9 e1.
40. Walhout RJ, Lekkerkerker JC, Oron GH, Hitchcock FJ, Meijboom EJ, Bennink GB. Comparison of polytetrafluoroethylene patch aortoplasty and end-to-end anastomosis for coarctation of the aorta. J Thorac Cardiovasc Surg. 2003;126(2):521–8.
41. Roselli EE, Qureshi A, Idrees J, Lima B, Greenberg RK, Svensson LG, et al. Open, hybrid, and endovascular treatment for aortic coarctation and postrepair aneurysm in adolescents and adults. Ann Thorac Surg. 2012;94(3):751–6; discussion 7–8.
42. Said SM, Burkhart HM, Dearani JA, Connolly HM, Schaff HV. Ascending-to-descending aortic bypass: a simple solution to a complex problem. Ann Thorac Surg. 2014;97(6):2041–7; discussion 7–8.
43. Idrees J, Arafat A, Svensson LG, Clair D, Roselli EE. Hybrid repair of aortic aneurysm in patients with previous coarctation. J Thorac Cardiovasc Surg. 2014;148(1):60–4.

44. Bacha EA, Scheule AM, Zurakowski D, Erickson LC, Hung J, Lang P, et al. Long-term results after early primary repair of tetralogy of Fallot. J Thorac Cardiovasc Surg. 2001;122(1):154–61.
45. Diller GP, Kempny A, Liodakis E, Alonso-Gonzalez R, Inuzuka R, Uebing A, et al. Left ventricular longitudinal function predicts life-threatening ventricular arrhythmia and death in adults with repaired tetralogy of fallot. Circulation. 2012;125(20):2440–6.
46. Liu H, Liu S, Zaki A, Wang X, Zhu K, Lu Y, et al. Pulmonary valve replacement in primary repair of tetralogy of Fallot in adult patients. J Thorac Dis. 2020;12(9):4833–41.
47. Ferraz Cavalcanti PE, Sa MP, Santos CA, Esmeraldo IM, de Escobar RR, de Menezes AM, et al. Pulmonary valve replacement after operative repair of tetralogy of Fallot: meta-analysis and meta-regression of 3,118 patients from 48 studies. J Am Coll Cardiol. 2013;62(23):2227–43.
48. Cuypers JA, Menting ME, Konings EE, Opic P, Utens EM, Helbing WA, et al. Unnatural history of tetralogy of Fallot: prospective follow-up of 40 years after surgical correction. Circulation. 2014;130(22):1944–53.
49. Patel ND, Levi DS, Cheatham JP, Qureshi SA, Shahanavaz S, Zahn EM. Transcatheter pulmonary valve replacement: a review of current valve technologies. J Soc Cardiovasc Angiogr Interv. 2022;1(6):100452.
50. Jones TK, McElhinney DB, Vincent JA, Hellenbrand WE, Cheatham JP, Berman DP, et al. Long-term outcomes after melody transcatheter pulmonary valve replacement in the US investigational device exemption trial. Circ Cardiovasc Interv. 2022;15(1):e010852.
51. Lugones I, Barbosa JD, Schvartz G, Ackerman J, Laudani V, Vitorino AM, et al. A hybrid strategy for geometrical reshaping of the main pulmonary artery and transcatheter pulmonary valve replacement. World J Pediatr Congenit Heart Surg. 2021;12(5):643–8.
52. Porras D, Gurvitz M, Marshall AC, Emani SM. Hybrid approach for off-pump pulmonary valve replacement in patients with a dilated right ventricular outflow tract. Ann Thorac Surg. 2015;100(5):e99–101.
53. Uretzky GPF, Danielson GK, Hagler DJ, McGoon DC. Reoperation after correction of tetralogy of Fallot. Circulation. 1982;66:I202.
54. Tirilomis T, Friedrich M, Zenker D, Seipelt RG, Schoendube FA, Ruschewski W. Indications for reoperation late after correction of tetralogy of Fallot. Cardiol Young. 2010;20(4):396–401.
55. Baspinar O, Kosger P, Aydin SD. Percutaneous closure of hemodynamically significant postoperative residual ventricular septal defects. Pediatr Cardiol. 2024;45(2):272–81.
56. Warnes CA. Transposition of the great arteries. Circulation. 2006;114(24):2699–709.
57. Bradley EA, Cai A, Cheatham SL, Chisolm J, Sisk T, Daniels CJ, et al. Mustard baffle obstruction and leak – how successful are percutaneous interventions in adults? Prog Pediatr Cardiol. 2015;39(2 Pt B):157–63.
58. Balzer DT, Johnson M, Sharkey AM, Kort H. Transcatheter occlusion of baffle leaks following atrial switch procedures for transposition of the great vessels (d-TGV). Catheter Cardiovasc Interv. 2004;61(2):259–63.
59. Poterucha JT, Taggart NW, Johnson JN, Cannon BC, Cabalka AK, Hagler DJ, et al. Intravascular and hybrid intraoperative stent placement for baffle obstruction in transposition of the great arteries after atrial switch. Catheter Cardiovasc Interv. 2017;89(2):306–14.
60. Dennis M, Kotchetkova I, Cordina R, Celermajer DS. Long-term follow-up of adults following the atrial switch operation for transposition of the great arteries – a contemporary cohort. Heart Lung Circ. 2018;27(8):1011–7.
61. Losay JTA, Serraf A, Litvinova A, Lambert V, Piot JD, Lacour-Gayet F, Capderou A, Planche C. Late outcome after arterial switch operation for transposition of the great arteries. Circulation. 2001;104(12):6.
62. Lee J, Abdullah Shahbah D, El-Said H, Rios R, Ratnayaka K, Moore J. Pulmonary artery interventions after the arterial switch operation: unique and significant risks. Congenit Heart Dis. 2019;14(2):288–96.

63. Vonder Muhll I, Alaklabi M. The fate of the aortic root after the arterial switch operation. JACC Adv. 2024;3(4):100881.
64. Jacquemyn X, Van den Eynde J, Schuermans A, van der Palen RLF, Budts W, Danford DA, et al. Neoaortic regurgitation detected by echocardiography after arterial switch operation: a systematic review and meta-analysis. JACC Adv. 2024;3(4):100878.
65. Kreutzer C, De Vive J, Oppido G, Kreutzer J, Gauvreau K, Freed M, et al. Twenty-five-year experience with rastelli repair for transposition of the great arteries. J Thorac Cardiovasc Surg. 2000;120(2):211–23.
66. Cheatham JP, Hellenbrand WE, Zahn EM, Jones TK, Berman DP, Vincent JA, et al. Clinical and hemodynamic outcomes up to 7 years after transcatheter pulmonary valve replacement in the US melody valve investigational device exemption trial. Circulation. 2015;131(22):1960–70.
67. Horer J, Schreiber C, Dworak E, Cleuziou J, Prodan Z, Vogt M, et al. Long-term results after the Rastelli repair for transposition of the great arteries. Ann Thorac Surg. 2007;83(6):2169–75.
68. Deng L, Xu J, Tang Y, Sun H, Liu S, Song Y. Long-term outcomes of tricuspid valve surgery in patients with congenitally corrected transposition of the great arteries. J Am Heart Assoc. 2018;7(6)
69. Zubrzycki M, Schramm R, Costard-Jackle A, Morshuis M, Grohmann J, Gummert JF, et al. Pathogenesis and surgical treatment of congenitally corrected transposition of the great arteries (ccTGA): part III. J Clin Med. 2024;13(18)
70. Egbe AC, Miranda WR, Katta RR, Goda AY, Andi K, Connolly HM. Determinants of aerobic capacity after tricuspid valve replacement in congenitally corrected transposition of great arteries. JACC Adv. 2022;1(2):100027.
71. Komori M, Benesch Vidal ML, Imai K, Tominaga Y, Shibagaki K, Kutsuzawa R, et al. Diagnosis, management, and outcome of heart failure in congenitally corrected transposition of the great arteries (ccTGA)-a narrative review. Cardiovasc Diagn Ther. 2025;15(2):500–8.
72. Alonso-Gonzalez R, Massarella D. Congenitally corrected transposition of the great arteries: long-term benefits of tricuspid valve replacement. JACC Adv. 2022;1(2):100044.
73. Hagler DJ, Miranda WR, Haggerty BJ, Anderson JH, Johnson JN, Cetta F, et al. Fate of the Fontan connection: mechanisms of stenosis and management. Congenit Heart Dis. 2019;14(4):571–81.
74. Galeano-Lovera SF, Pollak P, Phillips S, Gonzalez C, Cabalka AK, Bravo-Jaimes K. Intravascular lithotripsy in an adult with Fontan pathway obstruction. JACC Case Rep. 2024;29(9):102296.
75. Venkatesh P, Gao H, Abudayyeh I, Pai RG, Varadarajan P. Contemporary management of the failing Fontan. J Clin Med. 2024;13(11)
76. Kanakis M, Chatziantoniou A, Rorris FP, Chamogeorgakis T, Kostolny M, Bobos D. Converting the Fontan circulation: challenges and evolution. Heart Surg Forum. 2023;26(6):E917–E23.
77. Buratto E, Konstantinov IE. Atrioventricular valve repair in patients with a single ventricle: emulating the fibrous skeleton of the heart. Oper Tech Thorac Cardiovasc Surg. 2022;27(1):105–13.
78. Nakata T, Hoashi T, Shimada M, Ozawa H, Higashida A, Kurosaki K, et al. Systemic atrioventricular valve replacement in patients with functional single ventricle. Semin Thorac Cardiovasc Surg. 2019;31(3):526–34.
79. Stephens EH, Dearani JA. Management of the bad atrioventricular valve in Fontan...time for a change. J Thorac Cardiovasc Surg. 2019;158(6):1643–8.
80. Kamp AN, Nair K, Fish FA, Khairy P. Catheter ablation of atrial arrhythmias in patients Post-Fontan. Can J Cardiol. 2022;38(7):1036–47.
81. Deal BJ, Costello JM, Webster G, Tsao S, Backer CL, Mavroudis C. Intermediate-term outcome of 140 consecutive Fontan conversions with arrhythmia operations. Ann Thorac Surg. 2016;101(2):717–24.

82. Itkin MG, McCormack FX, Dori Y. Diagnosis and treatment of lymphatic plastic bronchitis in adults using advanced lymphatic imaging and percutaneous embolization. Ann Am Thorac Soc. 2016;13(10):1689–96.
83. Udink Ten Cate FEA, Tjwa E. Imaging the lymphatic system in Fontan patients. Circ Cardiovasc Imaging. 2019;12(4):e008972.
84. Vyas H, Driscoll DJ, Cabalka AK, Cetta F, Hagler DJ. Results of transcatheter Fontan fenestration to treat protein losing enteropathy. Catheter Cardiovasc Interv. 2007;69(4):584–9.
85. Itkin M, Rabinowitz D, Hur S. Liver lymphatic imaging and interventions: resurrection of the forgotten knowledge. Semin Intervent Radiol. 2020;37(3):318–23.
86. Rochelson E, Richmond ME, LaPar DJ, Torres A, Anderson BR. Identification of risk factors for early Fontan failure. Semin Thorac Cardiovasc Surg. 2020;32(3):522–8.

Cutting-Edge Technology and Tools 13

Alexandru Burlacu, Crischentian Brinza, and Adrian Covic

Introduction

Over the past two decades, structural cardiac interventions have undergone a significant transformation, transitioning from invasive open-heart surgeries to procedures involving minimal access, advanced imaging, and digitally enhanced platforms. This paradigm shift has been driven not only by technological innovation but also by a growing body of evidence supporting less invasive approaches in selected patients, which are associated with reduced perioperative morbidity, shorter hospital stays, and faster functional recovery [1, 2].

Among these technological innovations, robotic-assisted procedures have emerged as a central component in the evolution of minimally invasive cardiac surgery. The role of robotic-assisted procedures has expanded to include tricuspid valve surgery, atrial septal defect closures, and hybrid procedures that integrate surgical and catheter-based approaches. Compared to conventional surgical techniques, robotic platforms could offer superior instrument dexterity, tremor elimination, and better visualization. These features facilitate greater surgical precision and have

A. Burlacu
Interventional Cardiology, Cardiovascular Diseases Institute, Iasi & Grigore T. Popa University of Medicine and Pharmacy, Iasi, Romania
e-mail: alexandru.burlacu@umfiasi.ro

C. Brinza (✉)
Faculty of Medicine, University of Medicine and Pharmacy "Grigore T Popa", Iasi, Romania
e-mail: crischentian.brinza@d.umfiasi.ro

A. Covic
Faculty of Medicine, University of Medicine and Pharmacy "Grigore T Popa", Iasi, Romania

Nephrology Clinic, Dialysis, and Renal Transplant Center—"C.I. Parhon" University Hospital, Iasi, Romania
e-mail: adrian.covic@umfiasi.ro

G. Tinică, A. Burlacu (eds.), *Surgical, Hybrid and Minimally Invasive Structural Cardiac Interventions*, https://doi.org/10.1007/978-3-032-16676-0_13

been associated with improved intraoperative control and potentially better clinical outcomes in selected structural cardiac procedures [3–7]. Despite initial concerns related to cost, operative times, and learning curve, long-term data increasingly support the safety and efficacy of robotic surgery in experienced centers [8, 9].

In parallel, the adoption of immersive visualization technologies such as virtual reality (VR) and augmented reality (AR) is transforming how structural heart disease is assessed and managed. These platforms enable three-dimensional, interactive representations of patient-specific anatomy, facilitating preoperative planning, intraoperative anatomical orientation, and enhanced procedural visualization. VR and AR are particularly advantageous in the context of congenital heart disease and complex reinterventions, where anatomical variability poses considerable challenges to conventional planning modalities [10, 11].

The emergence of computational models that simulate individual cardiac physiology and three-dimensional (3D) printed anatomical replicas has further advanced personalized medicine in structural cardiology. These platforms enable clinicians to simulate device deployment and prosthesis positioning in patient-specific anatomical models, improving preoperative planning and reducing the likelihood of intraoperative complications. Also, they could support accurate sizing, access route selection, and anticipation of technical challenges, by providing a detailed, 3D representation of the cardiac structures [12]. Incorporating these technologies into hybrid operating rooms, where real-time imaging, robotic systems, and advanced planning tools are used in combination, could enhance procedural coordination, allowing a more precise execution of structural cardiac interventions [13, 14].

This chapter provides a comprehensive and evidence-based overview of robotic systems, virtual and augmented reality, digital simulation, and 3D printing in the field of structural cardiac interventions. It critically examines their current applications, benefits, limitations, and future perspectives. Also, this chapter aims to support practicing clinicians, researchers, and healthcare decision-makers in understanding and integrating these innovations into contemporary clinical practice.

Robotic Structural Cardiac Surgery

Robotic cardiac surgery represents one of the most significant technological advancements in the field of minimally invasive cardiovascular procedures. Unlike conventional open surgery, which typically requires a median sternotomy, robotic systems offer the ability to perform intricate structural interventions through small thoracic incisions, with enhanced dexterity, precision, and visualization. Surgical robotics transitioned from basic assistive devices to fully integrated telemanipulated systems. The AESOP device, a voice-activated robotic camera holder, was approved by the Food and Drug Administration (FDA) in 1994, marking an early milestone in robotic-assisted minimally invasive surgery [15]. This was followed by the ZEUS system, approved in 2001, which incorporated multiple robotic arms controlled remotely by the surgeon [16, 17].

The da Vinci Surgical System (Intuitive Surgical, Inc.), one of the most widely used robotic platform, features multi-articulating instruments, tremor filtration, and high-definition 3D visualization, allowing the surgeon to operate from a remote console with precise control over instrument motion [18].

The first substantial use of robotics in cardiac surgery occurred in the late 1990s. In 1998, the da Vinci system was utilized for a totally endoscopic coronary artery bypass graft (CABG) intervention in Paris [19]. Also, Boyd and colleagues described the first robot-assisted, beating-heart bypass on a closed-chest patient using the ZEUS system in September 1999 at London, Ontario. Their subsequent series confirmed that internal thoracic artery harvest could be safely performed [20].

While initially employed in mitral valve repairs, robotic systems are now used in a variety of structural cardiac procedures, including tricuspid valve repair, atrial septal defect (ASD) and ventricular septal defect (VSD) closure, left atrial appendage occlusion, and even selected aortic valve operations. The shift toward robotic techniques has been driven by patient demand for less invasive alternatives, reduced hospitalization, and faster recovery times, as well as by accumulating evidence supporting their safety and efficacy in experienced centers [5, 21, 22].

Robotic Mitral Valve Surgery—Evidence and Outcomes

Mitral valve repair remains the most common application of robotic surgery in structural cardiology. Numerous comparative studies have evaluated the clinical outcomes of robotic-assisted mitral valve repair versus conventional open or minimally invasive approaches. A recent systematic review and meta-analysis analyzed the clinical performance of robot-assisted mitral valve repair in comparison with conventional sternotomy, partial sternotomy, and right minithoracotomy. Based on 15 comparative studies, the analysis showed that robotic surgery achieved similar rates of key adverse outcomes, including stroke, renal dysfunction, bleeding, and mortality, when compared to both traditional and minimally invasive techniques. In addition, robot-assisted repair was associated with a lower incidence of postoperative atrial fibrillation, shorter intensive care unit (ICU) stay, reduced pain, earlier return to normal activities, and improved physical functioning at one-year follow-up compared to full sternotomy. However, robotic procedures required longer total operative times, including cardiopulmonary bypass and cross-clamp durations. The overall certainty of evidence was rated as low, and long-term outcome data were limited. Nevertheless, these findings suggest that robotic mitral repair is a safe and effective approach in appropriately selected patients and experienced surgical teams [23].

An extensive single-center analysis of robotic mitral valve repair over an 11-year period has provided valuable long-term echocardiographic and clinical outcome data. The study, conducted at the Mayo Clinic and involving 843 patients, demonstrated that robotic repair was associated with a low early mortality rate (0.4%) and a low incidence of early reoperation (2.8%). Most patients presented with posterior or bileaflet prolapse as the underlying mechanism of mitral regurgitation.

Longitudinal echocardiographic assessment revealed sustained reductions in left ventricular volumes, left atrial size, and pulmonary artery pressures up to two years post-surgery. At ten-year follow-up, overall survival was 93%, while freedom from reoperation reached 92.6% [24].

Another meta-analysis that included six retrospective studies comparing robotic and conventional mitral valve surgery in degenerative disease found that perioperative survival was higher in the robotic group. Nevertheless, the rates of stroke and reoperation for bleeding were similar between the two approaches. Also, robotic procedures were associated with longer cardiopulmonary bypass and aortic cross-clamp times, but no significant differences were observed in ICU or total hospital stay. Both surgical techniques resulted in acceptable echocardiographic outcomes. The authors noted that robotic mitral surgery can be performed safely in selected patients, provided it is carried out by experienced surgical teams working in centers with adequate case volumes and specialized training [25].

Robotic Tricuspid Valve Surgery and ASD Repair

Although less commonly performed, robotic tricuspid valve repair and congenital defect closures are gaining interest. A retrospective analysis from a single institution assessed the safety and outcomes of totally endoscopic robotic tricuspid valve surgery over a ten-year period. Seventy patients underwent tricuspid valve repair using the da Vinci robotic system, including both isolated and concomitant procedures. Most patients (97%) received an annuloplasty band, and there were no conversions to open surgery, with early mortality rate of 1.4%. Postoperative echocardiography showed mild residual tricuspid regurgitation in 93% of patients. At a mean follow-up of 45 months, moderate or greater recurrent regurgitation was observed in 9% of patients with available echocardiographic data. The majority of late deaths were not related to cardiac causes. These findings suggest that robot-assisted tricuspid valve repair can be performed safely and with satisfactory mid-term valve function in appropriately selected patients [26].

A retrospective study examined the safety and efficiency of robot-assisted atrial septal defect (ASD) repair performed with either a beating or non-beating heart approach. The analysis included 45 patients who underwent robotic ASD closure using the da Vinci system between 2010 and 2019. Of these, 27 cases were completed on a beating heart and 18 on an arrested or fibrillating heart. In all patients, cardiopulmonary bypass was established through femoral and jugular cannulation. Complete defect closure was confirmed intraoperatively in every case, and there were no conversions to open surgery or incidences of stroke or major complications. Neurological recovery was uneventful in all patients. In a subgroup of patients undergoing isolated patch repair, the beating-heart group had shorter cardiopulmonary bypass times compared to the non-beating-heart group. These findings suggest that robotic ASD repair can be safely performed using a beating-heart strategy without increasing the risk of cerebral embolic events [4].

Benefits and Limitations

Robotic surgery provides several distinct advantages in the context of structural cardiac procedures. These include reduced surgical trauma through smaller incisions, improved cosmetic results, and decreased postoperative pain. Multiple studies reported shorter hospital stays and faster return to normal activities following robotic surgery compared to conventional sternotomy, while maintaining comparable safety profiles in terms of stroke, renal failure, and mortality rates [2, 25]. Robotic systems also offer high-definition, three-dimensional visualization and articulated instruments that facilitate precise manipulation of cardiac structures. These technical attributes are especially beneficial in procedures involving complex valve anatomy [24, 26]. In tricuspid valve surgery, robotic technique was associated with favorable midterm valve competence and low perioperative morbidity, supporting the feasibility of a sternal-sparing technique in experienced centers [26]. Similarly, robotic ASD repair has shown reliable defect closure and shorter bypass times in beating-heart approaches [4].

Despite these advantages, some limitations should be addressed. Robotic procedures are consistently associated with longer cardiopulmonary bypass and aortic cross-clamp times, particularly in the early phases of adoption. These prolonged operative times are partly attributable to the setup process, as well as the need for precise coordination among the surgical team. Furthermore, the financial cost of acquiring and maintaining robotic platforms, along with limited access to emergency conversion options, poses logistical and institutional challenges. Robotic surgery presents a learning curve that can impact early performance. In a report from a high-volume center, total operative time decreased significantly after approximately 30 cases, indicating team adaptation to robotic workflows with advancing experience [8]. A prospective analysis of initial robotic mitral valve repair procedures at two European centers evaluated the number of cases required to reach technical proficiency. The study found that operative efficiency, measured by cardiopulmonary bypass and cross-clamp times, improved markedly as experience was gained. Specifically, the learning plateau occurred at the 60th and 50th cases at the two centers, respectively, indicating that structured experience can significantly reduce operative duration and improve outcomes in robotic mitral repair. Long-term success in robotic cardiac surgery, therefore, depends not only on technology but also on dedicated training, team experience, and appropriate patient selection [27].

Cost-Effectiveness

Economic analyses of robotic structural heart surgery remain nuanced, as the initial investment in robotic platforms, maintenance, and disposable instrumentation is substantial. A recent national study examined over 40,000 elective mitral valve repair procedures performed across the United States and compared outcomes and costs between robotic-assisted and conventional surgical approaches. The analysis found that both techniques yielded similar short-term clinical results, including mortality, stroke, and postoperative complications. Patients who underwent robotic repair had a shorter hospital stay by approximately 1.3 days. However, the robotic approach was associated with higher overall hospitalization costs, with a median of $46,800 compared to $38,500 for conventional surgery. Even after adjusting for clinical risk factors and hospital characteristics, robotic procedures remained more expensive by an average of $10,500. Notably, in hospitals performing the highest number of mitral valve repairs, this cost difference became smaller and was not statistically significant. These results suggest that while robotic-assisted surgery could be more expensive, programs with greater experience and higher case volumes can deliver robotic procedures at a similar cost level to traditional methods, supporting the concentration of robotic programs in well-established centers [28].

Extended Reality in Structural Cardiac Interventions

Virtual reality (VR), augmented reality (AR), and mixed reality (MR), together known as extended reality (XR), offer immersive, three-dimensional visualization environments that enhance understanding of complex cardiovascular anatomy. XR enables surgeons to interact with patient-specific cardiac models, facilitating both preoperative planning and intraoperative orientation. Real-time integration of imaging and procedural data within the XR environment helps address many of the limitations associated with standard visual platforms in structural heart interventions [29].

Extended Reality for Structural Heart Surgery Planning

Emerging evidence highlighted the potential of XR to enhance surgical planning in structural heart disease. In controlled studies, XR use has led to measurable intraoperative benefits. Notably, one study evaluated the impact of cinematic MR rendering in a cohort of 26 patients undergoing congenital heart surgery, showing that MR-guided planning reduced intraoperative preparation time compared to conventional approaches (24.5 ± 23 min versus 73 ± 43 min) [29, 30].

Another study explored the application of MR in the diagnosis and surgical planning of double outlet right ventricle, comparing it to conventional 3D image interpretation. Thirty-four patients had computed tomography (CT) angiography images, and were randomly allocated to either an MR-guided group or a control group. The MR holograms closely matched intraoperative findings and enabled correct classification of all double outlet right ventricle subtypes. Although the improvement in diagnostic accuracy over conventional 3D reconstruction was not statistically significant, the MR-guided approach significantly reduced surgical planning time. Moreover, in all cases within the MR group, the surgery proceeded exactly as initially planned. The findings suggest that MR holography enhances anatomical visualization and may facilitate more efficient and reliable preoperative decision-making in complex congenital heart disease [29, 31].

Other studies have documented the feasibility of XR across a variety of challenging procedures, including pulmonary artery reconstructions, aortic valve repairs, and reoperations in adults. Notably, surgeons consistently reported improved anatomical understanding and planning accuracy [29]. XR technologies showed a potential role in optimizing preoperative planning for structural heart surgery. XR can improve anatomical assessment, reduce planning time, and support procedural accuracy, including in complex congenital cases. While broader clinical validation is required, current findings support the integration of XR as a valuable adjunct in surgical strategy planning [29].

Limitations and Challenges

Despite growing enthusiasm, XR technologies continue to face several challenges that could limit their routine integration into structural heart interventions. First, some users experience visual discomfort during prolonged use of VR systems. Although newer-generation devices have improved comfort and responsiveness, these issues can influence user acceptance in high-volume centers [30, 32].

Moreover, integrating XR tools into existing clinical workflows remains technically and logistically complex. Image segmentation, model rendering, device calibration, and data transfer between systems often require time-intensive preparation and specialized personnel. Furthermore, the high cost of XR platforms, combined with unclear reimbursement pathways, poses additional barriers to widespread adoption, particularly in low- and middle-income settings [33, 34].

Lastly, while feasibility studies and case series have highlighted subjective benefits and encouraging short-term outcomes, the field still lacks large-scale randomized trials or multicenter registries to objectively evaluate clinical efficacy, safety, and cost-effectiveness. Without such data, it remains difficult to assess the true impact of XR integration on patient outcomes and resource utilization across diverse healthcare systems [33, 34].

Digital Simulation and 3D Printing in Structural Cardiac Interventions

Digital simulation and 3D printing technologies provided new dimensions to the preoperative planning of structural cardiac interventions. These technologies allow for the physical and virtual reproduction of individual cardiovascular anatomy, facilitating not only surgical planning, but also interdisciplinary collaboration and patient communication. Unlike traditional training models, digital simulations tailored to patient imaging could provide surgical teams with precise anatomical insights before the procedure [35, 36].

Digital Simulation

Simulation in this context refers to the virtual recreation of physiological structures and flow dynamics derived from CT, magnetic resonance imaging (MRI), or echocardiographic data. These can be embedded in software platforms that allow interactive manipulation of the heart, mimicking intraoperative views and responses to intervention. In some systems, these digital models are exported to 3D printers, producing tangible heart structures used for hands-on procedural planning or education [37, 38].

Patient-specific simulation has found application in the planning of complex mitral and tricuspid valve surgeries, left atrial appendage occlusion, septal defect repair, and transcatheter valve-in-valve procedures. The utility of such simulation lies in its ability to anticipate anatomical challenges, such as left ventricular outflow tract obstruction, device malposition, or the proximity of key conduction pathways [37, 39, 40].

CT, MRI, or echocardiography data could be used to construct virtual models of the patient's anatomy. These images can be explored interactively on screen or transformed into physical, three-dimensional printed models made from tissue-mimicking materials. Simulation enables procedural teams to assess landing zones, select appropriate device size and orientation, and test access strategies, reducing uncertainty and potentially minimizing complications like device embolization or paravalvular leak [37].

In the case of left atrial appendage closure (LAAC), the randomized PREDICT-LAA trial reported that computational modeling led to 12.9% fewer post-procedure leaks or thrombotic events and fewer device repositioning compared to standard planning [37].

In transcatheter aortic valve implantation (TAVI), both 3D-printing and computer simulation have demonstrated promising applications in procedural planning and risk assessment. When integrated into pulsatile flow loops, these models have shown realistic valve behavior, providing accurate evaluation of stenosis severity and prediction of paravalvular leak risk during valve sizing. In one study involving 16 patients, 3D-printed models correctly identified paravalvular leaks in six of nine cases and ruled them out in five of seven patients [37, 41].

While the technical and resource demands remain high, due to the need for image segmentation, model development, and printing expertise, simulation continues to evolve as a valuable tool in complex structural interventions, providing tailored planning that aims to reduce procedural complications and improve clinical outcomes [37].

Role of 3D Printing in Cardiac Surgery

Three-dimensional printing allows clinicians to hold and manipulate exact replicas of patient hearts. These are typically constructed from multi-material resin or silicone, which can replicate tissue compliance and offer insight into the interaction between devices and cardiac structures. The creation process involves segmentation of imaging data, computer-aided design (CAD) modeling, and finally additive manufacturing via polymer-based printers [42, 43].

One study demonstrated the practical application and clinical value of patient-specific 3D-printed cardiac prototypes in the surgical management of complex congenital heart defects. Utilizing high-resolution cardiac MRI and CT data, the authors generated life-sized models for five patients presenting with complex conditions, such as double-outlet right ventricle, criss-cross atrioventricular connections, and congenitally corrected transposition of the great arteries with pulmonary atresia. The use of 3D models enhanced the spatial understanding of the surgical team, enabling precise preoperative planning. The printed prototypes facilitated the identification of operative challenges and guided surgical strategies, which were subsequently implemented as planned, with favorable outcomes in all patients. This experience highlights the value of 3D printing not only as a visual aid but also as a critical tool for operative decision-making [35].

In case of mitral valve interventions, 3D printed replicas have been used to plan MitraClip deployment, guide the selection of occluder devices, and predict procedural challenges such as left ventricular outflow tract (LVOT) obstruction in transcatheter mitral valve replacement (TMVR). Models constructed with materials mimicking the elasticity and rigidity of valvular tissue offer insight into device–anatomy interaction that is difficult to achieve with digital imaging alone [36].

The utility of 3D printing extends to congenital heart disease, where unique structural anomalies often require highly individualized surgical approaches. Three-dimensional printed models have been used to plan repair of atrial or ventricular septal defects, Fontan reinterventions, and complex conduit placements. Also, 3D models have improved device sizing and reduced procedural times and complications in LAAC interventions. These models not only facilitate surgical planning but also enhance communication among multidisciplinary teams [36].

The integration of 3D printing into cardiac surgery represents a paradigm shift toward personalized intervention. These models bridge the gap between imaging and intervention by allowing teams to identify procedural difficulties, refine therapeutic approaches, and ultimately, improve patient outcomes. Moreover, as printing technologies and material sciences advance, their role in planning, simulation, and even intraoperative guidance is expected to expand significantly [36].

References

1. Galloway AC, et al. A decade of minimally invasive mitral repair: long-term outcomes. Ann Thorac Surg. 2009;88(4):1180–4.
2. Modi P, Hassan A, Chitwood WR Jr. Minimally invasive mitral valve surgery: a systematic review and meta-analysis. Eur J Cardiothorac Surg. 2008;34(5):943–52.
3. Vardas PN, et al. Safety and outcomes of reoperative robotic tricuspid valve surgery. Innovations (Phila). 2024;19(5):526–31.
4. Yun T, et al. Robot-assisted repair of atrial septal defect: a comparison of beating and non-beating heart surgery. J Chest Surg. 2022;55(1):55–60.

5. Balkhy HH, et al. Multi-spectrum robotic cardiac surgery: early outcomes. JTCVS Tech. 2022;13:74–82.
6. Hamandi M, et al. A review of robotic mitral valve surgery. Struct Heart. 2021;5(2):151–7.
7. Catelli C, et al. Satisfactory outcome with robotic-assisted chest wall resection and reconstruction: a case report. J Visual Surg. 2024;10:10.
8. Khairallah SM, Rahouma M, Mick SL. Transferring surgical expertise: analyzing the learning curve of robotic cardiac surgery operative time reduction when surgeon moves from one experienced center to another. J Cardiovasc Dev Dis. 2024;11(3)
9. Williams ML, et al. Systematic review and meta-analysis of mid-term survival, reoperation, and recurrent mitral regurgitation for robotic-assisted mitral valve repair. Ann Cardiothorac Surg. 2022;11(6):553–63.
10. Sadeghi AH, et al. Immersive 3D virtual reality imaging in planning minimally invasive and complex adult cardiac surgery. Eur Heart J Digit Health. 2020;1(1):62–70.
11. Valverde I, et al. Three-dimensional printed models for surgical planning of complex congenital heart defects: an international multicentre study. Eur J Cardiothorac Surg. 2017;52(6):1139–48.
12. Bernhard B, et al. Imaging-based, patient-specific three-dimensional printing to plan, train, and guide cardiovascular interventions: a systematic review and meta-analysis. Heart Lung Circ. 2022;31(9):1203–18.
13. Creazzo G, et al. Deployment of a digital twin using the coupled momentum method for fluid-structure interaction: a case study for aortic aneurysm. Comput Biol Med. 2025;190:110084.
14. Silaschi M, et al. Proposal for valve sizing, prosthesis simulation, and procedure planning based on computed tomography in endoscopic mitral valve surgery. Innovations (Phila). 2025:15569845251330863.
15. Pugin F, Bucher P, Morel P. History of robotic surgery: from AESOP® and ZEUS® to da Vinci®. J Visc Surg. 2011;148(5, Supplement):e3–8.
16. Rivero-Moreno Y, et al. Robotic surgery: a comprehensive review of the literature and current trends. Cureus. 2023;15(7):e42370.
17. Pugin F, Bucher P, Morel P. History of robotic surgery: from AESOP® and ZEUS® to da Vinci®. J Visc Surg. 2011;148:e3–8.
18. Ngu JC, Tsang CB, Koh DC. The da Vinci Xi: a review of its capabilities, versatility, and potential role in robotic colorectal surgery. Robot Surg. 2017;4:77–85.
19. Raja SG. New clinical advances in minimally invasive coronary surgery. J Clin Med. 2025;14(9)
20. Bonatti J. Historical landmarks in the development of robotic coronary bypass grafting. Ann Cardiothorac Surg. 2024;13(4):332–8.
21. Xiao C, et al. Totally robotic atrial septal defect closure: 7-year single-institution experience and follow-up. Interact Cardiovasc Thorac Surg. 2014;19(6):933–7.
22. Arslanhan G, et al. Concomitant tricuspid valve surgery is not associated with increased operative risk during robotic mitral valve surgery. Innovations (Phila). 2024;19(1):72–9.
23. Fatehi Hassanabad A, et al. A systematic review and meta-analysis of robot-assisted mitral valve repair. Innovations (Phila). 2022;17(6):471–81.
24. Arghami A, et al. Robotic mitral valve repair: a decade of experience with echocardiographic follow-up. Ann Thorac Surg. 2022;114(5):1587–95.
25. Cao C, et al. A meta-analysis of robotic vs. conventional mitral valve surgery. Ann Cardiothoracic Surg. 2015;4(4):305–14.
26. Bhasin R, et al. Robotic totally endoscopic tricuspid valve surgery: early results and midterm outcomes. Innovations. 2025;20(2):188–93.
27. Sandoval E, et al. Learning curve of robotic mitral repair: prospective two-Centre study of proficiency and clinical outcomes. Eur J Cardiothorac Surg. 2024;66(6)
28. Hadaya J, et al. Clinical outcomes and costs of robotic-assisted vs conventional mitral valve repair: a National Analysis. Ann Thorac Surg. 2025;119(5):1011–9.
29. Stephenson N, et al. Extended reality for procedural planning and guidance in structural heart disease—a review of the state-of-the-art. Int J Cardiovasc Imaging. 2023;39(7):1405–19.
30. Gehrsitz P, et al. Cinematic rendering in mixed-reality holograms: a new 3D preoperative planning tool in pediatric heart surgery. Front Cardiovasc Med. 2021;8:633611.

31. Ye W, et al. Mixed-reality hologram for diagnosis and surgical planning of double outlet of the right ventricle: a pilot study. Clin Radiol. 2021;76(3):237.e1–7.
32. Bhaskaran V, Mahbub U. Immersive user experiences: trends and challenges of using XR technologies. Computer Vision; 2024. p. 260–78.
33. Tsai T-Y, et al. Merging virtual and physical experiences: extended realities in cardiovascular medicine. Eur Heart J. 2023;44(35):3311–22.
34. Bui J, et al. The role of extended reality in enhancing surgical training: a narrative review. Curr Chall Thoracic Surg. 2025;7:7.
35. Kappanayil M, et al. Three-dimensional-printed cardiac prototypes aid surgical decision-making and preoperative planning in selected cases of complex congenital heart diseases: early experience and proof of concept in a resource-limited environment. Ann Pediatr Cardiol. 2017;10(2):117–25.
36. Vukicevic M, Filippini S, Little SH. Patient-specific modeling for structural heart intervention: role of 3D printing today and tomorrow (CME). Methodist Debakey Cardiovasc J. 2020;16(2):130–7.
37. Chandrasekhar J, Saw J. Simulation for procedural planning and intracardiac echo for enhancing precision in cardiac interventions with a focus on left atrial appendage closure. Structural Heart. 2025;9(5):100427.
38. Vukicevic M, et al. Patient-specific 3D valve modeling for structural intervention. Structural Heart. 2017;1(5):236–48.
39. Mendez K, et al. Design and validation of a high-Fidelity left atrial cardiac simulator for the study and advancement of left atrial appendage occlusion. Cardiovasc Eng Technol. 2025;16(3):279–95.
40. Ciobotaru V, et al. Left atrial appendage occlusion simulation based on three-dimensional printing: new insights into outcome and technique. EuroIntervention. 2018;14(2):176–84.
41. Ripley B, et al. 3D printing based on cardiac CT assists anatomic visualization prior to transcatheter aortic valve replacement. J Cardiovasc Comput Tomogr. 2016;10(1):28–36.
42. Goo HW, Park SJ, Yoo S-J. Advanced medical use of three-dimensional imaging in congenital heart disease: augmented reality, mixed reality, virtual reality, and three-dimensional printing. Korean J Radiol. 2020;21(2):133–45.
43. Fan Y, Wong RHL, Lee AP-W. Three-dimensional printing in structural heart disease and intervention. Ann Transl Med. 2019;7(20):579.

Valvular Dilated Cardiomyopathy: Modern Treatment Strategies Versus Heart Transplantation

14

Bhalinder Dhaliwal, Leonardo Paim da Costa, and Lucian Lozonschi

Introduction

Valvular dilated cardiomyopathy (DCM) represents a clinically significant subtype of heart failure where progressive left ventricular (LV) dysfunction arises secondary to chronic volume or pressure overload due to valvular lesions. Unlike idiopathic DCM, valvular DCM offers an opportunity for reversal if the primary mechanical cause is addressed in time. This chapter provides a comprehensive overview of the pathophysiological basis of valvular DCM, contemporary diagnostic modalities, and evolving management strategies, with a final focus on heart transplantation for end-stage disease.

Advanced Diagnostic Technologies

Artificial Intelligence in Cardiac Imaging

The integration of artificial intelligence (AI) into cardiac imaging is a major advancement in valvular DCM diagnosis, rivaling the impact of echocardiography [1]. Machine learning, especially deep neural networks, excels at analyzing complex imaging data, often outperforming human experts in specific diagnostic tasks. In echocardiography, AI enables automated chamber quantification and real-time

B. Dhaliwal
Division of Cardiothoracic Surgery & Transplantation, Tampa General Hospital, Tampa, FL, USA

L. P. da Costa · L. Lozonschi (✉)
Division of Cardiothoracic Surgery & Transplantation, Tampa General Hospital/University of South Florida, Tampa, FL, USA
e-mail: Lozonschi@usf.edu

G. Tinică, A. Burlacu (eds.), *Surgical, Hybrid and Minimally Invasive Structural Cardiac Interventions*, https://doi.org/10.1007/978-3-032-16676-0_14

segmentation with expert-level accuracy [2]. These systems identify standard views, assess image quality, and provide immediate feedback, while detecting subtle functional changes that may signal early remodeling.AI has shown strong performance in mitral regurgitation assessment, with deep learning models analyzing over 50,000 echocardiograms and achieving AUCs of 0.916 and 0.934 for moderate and severe cases, respectively, and even higher in external validation [3]. In cardiac magnetic resonance (CMR), AI automates valve tracking and parametric mapping, enhancing diagnostic precision and reproducibility [4].

Advanced Biomarker Discovery

The biomarker landscape in valvular DCM has expanded well beyond traditional markers like B-type natriuretic peptides and troponins [5]. New biomarkers now reflect diverse pathophysiological processes including inflammation, fibrosis, oxidative stress, and metabolic dysfunction, offering deeper insights into disease mechanisms and therapeutic targets. Soluble ST2 (sST2) has emerged as a key marker of mechanical stress and fibrotic remodeling, with elevated levels predicting mortality and heart failure hospitalization independently of other clinical variables [6]. Unlike traditional hemodynamic markers, sST2 provides information about the underlying remodeling process and may help identify patients who would benefit from early intervention. Galectin-3, a β-galactoside-binding lectin involved in fibrosis and inflammation, is associated with increased collagen deposition and adverse outcomes, making it a promising target for anti-fibrotic therapy [7].High-sensitivity troponin assays have revealed that subclinical myocardial injury is common in valvular DCM even in asymptomatic patients providing early warning of disease progression [8]. Circulating microRNAs (miRNAs) represent a particularly exciting class of biomarkers, with specific miRNAs linked to distinct aspects of cardiac remodeling: hypertrophy (miR-1, miR-133), fibrosis (miR-21, miR-29), and angiogenesis (miR-126, miR-210) [9].

Precision Imaging Approaches

Precision imaging in valvular DCM involves tailoring diagnostic protocols to individual patient characteristics, including genetic background, comorbidities, and specific disease mechanisms [10]. This personalized approach enhances diagnostic precision and supports more targeted therapeutic decisions. Strain imaging has become a clinical necessity, offering insights into myocardial function that are not captured by conventional measures. Global longitudinal strain (GLS) can detect early myocardial dysfunction before ejection fraction declines, while layer-specific strain analysis distinguishes between endocardial and epicardial impairment, providing deeper understanding of disease progression [11].

Machine learning further enhances strain imaging by automating measurements, reducing inter-observer variability, and generating standardized reports that support clinical workflows [12]. Three-dimensional echocardiography, powered by AI, has transformed the assessment of complex valvular pathology. These tools provide detailed anatomical models that improve surgical planning, predict procedural outcomes, and enable the development of patient-specific therapeutic strategies, including custom prosthetic devices and surgical techniques [13].

Surgical Decision-Making Framework

The Point of No Return: When the Ventricle Is Too Far Gone

The most critical decision facing cardiac surgeons in valvular DCM is determining when left ventricular dysfunction becomes irreversible despite valve correction. Traditional metrics like ejection fraction and end-systolic dimension provide limited guidance for this crucial determination.

Advanced Surgical Markers for Irreversibility

The concept of "reverse remodeling potential"has emerged as the key determinant of surgical success. Recent evidence from the CTSN trials demonstrates that patients who achieve reverse remodeling after mitral valve surgery show dramatic improvements in long-term survival, while those who fail to reverse remodel have outcomes similar to medical therapy [14].

Intraoperative Assessment Protocols

Transesophageal echocardiography during surgery provides critical real-time information that can alter surgical strategy. The "tethering distance" measured from the annular plane to the papillary muscle tips serves as a powerful predictor of repair durability. When this distance exceeds 10 mm, repair failure rates increase exponentially, favoring replacement over complex repair attempts [15].

Surgical Risk Stratification

The development of surgical risk calculators specific to valvular DCM has revolutionized preoperative planning. The EuroSCORE II and STS risk models, while useful for general cardiac surgery, underestimate risk in functional mitral regurgitation. Advanced centers now employ institution-specific algorithms that incorporate ventricular geometry, degree of tethering, and functional capacity to predict surgical outcomes with remarkable accuracy [16].

Repair Versus Replacement: The Evidence-Based Decision

The traditional surgical dogma of "repair whenever possible" has been challenged by compelling evidence from randomized controlled trials. The CTSN trial comparing repair versus replacement in severe ischemic mitral regurgitation revealed that repair, despite technical success, resulted in significantly higher rates of recurrent regurgitation without improvement in survival or reverse remodeling [14].

Technical Factors Favoring Repair

Complex neochordal reconstruction techniques have emerged as game-changers in mitral valve repair. The revolutionary approach described by EL-Andari and colleagues involves creating multiple neochordae of uniform length across the entire leaflet, establishing a new plane of coaptation that remains symmetric regardless of individual segment pathology [17]. This technique addresses the fundamental limitation of traditional repair methods that rely on precise individual measurements.

Technical Factors Favoring Replacement

Severe leaflet tethering, defined as a coaptation depth greater than 11 mm or tethering area exceeding 2.5 cm^2, represents a strong indication for valve replacement. In these cases, restrictive annuloplasty alone fails to address the underlying geometric distortion, leading to high rates of repair failure. Chordal-sparing replacement preserves ventricular geometry while providing definitive correction of regurgitation [18].

The Hybrid Approach

Advanced surgical centers have developed hybrid techniques that combine elements of repair and replacement. The "mitral complex remodeling" procedure involves division and reconstruction of secondary chords, undersized annuloplasty, and selective papillary muscle repositioning. This approach addresses both annular and subvalvular pathology while preserving native valve tissue where possible [19].

Concomitant Procedure Decision-Making

The management of concomitant pathology in valvular DCM requires sophisticated surgical judgment that extends beyond individual valve pathology. The decision to address tricuspid regurgitation, perform coronary revascularization, or ablate atrial fibrillation significantly impacts operative risk and long-term outcomes.

Tricuspid Valve Intervention Thresholds

Recent guidelines have lowered the threshold for concomitant tricuspid valve intervention, recognizing that functional tricuspid regurgitation in the setting of left-sided valve disease represents a progressive condition that rarely improves with mitral correction alone. The presence of moderate or greater tricuspid regurgitation with annular dilation exceeding 40 mm constitutes a Class I indication for concomitant repair [20].

Coronary Revascularization Strategy

The decision to perform coronary revascularization in functional mitral regurgitation remains controversial. The CTSN trial demonstrated that adding mitral valve repair to coronary bypass surgery reduced recurrent regurgitation but increased neurologic complications without improving survival [14]. This finding has led to more selective approaches, with revascularization reserved for patients with significant viable myocardium in the distribution of stenotic vessels.

Atrial Fibrillation Management

Concomitant surgical ablation for atrial fibrillation in valvular DCM patients shows excellent success rates when performed with appropriate technique. The Cox-Maze IV procedure, utilizing bipolar radiofrequency and cryoablation, achieves freedom from atrial fibrillation in over 90% of patients at 1 year. The decision to perform ablation should consider patient age, atrial size, and duration of fibrillation [21].

Advanced Surgical Techniques

Complex Neochordal Reconstruction: The New Gold Standard

The evolution of neochordal techniques represents one of the most significant advances in mitral valve surgery over the past decade. Traditional approaches that relied on individual segment repair and intraoperative measurement have given way to sophisticated preoperative planning and standardized reconstruction methods that achieve superior and reproducible results.

Preoperative Planning and Measurement

The foundation of successful neochordal reconstruction begins with high-quality preoperative imaging. Three-dimensional echocardiography provides precise measurements of leaflet geometry, papillary muscle position, and the extent of prolapse or restriction. These measurements guide the preoperative preparation of neochordae, eliminating the guesswork and time-consuming adjustments that characterize traditional approaches [17].

Standard neochord lengths have been established through extensive clinical experience: 20–25 mm for anterior leaflet reconstruction and 10–15 mm for posterior leaflet procedures. These measurements can be adjusted based on individual patient anatomy, but the standardized approach provides a reliable starting point that reduces operative time and improves consistency [17].

Technical Execution of Complex Reconstruction

The surgical technique begins with the preparation of multiple neochordae using CV-5 polytetrafluoroethylene Gore-Tex suture and PCP 20 Gore-Tex pledgets. The key innovation lies in creating multiple neochordae of identical length that span the entire affected leaflet, rather than attempting to repair individual segments with varying lengths [17].

The caliper-based preparation method ensures precise length control while addressing the notorious slipperiness of Gore-Tex sutures that has plagued traditional techniques. The Mohr loop technique, which involves looping the suture around a caliper and securing it with multiple knots, provides reliable fixation that maintains length during implantation [17].

Implantation Strategy

Once the mitral valve is exposed and inspected, the free needle from the prepared neochords is placed into either the anterolateral or posteromedial papillary muscle, depending on the leaflet pathology. The choice of papillary muscle attachment site requires understanding of the complex three-dimensional anatomy and blood flow patterns within the left ventricle [17].

The leaflet attachment involves passing 2-0 ETHIBOND sutures through the mitral valve leaflet at predetermined locations that correspond to the areas of maximum prolapse or restriction. The uniform length of the neochordae creates a new plane of coaptation that remains symmetric across the entire leaflet, preventing the misalignment that commonly occurs with traditional segment-specific repairs [17].

Restrictive Annuloplasty: Beyond Simple Ring Placement

While annuloplasty remains a cornerstone of mitral valve repair, the approach in functional mitral regurgitation requires sophisticated understanding of annular dynamics and ventricular geometry. Simple ring placement without consideration of subvalvular pathology often leads to repair failure and recurrent regurgitation.

Ring Selection and Sizing Strategy

The choice between rigid, semi-rigid, and flexible rings significantly impacts repair durability in functional mitral regurgitation. Rigid rings provide maximum reduction in annular area but may increase leaflet stress and tethering. Semi-rigid rings offer a compromise between reduction and flexibility, while complete flexible rings may provide insufficient correction in severely dilated annuli [22].

Undersizing strategy has evolved from aggressive downsizing to more nuanced approaches based on leaflet geometry. The traditional practice of downsizing by two sizes has been replaced by individualized sizing based on anterior leaflet area and the degree of posterior leaflet restriction. Excessive downsizing can paradoxically increase tethering and reduce repair durability [23].

Advanced Annuloplasty Techniques

The concept of "asymmetric annuloplasty" has emerged as a refinement of traditional techniques. This approach involves selective reduction of the posterior annulus while preserving anterior annular geometry, reducing the risk of increased tethering while maintaining effective regurgitation control [24].

Suture technique for annuloplasty placement requires careful attention to tissue handling and knot security. The use of pledgeted sutures in friable tissue and the incorporation of trigonal tissue into the repair provide enhanced durability. The sequence of suture placement and tying can significantly impact the final annular geometry and should follow established protocols [25].

Papillary Muscle Procedures: Addressing Subvalvular Pathology

The recognition that functional mitral regurgitation results primarily from subvalvular pathology rather than leaflet disease has led to the development of sophisticated papillary muscle procedures that address the root cause of valve dysfunction.

Papillary Muscle Approximation Techniques

The "papillary muscle sling" procedure involves placing a CV-4 Gore-Tex suture between the heads of the papillary muscles to reduce the interpapillary distance and decrease leaflet tethering. This technique requires precise understanding of papillary muscle anatomy and the relationship between muscle position and leaflet coaptation [26].

The suture placement must avoid injury to the papillary muscle blood supply while achieving sufficient approximation to improve leaflet geometry. Intraoperative echocardiography guides the degree of approximation, with the goal of achieving leaflet coaptation without creating stenosis [26].

Papillary Muscle Relocation

For patients with severe papillary muscle displacement, particularly those with posterior or lateral wall infarction, papillary muscle relocation offers a more definitive solution. This technique involves mobilizing the displaced papillary muscle and securing it to a more anatomically appropriate position using Gore-Tex sutures [27].

The relocation procedure requires careful assessment of papillary muscle viability and blood supply. The use of 4-mm Gore-Tex tubes to encircle the papillary muscle bodies provides secure fixation while preserving muscle integrity. The technique is particularly effective for type III, IV, and V papillary muscle displacement patterns [17].

Minimally Invasive and Robotic Approaches

The evolution of minimally invasive cardiac surgery has reached remarkable sophistication, with robotic assistance now providing outcomes that match or exceed traditional sternotomy approaches in carefully selected patients.

Patient Selection for Robotic Surgery

The Cleveland Clinic algorithm for robotic mitral valve surgery represents the gold standard for patient selection, having been validated across over 2400 procedures with exceptional outcomes. The algorithm requires specific criteria from both transthoracic echocardiography and computed tomography to ensure safe and effective robotic intervention [16].

The echocardiographic requirements include mild or no aortic regurgitation, absence of significant mitral annular calcification, good left ventricular function, and no significant pulmonary hypertension. These criteria ensure that the technical limitations of robotic surgery do not compromise repair quality or patient safety [16].

The computed tomography requirements focus on vascular access, requiring minimal aortoiliac atherosclerosis, femoral artery diameter of at least 7 mm, and absence of severe pectus excavatum. These anatomical considerations are critical for safe peripheral cannulation and adequate surgical exposure [16].

Technical Execution of Robotic Repair

Robotic mitral valve repair involves the placement of three robotic arm ports and one working incision of 3–4 cm between the ribs. The robotic system provides 10× magnification with 360-degree visualization, enabling precise manipulation of delicate cardiac structures [16].

The articulation of robotic instruments mimics the surgeon's hand movements with enhanced precision, allowing for complex repairs that would be challenging through traditional minimally invasive approaches. The learning curve for robotic surgery is significant, requiring specialized training beyond standard cardiac surgery residency [16].

Outcomes and Limitations

The Cleveland Clinic experience demonstrates that robotic mitral valve repair can achieve a 99.7% repair rate with 0.04% mortality in appropriately selected patients. These outcomes rival or exceed those achieved with traditional sternotomy approaches while providing significant benefits in terms of recovery time and cosmetic results [16].

However, the conservative selection criteria mean that only 70% of patients with isolated degenerative mitral valve disease qualify for robotic surgery. The remaining 30% require alternative approaches due to anatomical or technical factors that preclude safe robotic intervention [16].

Surgical Outcomes and Complications Management

Immediate Postoperative Management

The immediate postoperative period following valvular DCM surgery requires sophisticated monitoring and management strategies that differ significantly from routine cardiac surgery protocols. The compromised ventricular function and altered loading conditions necessitate careful attention to hemodynamic optimization and early recognition of complications.

Hemodynamic Optimization Strategies

Patients with valvular DCM often experience dramatic changes in loading conditions following valve repair or replacement. The sudden reduction in regurgitant volume can unmask underlying systolic dysfunction, requiring careful titration of inotropic support and afterload reduction. The use of milrinone as a first-line inotrope provides both positive inotropic and vasodilatory effects that are particularly beneficial in this population [28].

Monitoring of pulmonary artery pressures and cardiac output provides essential information for hemodynamic management. The goal is to maintain adequate cardiac output while avoiding excessive preload that could precipitate right heart failure. Early extubation protocols, when safely achievable, reduce the risk of ventilator-associated complications and facilitate early mobilization [29].

Quality Metrics and Outcome Assessment

The assessment of surgical quality in valvular DCM requires sophisticated metrics that go beyond traditional measures of mortality and morbidity. The unique challenges of this patient population necessitate specialized outcome measures that capture the complexity of the disease and treatment.

Repair Rate and Durability

The repair rate in valvular DCM surgery varies significantly based on patient selection and surgical expertise. Centers of excellence achieve repair rates exceeding 95% in carefully selected patients, while general cardiac surgery programs may have repair rates below 70%. The durability of repair, measured as freedom from reoperation or recurrent regurgitation, provides a more meaningful assessment of surgical quality [30].

Functional Improvement Measures

Traditional measures of surgical success such as mortality and morbidity fail to capture the functional improvement that represents the primary goal of valvular DCM surgery. Patient-reported outcome measures, exercise capacity testing, and quality of life assessments provide more meaningful evaluation of surgical success [31].

The use of standardized assessment tools such as the Kansas City Cardiomyopathy Questionnaire and six-minute walk test enables comparison of outcomes across institutions and surgical approaches. These measures should be incorporated into routine follow-up protocols to assess the effectiveness of surgical intervention [32].

Multidisciplinary Care Coordination

The Heart Team Approach

The complexity of valvular DCM management necessitates a multidisciplinary approach that brings together specialists from multiple disciplines [33]. The heart team model, originally developed for complex coronary artery disease, has been adapted for valvular heart disease and represents the standard of care for complex cases.

The heart team composition for valvular DCM typically includes cardiac surgeons, interventional cardiologists, heart failure specialists, cardiac imaging specialists, and cardiac anesthesiologists [34]. Additional specialists may be included based on patient-specific needs, including electrophysiologists for patients with arrhythmias, nephrologists for patients with renal dysfunction, and geriatricians for elderly patients with multiple comorbidities.

Standardized Decision-Making Protocols

The development of standardized protocols for heart team decision-making has improved care consistency and quality [35]. These protocols typically include structured case presentation formats, standardized risk assessment tools, and clear criteria for different therapeutic options. Decision support tools that integrate complex clinical data may facilitate heart team discussions and improve decision-making quality.

Patient and family engagement in heart team discussions is crucial for ensuring treatment decisions align with patient values and preferences [34]. This requires effective communication of complex medical information and shared decision-making processes that involve patients and families in treatment planning.

Quality Improvement Initiatives

Quality improvement initiatives within heart teams are essential for maintaining high care standards and identifying improvement opportunities [35]. This includes regular outcomes data review, complications and adverse events analysis, and evidence-based quality improvement measures implementation. Participation in national quality registries and clinical trials may provide additional insights into best practices and emerging therapies.

Advanced Expert Strategies

The Repair Paradox: When Replacement Is Superior to Repair

One of the most challenging paradigm shifts in modern cardiac surgery involves recognizing when valve replacement provides superior outcomes to repair, despite the traditional surgical dogma favoring repair whenever technically feasible. This counterintuitive concept has emerged from rigorous analysis of long-term outcomes and represents a fundamental evolution in surgical thinking.

The CTSN Revelation

The Cardiothoracic Surgical Trials Network studies fundamentally challenged the repair-first mentality by demonstrating that technically successful repairs often fail to provide clinical benefit. In patients with severe functional mitral regurgitation, repair achieved a 58% rate of recurrent regurgitation compared to only 3.8% for replacement, without any difference in survival or reverse remodeling [14].

The implications extend beyond simple recurrence rates. Patients who develop recurrent regurgitation after repair face the prospect of reoperation with significantly higher risk than the initial procedure. The psychological impact of repair failure, combined with the progressive nature of recurrent regurgitation, often results in worse outcomes than if replacement had been performed initially [36].

Advanced Geometric Considerations

The decision between repair and replacement should be based on sophisticated geometric analysis rather than traditional measures of valve pathology. The concept of "geometric futility" describes situations where the underlying ventricular distortion is so severe that repair cannot achieve durable results regardless of technical execution [37].

Specific geometric parameters that predict repair failure include a coaptation depth greater than 11 mm, tethering area exceeding 2.5 cm^2, and interpapillary distance greater than 20 mm. When these parameters are present, replacement with chordal preservation provides superior long-term outcomes despite the theoretical advantages of repair [38].

The Timing Paradox: Operating Too Early Can Be as Harmful as Too Late

The optimal timing of surgical intervention in valvular DCM represents one of the most nuanced decisions in cardiac surgery. While delayed intervention clearly leads to irreversible ventricular damage, emerging evidence suggests that premature intervention may also compromise outcomes through mechanisms that are only beginning to be understood.

The Preload Dependency Phenomenon

Patients with chronic mitral regurgitation develop adaptive mechanisms that optimize cardiac output in the presence of volume overload. The sudden elimination of regurgitation through surgical intervention can unmask underlying systolic dysfunction that was previously compensated by the low-impedance regurgitant pathway [39].

This phenomenon is particularly pronounced in patients with preserved ejection fraction who undergo early intervention. The acute increase in afterload following valve repair can precipitate heart failure in patients who appeared to have normal ventricular function preoperatively [40].

The Reverse Remodeling Window

Recent research has identified a critical window for reverse remodeling that challenges traditional timing recommendations. Patients who undergo surgery too early, before significant ventricular dilation has occurred, may not achieve the dramatic reverse remodeling that characterizes successful intervention. Conversely, patients who wait too long lose the capacity for reverse remodeling entirely [41].

The optimal timing appears to occur when ventricular dilation is moderate but not severe, typically corresponding to an end-systolic dimension of 45–55 mm. This narrow window requires careful monitoring and sophisticated decision-making that balances the risks of premature intervention against the consequences of delayed surgery [42].

Future Directions and Emerging Paradigms

Digital Health Technologies Integration

The future of valvular DCM management will be increasingly shaped by digital health technologies enabling continuous monitoring, predictive analytics, and personalized interventions [1]. Wearable devices capable of monitoring cardiac rhythm, activity levels, and hemodynamic parameters may provide real-time insights into disease progression and therapeutic response.

Remote monitoring technologies are particularly promising for valvular DCM patients who require frequent assessment but may have difficulty accessing specialized care [43]. Smartphone-based echocardiography, remote biomarker monitoring, and telemedicine consultations may improve access to expert care while reducing healthcare costs.

Artificial intelligence application to digital health data represents an exciting frontier that may transform valvular DCM care [44]. Machine learning algorithms can analyze patterns in continuous monitoring data to predict adverse events, optimize medication dosing, and guide therapeutic interventions. AI-powered clinical decision support systems may democratize access to expert-level care by providing sophisticated analysis and recommendations to clinicians at all experience levels.

Precision Medicine and Personalized Therapeutics

The future of valvular DCM treatment will be increasingly personalized, with therapeutic decisions based on individual patient characteristics including genetic background, molecular profiles, and disease phenotypes [45]. Companion diagnostics development that can predict therapeutic response may enable more precise intervention selection and improve outcomes while reducing adverse effects.

Pharmacogenomics will play an increasingly important role in valvular DCM management, with genetic variants influencing drug metabolism, efficacy, and toxicity [45]. Genetic variants identification that affect response to heart failure medications, anticoagulants, and other therapies may enable personalized dosing strategies that optimize efficacy while minimizing adverse effects.

Personalized therapeutic targets development based on individual molecular profiles represents the ultimate goal of precision medicine in valvular DCM [45]. This may include patient-specific anti-fibrotic strategies, personalized metabolic interventions, and individualized approaches to neurohormonal modulation.

Regenerative Medicine and Tissue Engineering

Regenerative medicine approaches application to valvular DCM represents one of the most exciting frontiers in cardiovascular therapeutics [46]. Advances in stem cell biology, tissue engineering, and gene therapy may provide solutions for patients with end-stage disease who are not candidates for conventional interventions.

Tissue engineering approaches for valve replacement and repair are advancing rapidly, with several products in clinical development [47]. These approaches may provide durable solutions that grow with the patient and avoid complications associated with prosthetic devices. Tissue engineering integration with precision medicine approaches may enable patient-specific valve replacements development tailored to individual anatomical and physiological characteristics.

Gene therapy and gene editing technologies offer potential for permanent correction of genetic defects that contribute to valvular DCM [48]. Safe and effective delivery systems development for cardiac gene therapy remains a major challenge, but recent advances in adeno-associated virus vectors and lipid nanoparticles are promising.

Heart Transplantation in End-Stage Valvular DCM

Patient Selection and Timing

Heart transplantation remains the definitive treatment for patients with end-stage valvular DCM who are not candidates for surgical correction or who have failed previous interventions. The decision to proceed with transplantation requires careful consideration of multiple factors including patient age, comorbidities, social support, and likelihood of successful outcomes.

The timing of transplantation referral is critical, as patients who are referred too late may develop irreversible complications that preclude successful transplantation. Early referral to transplant centers allows for comprehensive evaluation and optimization of medical therapy while the patient remains a suitable candidate.

Contraindications and Risk Assessment

Absolute contraindications to heart transplantation include active malignancy, severe irreversible pulmonary hypertension, active substance abuse, and severe psychiatric illness that would preclude compliance with post-transplant care. Relative contraindications include advanced age, diabetes with end-organ damage, and significant renal dysfunction.

The development of sophisticated risk assessment tools has improved patient selection for heart transplantation. These tools incorporate multiple variables including hemodynamic parameters, biomarker levels, functional capacity, and psychosocial factors to predict post-transplant outcomes.

Bridge-to-Transplant Strategies

For patients with end-stage valvular DCM who are not immediate transplant candidates, bridge-to-transplant strategies may provide life-sustaining support while awaiting organ availability. These strategies include mechanical circulatory support devices, inotropic therapy, and aggressive medical management.

Mechanical Circulatory Support

Left ventricular assist devices (LVADs) have revolutionized the management of patients with end-stage heart failure awaiting transplantation. Modern continuous-flow devices provide excellent hemodynamic support with acceptable complication rates, enabling patients to survive extended waiting periods for organ availability.

The decision to implant an LVAD as a bridge to transplantation requires careful consideration of patient factors, device-related complications, and the likelihood of successful transplantation. Patients with valvular DCM may be particularly good candidates for LVAD support due to the absence of significant right heart dysfunction in many cases.

Post-transplant Management

The management of heart transplant recipients requires specialized expertise in immunosuppression, infection prevention, and surveillance for complications. The unique challenges of patients with valvular DCM may require modifications to standard post-transplant protocols.

Immunosuppression Strategies

Modern immunosuppressive protocols typically include a combination of calcineurin inhibitors, antiproliferative agents, and corticosteroids. The selection and dosing of these agents must be individualized based on patient factors, risk of rejection, and potential complications.

The development of personalized immunosuppression based on genetic factors and biomarker profiles represents an active area of research that may improve outcomes while reducing complications.

Long-Term Surveillance

Long-term surveillance of heart transplant recipients includes regular monitoring for rejection, infection, malignancy, and cardiac allograft vasculopathy. The use of advanced imaging techniques and biomarker monitoring may enable earlier detection of complications and improved outcomes.

Clinical Vignettes: Institutional Approach to Valvular Dilated Cardiomyopathy

The following cases from our institution illustrate how tailored surgical interventions can effectively address complex structural pathology in valvular cardiomyopathy. By correcting hemodynamic compromise, these strategies support clinical stabilization and facilitate recovery or transition to definitive therapies, including transplantation when indicated.

Case 1: Functional MR Bridging to Transplant

A 54-year-old man with ischemic cardiomyopathy presented with NYHA class IV symptoms and severe functional MR. LV ejection fraction was 25%, pulmonary artery systolic pressure was 60 mm Hg, and PVR 3.5 WU. He was initiated on Sacubitril/Valsartan, Carvedilol, Spironolactone, and Dapagliflozin. However, despite medical therapy the patient remained symptomatic. Given the high surgical risk (EuroSCORE II 8%) and moderately dilated LV (end systolic dimension 55 mm), the heart team opted for MitraClip placement. Subsequent to the procedure, the MR reduced to mild, and NT proBNP dropped from 1500 to 400 pg/mL. Over the next 6 months, LV end diastolic volume decreased by 15%, PVR fell to 2.0 WU, and the patient achieved NYHA class II. Unfortunately, the residual LV systolic function remained poor. He was listed for heart transplantation and in the interim bridged with HeartMate 3 LVAD as waitlist timing extended beyond 9 months. The reduction of PVR following the LVAD implantation consequently allowed successful transplantation with minimal right ventricular support. This case illustrates the use of sequential therapy: GDMT, TEER, then LVAD to stabilize hemodynamics and optimize transplant candidacy.

Case 2: Pseudoaneurysm Repair with Concomitant Mitral Valve Intervention

A 69-year-old man presented with symptoms of advanced heart failure and was found to have a large inferoposterior left ventricular pseudoaneurysm with associated mitral regurgitation. Prior medical history included prior myocardial infarction, long-standing tobacco use, recent percutaneous coronary intervention, and a coronary artery bypass grafting (CABG) surgery performed 10 years ago. At the time of presentation, all the previous coronary grafts were occluded. Surgical exploration revealed a sizable pseudoaneurysm originating from the inferoposterior LV wall. A ventriculotomy approach was employed to excise the pseudoaneurysm. The mitral regurgitation was addressed with an edge-to-edge (Alfieri) repair to improve leaflet coaptation (see Fig. 14.1). The patient recovered uneventfully, was discharged 6 days postoperatively, and was found with improved EF to 40–45% at 6 months follow-up. This case illustrates the feasibility and durability of single-stage repair in complex post-infarction mechanical complications, emphasizing the role of timely surgical intervention in anatomically favorable candidates.

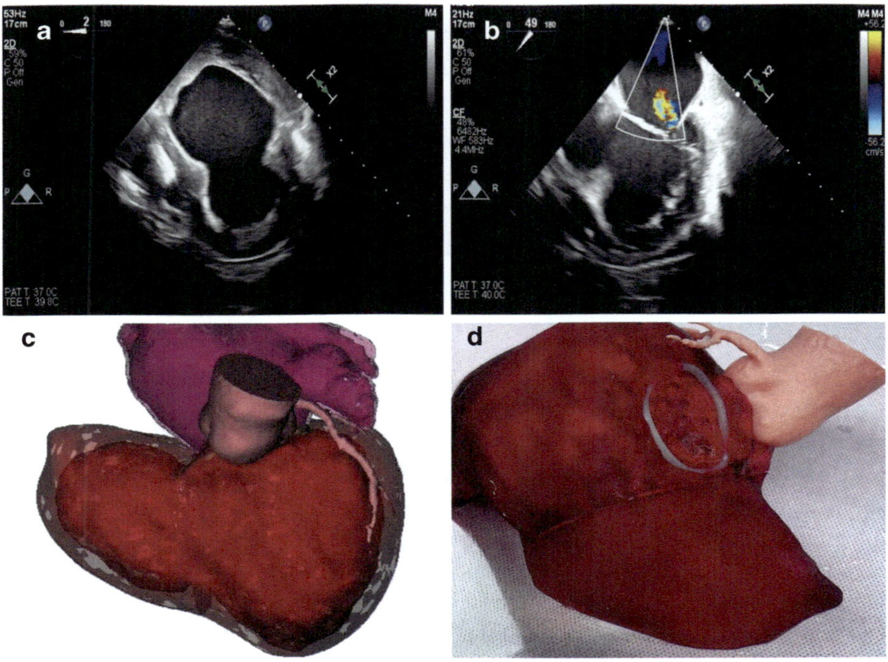

Fig. 14.1 (**a** and **b**) TEE images demonstrating a large inferoposterior left ventricular pseudoaneurysm (**a**), with color Doppler in systole (**b**) showing turbulent flow into the cavity, consistent with communication between the LV and pseudoaneurysm. (**c**) 3D reconstruction showing a large left ventricular pseudoaneurysm adjacent to a dilated LV cavity. (**d**) 3D-printed cardiac model illustrating the left ventricular pseudoaneurysm and its relation to the mitral valve and aortic root. (**e**) Intraoperative view of pseudoaneurysm cavity following ventriculotomy. (**f**) Alfieri stitch (arrow) placed to improve mitral leaflet coaptation. (**g**) Reconstructed pseudoaneurysm neck following patch closure and reinforcement. (**h**) Completed ventricular reconstruction with external reinforcement over the repair site

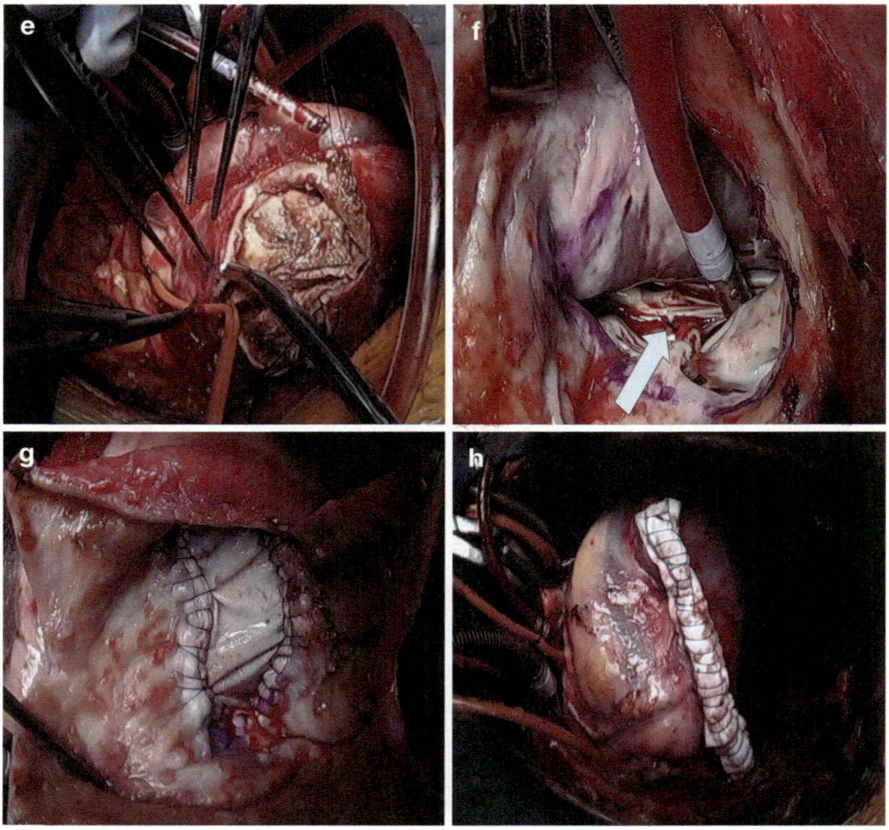

Fig. 14.1 (continued)

Conclusion

Valvular dilated cardiomyopathy represents a complex clinical entity that requires sophisticated diagnostic and therapeutic approaches. The integration of advanced imaging technologies, artificial intelligence, and precision medicine approaches is revolutionizing the diagnosis and management of this condition. Surgical techniques continue to evolve, with increasing emphasis on patient-specific approaches and multidisciplinary care coordination.

The future of valvular DCM management will be characterized by increasingly personalized approaches that integrate multiple data sources to optimize therapeutic decision-making. Digital health technologies, regenerative medicine, and precision therapeutics offer exciting possibilities for improving outcomes in this challenging patient population.

For patients with end-stage disease, heart transplantation remains a viable option that can provide excellent long-term outcomes when appropriate patient selection and post-transplant management protocols are employed. The continued evolution of bridge-to-transplant strategies and post-transplant care will further improve outcomes for these complex patients.

References

1. Krittanawong C, Zhang H, Wang Z, Aydar M, Kitai T. Artificial intelligence in precision cardiovascular medicine. J Am Coll Cardiol. 2017;69(21):2657–64. https://www.jacc.org/doi/10.1016/j.jacc.2017.03.571
2. Ouyang D, He B, Ghorbani A, et al. Video-based AI for beat-to-beat assessment of cardiac function. Nature. 2020;580(7802):252–6. https://www.nature.com/articles/s41586-020-2145-8
3. Zhang J, Gajjala S, Agrawal P, et al. Fully automated echocardiogram interpretation in clinical practice. Circulation. 2018;138(16):1623–35. https://www.ahajournals.org/doi/10.1161/CIRCULATIONAHA.118.034338
4. Bai W, Sinclair M, Tarroni G, et al. Automated cardiovascular magnetic resonance image analysis with fully convolutional networks. J Cardiovasc Magn Reson. 2018;20(1):65. https://jcmr-online.biomedcentral.com/articles/10.1186/s12968-018-0471-x
5. Januzzi JL Jr, Felker GM. Surfing the biomarker tsunami at JACC: heart failure. JACC Heart Fail. 2013;1(3):213–5. https://www.jacc.org/doi/10.1016/j.jchf.2013.04.003
6. Januzzi JL Jr, Peacock WF, Maisel AS, et al. Measurement of the interleukin family member ST2 in patients with acute dyspnea: results from the PRIDE (Pro-Brain Natriuretic Peptide Investigation of Dyspnea in the Emergency Department) study. J Am Coll Cardiol. 2007;50(7):607–13. https://www.jacc.org/doi/10.1016/j.jacc.2007.05.014
7. de Boer RA, Lok DJ, Jaarsma T, et al. Predictive value of plasma galectin-3 levels in heart failure with reduced and preserved ejection fraction. Ann Med. 2011;43(1):60–8. https://www.tandfonline.com/doi/full/10.3109/07853890.2010.538080
8. Sato Y, Yamada T, Taniguchi R, et al. Persistently increased serum concentrations of cardiac troponin t in patients with idiopathic dilated cardiomyopathy are predictive of adverse outcomes. Circulation. 2001;103(3):369–74. https://www.ahajournals.org/doi/10.1161/01.CIR.103.3.369
9. Vegter EL, van der Meer P, de Windt LJ, Pinto YM, Voors AA. MicroRNAs in heart failure: from biomarker to target for therapy. Eur J Heart Fail. 2016;18(5):457–68. https://onlinelibrary.wiley.com/doi/10.1002/ejhf.495
10. Sengupta PP, Chandrashekhar Y. The chicken or egg causality dilemma in heart failure: propelling the field forward with artificial intelligence. JACC Heart Fail. 2020;8(3):244–8. https://www.jacc.org/doi/10.1016/j.jchf.2019.12.005
11. Kalam K, Otahal P, Marwick TH. Prognostic implications of global LV dysfunction: a systematic review and meta-analysis of global longitudinal strain and ejection fraction. Heart. 2014;100(21):1673–80. https://heart.bmj.com/content/100/21/1673
12. Sengupta PP, Korinek J, Belohlavek M, et al. Left ventricular structure and function: basic science for cardiac imaging. J Am Coll Cardiol. 2006;48(10):1988–2001. https://www.jacc.org/doi/10.1016/j.jacc.2006.08.030
13. Lang RM, Badano LP, Mor-Avi V, et al. Recommendations for cardiac chamber quantification by echocardiography in adults: an update from the American Society of Echocardiography and the European Association of Cardiovascular Imaging. J Am Soc Echocardiogr. 2015;28(1):1–39.e14. https://www.onlinejase.com/article/S0894-7317(14)00746-2/fulltext
14. Nappi F, Singh SS, Santana O, Mihos CG. Functional mitral regurgitation: an overview for surgical management framework. J Thorac Dis. 2018;10(7):4540–55. Available at: https://pmc.ncbi.nlm.nih.gov/articles/PMC6106031/

15. Grigioni F, Enriquez-Sarano M, Zehr KJ, et al. Ischemic mitral regurgitation: long-term outcome and prognostic implications with quantitative Doppler assessment. Circulation. 2001;103(13):1759–64.
16. Gillinov AM, Malas T, Griffin B. Robotic mitral valve repair: reflections after 2,400-plus cases. Cleveland Clinic ConsultQD; 2024. Available at: https://consultqd.clevelandclinic.org/robotic-mitral-valve-repair-reflections-after-2400-plus-cases
17. EL-Andari R, Kang J, Bozso S, Moon M, Nagendran J. Minimally invasive complex neochordal reconstruction for mitral valve regurgitation. JTCVS Tech. 2024;27:91–5. Available at: https://pmc.ncbi.nlm.nih.gov/articles/PMC11518925/
18. David TE, Burns RJ, Bacchus CM, Druck MN. Mitral valve replacement for mitral regurgitation with and without preservation of chordae tendineae. J Thorac Cardiovasc Surg. 1984;88(5 Pt 1):718–25.
19. Kron IL, Green GR, Cope JT. Surgical relocation of the posterior papillary muscle in chronic ischemic mitral regurgitation. Ann Thorac Surg. 2002;74(2):600–1.
20. Otto CM, Nishimura RA, Bonow RO, et al. 2020 ACC/AHA guideline for the management of patients with valvular heart disease. Circulation. 2021;143(5):e72–e227.
21. Ad N, Damiano RJ Jr, Badhwar V, et al. Expert consensus guidelines: examining surgical ablation for atrial fibrillation. J Thorac Cardiovasc Surg. 2017;153(6):1330–54.
22. Carpentier AF, Lessana A, Relland JY, et al. The "physio-ring": an advanced concept in mitral valve annuloplasty. Ann Thorac Surg. 1995;60(5):1177–85.
23. McGee EC, Gillinov AM, Blackstone EH, et al. Recurrent mitral regurgitation after annuloplasty for functional ischemic mitral regurgitation. J Thorac Cardiovasc Surg. 2004;128(6):916–24.
24. Kuwahara E, Otsuji Y, Iguro Y, et al. Mechanism of recurrent/persistent ischemic/functional mitral regurgitation in the chronic phase after surgical annuloplasty. Circulation. 2006;114(1 Suppl):I529–34.
25. Cohn LH, Couper GS, Aranki SF, Rizzo RJ, Kinchla NM, Collins JJ Jr. Long-term results of mitral valve reconstruction for regurgitation of the myxomatous mitral valve. J Thorac Cardiovasc Surg. 1994;107(1):143–50.
26. Kron IL, Hung J, Overbey JR, et al. Predicting recurrent mitral regurgitation after mitral valve repair for severe ischemic mitral regurgitation. J Thorac Cardiovasc Surg. 2015;149(3):752–61.
27. Langer F, Kunihara T, Hell K, Schramm R, Schmidt KI, Aicher D, Schäfers HJ. RING+STRING: successful repair technique for ischemic mitral regurgitation with severe leaflet tethering. Circulation. 2009;120(11 Suppl):S85–91.
28. Fellahi JL, Parienti JJ, Hanouz JL, Plaud B, Riou B, Ouattara A. Perioperative use of dobutamine in cardiac surgery and adverse cardiac outcome: propensity-adjusted analyses. Anesthesiology. 2008;108(6):979–87.
29. Cheng DC, Karski J, Peniston C, et al. Early tracheal extubation after coronary artery bypass graft surgery reduces costs and improves resource use. Anesthesiology. 1996;85(6):1300–10.
30. Suri RM, Schaff HV, Dearani JA, et al. Recovery of left ventricular function after surgical correction of mitral regurgitation caused by leaflet prolapse. J Thorac Cardiovasc Surg. 2009;137(5):1071–6.
31. Spertus J, Peterson E, Conard MW, et al. Monitoring clinical changes in patients with heart failure: a comparison of methods. Am Heart J. 2005;150(4):707–15.
32. Green CP, Porter CB, Bresnahan DR, Spertus JA. Development and evaluation of the Kansas City Cardiomyopathy Questionnaire: a new health status measure for heart failure. J Am Coll Cardiol. 2000;35(5):1245–55.
33. Holmes DR Jr, Rich JB, Zoghbi WA, Mack MJ. The heart team of cardiovascular care. J Am Coll Cardiol. 2013;61(9):903–7. https://www.jacc.org/doi/10.1016/j.jacc.2013.01.040
34. Vahanian A, Beyersdorf F, Praz F, et al. 2021 ESC/EACTS guidelines for the management of valvular heart disease. Eur Heart J. 2022;43(7):561–632. https://academic.oup.com/eurheartj/article/43/7/561/6358470
35. Otto CM, Nishimura RA, Bonow RO, et al. 2020 AHA/ACC guideline for the management of patients with valvular heart disease. Circulation. 2021;143(5):e72–e227. https://www.ahajournals.org/doi/10.1161/CIR.0000000000000923

36. Enriquez-Sarano M, Tajik AJ, Schaff HV, Orszulak TA, Bailey KR, Frye RL. Echocardiographic prediction of survival after surgical correction of organic mitral regurgitation. Circulation. 1994;90(2):830–7.
37. Borger MA, Alam A, Murphy PM, Doenst T, David TE. Chronic ischemic mitral regurgitation: repair, replace or rethink? Ann Thorac Surg. 2006;81(3):1153–61.
38. Yiu SF, Enriquez-Sarano M, Tribouilloy C, Seward JB, Tajik AJ. Determinants of the degree of functional mitral regurgitation in patients with systolic left ventricular dysfunction: a quantitative clinical study. Circulation. 2000;102(12):1400–6.
39. Enriquez-Sarano M, Tajik AJ, Schaff HV, Orszulak TA, McGoon MD, Bailey KR. Echocardiographic prediction of left ventricular function after correction of mitral regurgitation: results and clinical implications. J Am Coll Cardiol. 1994;24(6):1536–43.
40. Crawford MH, Souchek J, Oprian CA, et al. Determinants of survival and left ventricular performance after mitral valve replacement. Circulation. 1990;81(4):1173–81.
41. Rosenhek R, Rader F, Klaar U, et al. Outcome of watchful waiting in asymptomatic severe mitral regurgitation. Circulation. 2006;113(18):2238–44.
42. Enriquez-Sarano M, Avierinos JF, Messika-Zeitoun D, et al. Quantitative determinants of the outcome of asymptomatic mitral regurgitation. N Engl J Med. 2005;352(9):875–83.
43. Abraham WT, Adamson PB, Bourge RC, et al. Wireless pulmonary artery haemodynamic monitoring in chronic heart failure: a randomised controlled trial. Lancet. 2011;377(9766):658–66. https://www.thelancet.com/journals/lancet/article/PIIS0140-6736(11)60101-3/fulltext
44. Krittanawong C, Zhang H, Wang Z, Aydar M, Kitai T. Artificial intelligence in pecision cardiovascular medicine. J Am Coll Cardiol. 2017;69(21):2657–64. https://www.jacc.org/doi/10.1016/j.jacc.2017.03.571
45. Hershberger RE, Givertz MM, Ho CY, et al. Genetic evaluation of cardiomyopathy-a heart failure society of America practice guideline. J Card Fail. 2018;24(5):281–302. https://www.onlinejcf.com/article/S1071-9164(18)30056-9/fulltext
46. Sanganalmath SK, Bolli R. Cell therapy for heart failure: a comprehensive overview of experimental and clinical studies, current challenges, and future directions. Circ Res. 2013;113(6):810–34. https://www.ahajournals.org/doi/10.1161/CIRCRESAHA.113.300219
47. Takahashi K, Yamanaka S. Induction of pluripotent stem cells from mouse embryonic and adult fibroblast cultures by defined factors. Cell. 2006;126(4):663–76. https://www.cell.com/cell/fulltext/S0092-8674(06)00976-7
48. Hulot JS, Ishikawa K, Hajjar RJ. Gene therapy for the treatment of heart failure: promise postponed. Eur Heart J. 2016;37(21):1651–8. https://academic.oup.com/eurheartj/article/37/21/1651/1748966

15 The Artificial Heart and Beyond: Evolving Frontiers in Mechanical Circulatory Support

Alexandru Plesoianu and Carmen Elena Plesoianu

The Genesis of Mechanical Circulatory Support

Early Concepts and the Dawn of Cardiopulmonary Bypass

The intellectual origins of mechanical circulatory support predate its clinical feasibility by several decades. The foundational concept of maintaining organ viability outside the body was demonstrated in the 1930s through the in-vitro perfusion apparatus developed by Alexis Carrel and Charles Lindbergh, which successfully sustained animal organs for days [1]. Concurrently, in 1937, Vladimir Demikhov conducted audacious experiments in which he replaced a dog's heart with a set of piston pumps, achieving short-term survival and providing an early, albeit rudimentary, proof of concept for a total artificial heart [1].

However, the meaningful origin of the modern MCS era is inextricably linked to the development of the heart-lung machine. The first successful clinical use of cardiopulmonary bypass (CPB) by Dr. John Gibbon in 1953 to close an atrial septal defect was a watershed moment that inaugurated the age of open-heart surgery [1]. This breakthrough technology was not only a prerequisite for complex intracardiac repairs but also the primary catalyst for the development of MCS. The success of CPB created a new clinical dilemma: patients who, after a successful operation, suffered from postcardiotomy cardiogenic shock and could not be weaned from the heart-lung machine [2]. This clinical reality established a direct and urgent need for

A. Plesoianu (✉) · C. E. Plesoianu
University of Medicine and Pharmacy Gr T Popa Iasi, Iaşi, Romania
e-mail: alexandru.plesoianu@umfiasi.ro

G. Tinică, A. Burlacu (eds.), *Surgical, Hybrid and Minimally Invasive Structural Cardiac Interventions*, https://doi.org/10.1007/978-3-032-16676-0_15

a device that could provide prolonged circulatory support, extending beyond the hours-long capability of a CPB circuit. The development of MCS, therefore, was not initially a linear pursuit of a permanent artificial heart but a direct, reactive solution to a critical problem created by another revolutionary technology. This symbiotic relationship, where the advance in cardiac surgery created the clinical niche for MCS, shaped the entire trajectory of the field.

The First Wave: Pioneering VADs and the Total Artificial Heart

The 1960s and 1970s represented a period of intense optimism and rapid progress, fueled by significant government investment. The establishment of the National Institutes of Health (NIH) Artificial Heart Program in 1964, with a mandate to develop both temporary assist devices and permanent replacement hearts, provided the institutional and financial backbone for this pioneering era [3]. This period saw the first landmark clinical applications that would define the field for decades to come. In 1963, Dr. Michael DeBakey implanted the first successful Left Ventricular Assist Device (LVAD) in a human, a pneumatically driven paracorporeal pump that supported a patient for 4 days [4]. In 1966, he used a similar device to support a patient for 10 days, leading to full recovery and discharge, demonstrating the potential of MCS as a "bridge to recovery" [5].

In 1969, Dr. Denton Cooley implanted the first total artificial heart (TAH), a device developed by Dr. Domingo Liotta, into a patient who could not be weaned from CPB. The device sustained the patient for 64 hours until a donor heart became available, establishing the concept of "bridge to transplant" [6]. While these early devices were extracorporeal and intended for short-term use, they proved that mechanical pumps could successfully sustain human circulation.

This era of exploration culminated in one of the most publicized medical events of the twentieth century: the implantation of the Jarvik-7 TAH into retired dentist Barney Clark on December 2, 1982, by a team at the University of Utah led by Dr. William DeVries. The Jarvik-7, a pneumatically driven TAH, was the first device intended for permanent circulatory support. Clark survived for 112 days, capturing worldwide attention and sparking intense public and ethical debate [7]. While a monumental feat of engineering and surgical courage, the Barney Clark case and subsequent implantations also exposed the severe limitations of the technology. Patients suffered from devastating complications, including life-threatening infections, hemolysis, and high rates of thromboembolism and stroke, which ultimately led the U.S. government to issue a moratorium on the device's use for permanent support in the mid-1980s [8].

This period revealed a critical divergence between public perception and technical reality. The ambitious, high-profile TAH projects captured the imagination but stalled due to intractable clinical failures. In parallel, the less glamorous but more pragmatic development of VADs, which assisted rather than replaced the native heart, was making steadier and more sustainable progress away from the spotlight. The stark clinical failures of the early TAHs directly catalyzed a strategic pivot in the field, shifting research focus and funding toward the development of more reliable, long-term VADs, which were proving to be a more viable therapeutic pathway [2].

The Paradigm Shift: From Pulsatile Pumps to Continuous-Flow Technology

The pivot toward VADs bore fruit with the development of the first generation of fully implantable, electrically powered devices. These were large, pulsatile, volume-displacement pumps, such as the Thoratec HeartMate XVE, which were designed to mimic the natural heartbeat by alternately filling and ejecting blood from a flexible chamber [9]. The landmark Randomized Evaluation of Mechanical Assistance for the Treatment of Congestive Heart Failure (REMATCH) trial, published in 2001, was a pivotal moment for the field. The trial demonstrated that the HeartMate XVE significantly improved survival compared to optimal medical therapy in patients with end-stage heart failure who were ineligible for transplantation [10]. This trial definitively established "Destination Therapy" (DT) as a viable clinical strategy and uncoupled MCS therapy from transplant eligibility, opening the door for a much larger patient population [10].

Despite their clinical success, first-generation pulsatile pumps had significant limitations. Their large size precluded implantation in smaller adults and children, and their mechanical complexity, with flexing membranes and valves cycling over 100,000 times per day, led to issues with long-term durability and device failure. These engineering challenges spurred the development of a new class of devices that represented the most significant technological leap in the history of MCS: continuous-flow (CF) rotary pumps.

Instead of mimicking a pulse, these second- and third-generation devices use a rapidly spinning impeller to propel blood in a continuous, non-pulsatile stream. This design innovation allowed for a dramatic reduction in size, weight, and mechanical complexity, as the pumps had only one moving part [11]. The first CF pumps were axial-flow devices, such as Hemopump and HeartMate II, which use a screw-like impeller within a tube housing [12, 13]. These were followed by even more compact centrifugal-flow pumps, such as the HeartWare HVAD and the HeartMate 3, which use a spinning disc-shaped impeller to accelerate blood radially [14, 15]. This transition to smaller, silent, and far more durable rotary pumps revolutionized the field, enabling less invasive surgical techniques, broader patient applicability, and vastly improved long-term outcomes, setting the stage for the contemporary era of MCS.

The Contemporary Landscape of MCS Technology

The modern era of mechanical circulatory support is dominated by sophisticated, durable, third-generation rotary pumps that have become the standard of care for advanced heart failure. These devices, alongside the sole clinical available worldwide total artificial heart, offer a spectrum of support tailored to specific clinical scenarios.

Ventricular Assist Devices: A Profile of Current-Generation Systems

Centrifugal-Flow LVADs: The HeartMate 3

The Abbott HeartMate 3 is the current market-leading LVAD, representing the pinnacle of third-generation centrifugal-flow technology. Its design incorporates several key innovations aimed at mitigating the complications that plagued earlier devices. The core of the HeartMate 3 is its "Full MagLev" technology, a fully magnetically levitated rotor that is suspended within the pump housing without any mechanical bearings. This contact-free design, combined with wide blood-flow gaps, is engineered to minimize shear stress on blood cells, thereby reducing the risk of hemolysis and thrombosis [16].

Another defining feature is its intrinsic "artificial pulse," where the pump's rotational speed is modulated once every 2 s to create momentary changes in flow. This is designed to wash out areas of potential stasis within the pump and the patient's ventricle, further reducing the risk of thrombus formation [16]. The device is compact and implanted within the chest, with an inflow cannula inserted into the apex of the left ventricle and an outflow graft anastomosed to the aorta.

The clinical superiority of the HeartMate 3 was established in the landmark Multicenter Study of MagLev Technology in Patients Undergoing Mechanical Circulatory Support Therapy With HeartMate 3 (MOMENTUM 3) trial. This trial demonstrated significantly lower rates of pump thrombosis and disabling stroke at 2 years compared to its predecessor, the axial-flow HeartMate II [17]. Based on these robust data, the HeartMate 3 has received FDA approval for both short-term use as a bridge to transplant (BTT) or myocardial recovery, and long-term use as destination therapy (DT) in adult and pediatric patients [18].

Axial-Flow LVADs: The Jarvik 2000

The Jarvik 2000 FlowMaker® represents a distinct design philosophy within the continuous-flow paradigm. As an axial-flow pump, it is exceptionally small and lightweight, approximately the size of a C-battery, weighing only 90 g. Its defining feature is its unique implantation method, where the pump itself is placed directly inside the left ventricle, eliminating the need for a surgical pump pocket in the abdomen or chest wall.

The device consists of a welded titanium shell containing a small, spinning impeller supported by ceramic bearings. This impeller rotates at speeds of 8000–12,000 rpm, capable of generating blood flow up to 8.5 L/min. Rather than completely taking over the heart's function, the Jarvik 2000 is designed to augment the weakened ventricle's output, allowing the native heart to continue to work and potentially recover. Due to its small size, it is a viable option for smaller adults and has been used successfully in pediatric patients as young as 11. It is primarily used as a bridge to transplantation [19].

A Note on the HeartWare HVAD

The Medtronic HeartWare HVAD was a historically significant third-generation centrifugal pump that competed directly with the HeartMate series. Its primary advantage was its extremely small size, which allowed for implantation entirely within the pericardial space, avoiding the need for an abdominal pump pocket and facilitating less invasive surgical approaches [14]. However, in June 2021, Medtronic stopped the sale and distribution of the HVAD system. This decision was based on a growing body of observational clinical data demonstrating a higher frequency of neurological adverse events, particularly stroke, and increased mortality compared to other commercially available LVADs. The HVAD's withdrawal serves as a critical case study in the importance of post-market surveillance and underscores the unforgiving nature of blood-device biocompatibility, where even subtle design differences can have profound clinical consequences [20].

Specialized and Temporary Support: The Impella Platform and Pediatric Devices

For short-term support, particularly in the setting of high-risk percutaneous coronary intervention (PCI) or acute cardiogenic shock, the Abiomed Impella platform is widely used. These are percutaneously inserted, catheter-based microaxial flow pumps [21]. Devices like the Impella 2.5, CP, and 5.5 are typically advanced via the femoral artery, across the aortic valve, and into the left ventricle. Once in place, the tiny internal motor pumps blood from the LV directly into the ascending aorta, unloading the ventricle and supporting systemic circulation. They are approved by the FDA for temporary support (up to 14 days for some models) and are a crucial tool in the interventional cardiology and critical care settings.

For the pediatric population, the Berlin Heart EXCOR® Pediatric is the only VAD system approved worldwide for infants and children. Unlike modern adult devices, the EXCOR is a paracorporeal (external), pulsatile pump. This design allows for a wide range of pump sizes (from 10 to 60 ml) to accommodate patients from newborns to adolescents. The pumps are located outside the body and connected to the heart via transcutaneous cannulae. The system can provide univentricular or biventricular support and serves as an essential life-saving bridge to transplantation for children with end-stage heart failure [22].

Total Artificial Hearts: The SynCardia TAH and the Pursuit of Biventricular Replacement

For patients with irreversible, end-stage biventricular failure, where both ventricles are failing, an LVAD alone is insufficient. In this scenario, the SynCardia temporary Total Artificial Heart (TAH-t) is the only FDA and CE-marked approved device [23]. The SynCardia TAH is a direct technological descendant of the original Jarvik-7, refined over decades of clinical use.

The device is a pneumatically driven, pulsatile pump that completely replaces the patient's native ventricles, which are surgically excised during implantation. It consists of two artificial ventricles with four mechanical valves, capable of generating a cardiac output of up to 9.5 L/min. The device is powered by an external pneumatic driver console connected via percutaneous drivelines. Its sole approved indication is as a bridge to heart transplantation. Clinical data from over 1800 implants show that it is an effective means of support, with over 50% of patients successfully bridged to transplant. A major advance in quality of life for these patients was the development of the 13.5-pound "Freedom® Portable Driver," which replaced the large, hospital-bound "Big Blue" console and allows stable patients to be discharged from the hospital while awaiting a donor heart [24].

Clinical Indications and Patient Selection: The INTERMACS Framework

The decision of when to implant an MCS device is critical and has been standardized by the Interagency Registry for Mechanically Assisted Circulatory Support (INTERMACS). Established in the mid-2000s, INTERMACS is a North American registry that tracks patients receiving durable MCS devices, providing invaluable data on outcomes and adverse events. A key contribution of INTERMACS is its patient profile scale, which classifies patients from Profile 1 ("Critical cardiogenic shock") to Profile 7 ("Advanced NYHA Class III"). This framework provides clinicians with a common language to define illness severity and has become the standard for guiding the timing of MCS implantation. Early intervention in sicker patients (e.g., Profiles 1–3) is often necessary but carries higher risk, while elective implantation in more stable patients (e.g., Profile 4–5) is associated with better outcomes. This classification system has been instrumental in refining clinical indications, which have expanded from the initial bridge-to-transplant to include destination therapy and bridge-to-recovery, reflecting the growing role of MCS as a definitive therapy for advanced heart failure (Table 15.1) [25].

Table 15.1 Comparative analysis of current-generation durable MCS devices

Feature	HeartMate 3	Jarvik 2000 FlowMaker®	SynCardia temporary TAH
Manufacturer	Abbott	Jarvik Heart, Inc.	SynCardia systems, LLC
Pump type	Centrifugal, continuous-flow	Axial, continuous-flow	Biventricular, pneumatic pulsatile
Key design features	Fully magnetically levitated rotor (full MagLev); engineered artificial pulse	Intraventricular placement; ceramic bearings; valveless design	Complete ventricular replacement; 4 mechanical valves; external pneumatic driver
Size/weight	Compact, intrathoracic pump	90 g, 25 ml displacement volume (size of a C-battery)	160 g, 70 cc or 50 cc models available
Max flow rate	>10 L/min	Up to 8.5 L/min	Up to 9.5 L/min
FDA approved indications	Bridge-to-transplant (BTT), destination therapy (DT), bridge-to-recovery	Bridge-to-transplant (BTT)	Bridge-to-transplant (BTT)
Key clinical data source	MOMENTUM 3 Trial [17]	Clinical Trials [19]	Registry Data [25]

The Enduring Clinical Challenges of Mechanical Support

Despite decades of technological refinement, the use of MCS devices is accompanied by a formidable profile of clinical complications. These challenges stem from the fundamental incompatibility of a mechanical pump with human biology and physiology, creating a persistent set of problems that define the limits of current therapy and drive the next wave of innovation.

The Blood-Device Interface: Biocompatibility, Hemolysis, and Thromboembolism

The most profound and persistent challenge in MCS is managing the interaction at the blood-device interface. Hemocompatibility refers to the property of a material to exist in contact with blood without inducing undesirable effects. The artificial surfaces of pumps and cannulae, typically made of materials like titanium and polyurethane, inevitably activate the body's coagulation cascade. Furthermore, the high rotational speeds of continuous-flow pumps generate non-physiological shear stresses that can damage blood cells (hemolysis) and activate platelets [26].

This constant prothrombotic stimulus creates a dual-edged sword of complications. On one side is the risk of *thrombosis*, where clots form within the device (pump thrombosis) or are ejected into the circulation, causing a devastating embolic stroke. Pump thrombosis can lead to device failure and requires high-risk surgical exchange [27].

On the other side is the risk of bleeding. To mitigate thrombosis, patients require lifelong, aggressive anticoagulation therapy (e.g., warfarin) and antiplatelet agents. This therapy, however, significantly increases the risk of major bleeding events, most commonly in the gastrointestinal (GI) tract and intracranially. This risk is further compounded by an acquired von Willebrand syndrome (AvWS), a condition where high shear stress breaks down a key clotting protein (von Willebrand factor), impairing normal platelet function. The clinical management of an MCS patient is thus a continuous, precarious balancing act between preventing clots and causing hemorrhage, a dilemma that remains the central, unresolved challenge of the field [27, 28].

For TAH patients, the adverse event profile is similarly daunting. Analysis of the FDA's MAUDE database reveals that the most common adverse events are infection (20.2%) and device malfunction (20.1%), followed by bleeding (16.5%), respiratory failure (10.1%), and neurological events (8.7%). Multiorgan failure and stroke are the leading causes of death in this population [29].

The Achilles' Heel: Driveline Infection and Biofilm Pathogenesis

For VADs, the single greatest source of morbidity is infection related to the percutaneous driveline [30]. This cable, which exits the skin of the abdomen to connect the internal pump to the external controller and batteries, serves as a permanent breach in the body's primary defense against pathogens. The driveline exit site creates a direct conduit for skin flora, most commonly *Staphylococcus aureus* and *Pseudomonas aeruginosa*, to invade the subcutaneous tissue [31].

The velour-covered surface of the driveline, designed to promote tissue integration, also provides an ideal scaffold for the formation of bacterial biofilms—complex, slime-encased microbial communities that are highly resistant to both antibiotics and the host immune system [32]. An infection that begins as a superficial exit-site issue can migrate along the driveline tunnel, leading to a deep, difficult-to-treat pump pocket infection, sepsis, and endocarditis. Driveline infections are a major cause of rehospitalization, significantly impair quality of life, and can jeopardize a patient's candidacy for a heart transplant [33].

The Power Problem: Drivelines, Batteries, and Device Durability

The necessity of an external power source creates significant practical and lifestyle limitations for VAD patients. The driveline itself is a constant source of concern, requiring meticulous daily care and subject to trauma or mechanical failure [30].

While the durability of third-generation continuous-flow pumps is vastly superior to their pulsatile predecessors, device failure remains a long-term risk [34]. A systematic review found that the overall incidence of device failure was approximately 3.9%, with pump thrombosis being the most common cause (50.5%), followed by lead or cable damage (21.7%). Although relatively infrequent, device failure is a catastrophic event that often necessitates an urgent, high-risk pump exchange surgery, which carries its own significant morbidity and mortality [35].

Systemic Complications: Right Heart Failure, Bleeding, and Neurological Events

Implanting an MCS device can have profound systemic physiological consequences. A common and serious complication following LVAD implantation is *right heart failure (RHF)*. By effectively unloading the left ventricle, the LVAD dramatically increases blood flow returning to the right side of the heart. If the right ventricle is already weakened, it may be unable to handle this increased preload, leading to RHF, systemic congestion, and end-organ dysfunction. Severe RHF may necessitate temporary or even durable right ventricular support (an RVAD) [36].

As previously mentioned, *neurological events* are a leading cause of death and long-term disability in the MCS population [29]. Both ischemic strokes, caused by thrombi originating from the device, and hemorrhagic strokes, often a consequence of intensive anticoagulation and hypertension, occur at alarmingly high rates [37]. The management of these complex, multifaceted complications requires a dedicated, multidisciplinary team and adherence to evolving clinical guidelines for blood pressure control, anticoagulation monitoring, and infection surveillance.

The history of MCS development reveals a pattern where solving one major problem often introduces or exacerbates another. The first-generation pulsatile pumps were plagued by mechanical failure due to the constant wear on their moving parts. This was a predictable, engineering-centric problem. The development of continuous-flow pumps, with their single moving part, brilliantly solved the issue of mechanical durability. However, the non-physiological, high-shear flow they produced created a new, more complex set of biological problems, including higher rates of GI bleeding, acquired von Willebrand syndrome, and stroke. The burden of complication was effectively transferred from the domain of mechanical engineering to that of hematology and fluid dynamics. This "conservation of complication" suggests that true progress in the field requires a holistic approach that simultaneously addresses both the engineering and biological challenges, rather than solving them sequentially [38].

The Near Future: Engineering Solutions for Current Limitations

The next generation of MCS technology is being engineered specifically to address the enduring clinical challenges of the current era. Innovations in miniaturization, wireless power, biomaterials, and control systems are poised to significantly improve patient outcomes and quality of life.

The Drive for Miniaturization and Minimally Invasive Implantation

The relentless trend toward device miniaturization is a central theme in next-generation MCS development. Smaller, more compact pumps offer numerous advantages. They can be implanted in a wider range of patients, including smaller adults and children, who were previously excluded due to anatomical constraints. Miniaturization is also a key enabler of less invasive surgical techniques. As pumps become smaller, surgeons can move from a full median sternotomy to less traumatic approaches like a thoracotomy or a subcostal incision, which can lead to reduced bleeding, shorter recovery times, and lower rates of right heart failure. This drive for smaller, less invasive devices aims to reduce the upfront surgical morbidity of MCS therapy, making it a more accessible and less daunting option for patients [39].

Severing the Connection: Wireless Power via Transcutaneous Energy Transfer (TET)

Arguably, the most sought-after innovation in the VAD field is the elimination of the percutaneous driveline. This would effectively solve the problem of driveline infection, the leading cause of morbidity. The enabling technology is the Transcutaneous Energy Transfer (TET) system, which uses the principle of magnetic inductive coupling to transfer power across intact skin from an external transmitter coil to a surgically implanted receiver coil [40]. This would allow for a fully implantable LVAD (FILVAS), freeing patients from the external driveline and its associated burdens and risks [40].

Significant engineering challenges remain in perfecting TET systems. These include maximizing power transfer efficiency across variable skin thicknesses and coil alignments, managing heat generation in the subcutaneous tissue to prevent burns, and developing a small, reliable, and long-lasting internal battery to provide backup power and allow the patient to be untethered from the external transmitter for short periods [40]. Despite these hurdles, multiple companies are actively developing and testing FILVAS platforms, and this technology represents the next major leap forward in VAD therapy.

Engineering Hemocompatibility: Advanced Biomaterials and Surface Coatings

Addressing the fundamental problem of blood-device incompatibility requires solutions at the materials science level. Research is focused on developing advanced biomaterials and surface modifications that can render the device surfaces less thrombogenic [41]. One established strategy is the use of textured surfaces, such as the sintered microspheres on HeartMate devices, which are designed to promote the growth of a stable, living layer of endothelial cells (a neointima) that passivates the artificial surface [42].

Another major area of innovation is the development of active and passive surface coatings. These include covalently bonding anticoagulant molecules like heparin directly to the device surface, creating a localized antithrombotic effect without requiring systemic anticoagulation. Other approaches involve coating surfaces with highly hydrophilic polymers (e.g., polyethylene glycol) that create a hydration layer to repel protein and platelet adhesion, or developing biomimetic surfaces that mimic the natural, anti-thrombotic properties of the vascular endothelium [43]. These materials-based solutions aim to fundamentally improve the device's biocompatibility, potentially reducing the need for aggressive anticoagulation and tipping the delicate balance away from bleeding and thrombosis.

Intelligent Adaptation: The Rise of Physiologic Control Systems

Current-generation VADs typically operate at a constant, fixed speed set by a clinician. This is a major limitation, as the pump cannot automatically adapt to the body's changing circulatory demands during activities like exercise, sleep, or changes in posture [44]. This mismatch can lead to inadequate support during exertion or over-pumping and ventricular suction during rest. The future of MCS control lies in the development of "smart" physiologic control systems that can automatically adjust pump speed in real-time.

These systems consist of two key components. First, a method for sensing the patient's hemodynamic state is required. This can be achieved through implantable sensors that directly measure parameters like left ventricular end-diastolic pressure (LVEDP), or through sophisticated "sensorless" algorithms that infer these parameters from the pump's own power consumption and flow waveforms. Second, an advanced control algorithm is needed to interpret this data and modulate the pump speed accordingly. Researchers are moving beyond simple proportional-integral-derivative (PID) controllers to more robust adaptive algorithms, such as Model Free Adaptive Control (MFAC), which can learn and respond to both inter-patient and intra-patient variations to maintain optimal support across a wide range of clinical scenarios [45]. The goal is to create a truly responsive system that seamlessly integrates with the patient's native physiology, maximizing cardiac output when needed and minimizing complications.

Investigational and Next-Generation TAHs and VADs

Several innovative devices currently in development or early clinical trials exemplify the engineering principles of the near future, aiming to provide more durable, biocompatible, and physiologically responsive biventricular support.

BiVACOR Total Artificial Heart

The BiVACOR TAH represents a significant shift from traditional pulsatile TAHs to a compact, electro-mechanical rotary blood pump. Its core is a single, magnetically levitated (MAGLEV) dual-sided rotor that simultaneously pumps blood to both the systemic and pulmonary circulations, making it a valveless device with only one moving part. This design, housed in titanium, is intended to enhance durability by eliminating mechanical wear and to improve biocompatibility by minimizing blood trauma. The device is small enough for most adults and is capable of producing high flows (>12 L/min) that adapt to patient activity via a smart controller. The BiVACOR TAH is currently being evaluated in an FDA-approved Early Feasibility Study (EFS) as a bridge to transplant. The initial phase of the study successfully bridged all five patients to a donor heart, leading the FDA to approve an expansion of the trial. The device has also received FDA Breakthrough Device Designation, which may accelerate its development pathway [46].

Scandinavian Realheart TAH

The Realheart TAH is being developed with a unique design philosophy: to closely mimic the form and function of the native human heart. It is the only TAH design that incorporates two atria and two ventricles, aiming to produce a physiological pulsatile flow that minimizes the risk of common complications like stroke and bleeding [47]. The device is currently in the preclinical development phase, where it has demonstrated success in animal studies by providing adequate cardiac function, automatically adapting to changes in activity, and maintaining good blood biochemistry with low levels of hemolysis [48]. In recognition of its potential to treat a small patient population with limited options, the FDA has granted the Realheart TAH a Humanitarian Use Device (HUD) designation, making it eligible for an expedited regulatory pathway in the United States [49].

Carmat Aeson® Total Artificial Heart

The Carmat Aeson® is an electro-hydraulically driven, pulsatile TAH that features blood-contacting surfaces made from bovine pericardial tissue, a biological material intended to enhance hemocompatibility and reduce the risk of thrombosis [50]. The device is designed for autoregulation, using embedded sensors and microprocessors to automatically adjust its output in response to the patient's physiological demands [51]. The Aeson® TAH is CE-marked in Europe and is commercially available as a bridge to transplant in several countries. It is also the subject of major clinical trials, including the EFICAS study in France and an Early Feasibility Study (EFS) in the United States [52]. Clinical data has shown a 90% survival rate at 6 months in cardiogenic shock patients and has demonstrated that the device can successfully bridge dozens of patients to heart transplantation [53].

Continuous-Flow Total Artificial Heart (CFTAH)

The concept of a CFTAH involves using two continuous-flow rotary pumps to provide biventricular support, similar to BIVACOR. Cleveland Clinic has been at the forefront of this research, developing both an adult CFTAH and a scaled-down pediatric version (P-CFTAH). The design features a unified dual-pump system with a single motor and a rotor supported by a hydrodynamic bearing. This sensorless design can automatically balance flow between the left and right circulations and can create pulsatility through speed modulation. The P-CFTAH is significantly smaller, designed to fit infants weighing as little as 5 kg, addressing a critical unmet need in pediatric cardiac care [54]. Preclinical in vivo studies have confirmed the feasibility, anatomical fit, and stable hemodynamic performance of the devices [55].

CH-VAD (China Heart)

The CH-VAD is a fully magnetically levitated, centrifugal-flow LVAD developed in China. It features a compact design with an optimized blood flow path to enhance hemocompatibility and a narrow, flexible driveline [56]. The device was approved for marketing in China by the National Medical Products Administration (NMPA) in 2021 [57]. A post-market, multicenter study of 77 patients in China demonstrated excellent clinical outcomes, with a 1-year survival rate of 91.6%. Notably, the study reported very low rates of adverse events, including no instances of pump thrombosis, ischemic stroke, or device failure, suggesting the CH-VAD is a safe and reliable option for long-term mechanical support [58].

Case Study in Innovation: The Work of the UMF Iasi Group

The research contributions of UMF Iași group led by Prof. Dr. Grigore Tinica and Dr. Alexandru Plesoianu materialized in Innovative LVADs & MAVIS Artificial Heart project serve as a compelling case study, embodying the next-generation principles of MCS design. This work is characterized by a holistic, problem-focused approach that directly targets the key limitations of current devices: cost, invasiveness, and infection risk.

A Holistic Design Philosophy: Low-Cost, Fully Implantable VAD Concepts

The core objective of "Innovative Solutions for Mechanical Circulatory Support in Heart Failure" doctoral research was to develop innovative MCS solutions that are not only technologically advanced but also affordable and accessible, particularly for healthcare systems with limited resources. This philosophy is a direct response to the high costs and significant complication profiles that currently limit the widespread application of MCS therapy. This work integrates a multidisciplinary perspective, drawing from engineering, medicine, and design thinking to address the needs of the patient, the manufacturer, and the clinician simultaneously.

Several innovative VAD architectures have been proposed and developed through this research. One patented concept features an integrated, monobloc design with an axial pump located *inside* the motor's rotor, intended for minimally invasive implantation in a subcutaneous pectoral pocket. Another concept utilizes an electric motor positioned coaxially around the pump impeller, which is suspended by magnetic bearings. This design aims to reduce blood trauma by minimizing mechanical contact, thereby lowering the risk of hemolysis and thrombosis. The development process for these concepts leverages modern engineering tools, including mathematical modeling to define pump characteristics, computational fluid dynamics (CFD) for in-silico performance testing and optimization, and 3D printing for rapid prototyping of both virtual and physical models [59]. This approach focuses on creating devices that are fully implantable, minimally traumatic to blood, energy-efficient, and free from the infectious risk of a percutaneous driveline.

The MAVIS Artificial Heart: Pushing the Boundaries of Miniaturization and Wireless Integration

The MAVIS Artificial Heart is a student project, initiative coordinated by Dr. A. Plesoianu at the "Gr. T. Popa" University of Medicine and Pharmacy from Iasi, Romania, representing the practical application of this group innovative design philosophy. The project has gained international recognition, winning the "Most Advanced Design" award at the global HeartHackathon competition for two consecutive years.

The MAVIS TAH is a testament to next-generation design principles. It is described as the world's smallest artificial heart, a critical feature for implantation, especially in smaller patients and newborns. The device features a central motor that electromagnetically levitates within the blood path, driving two pumps (left and right) at either end of a cylindrical housing. This design is intended to be highly biocompatible and durable, aiming for a lifespan of at least 10 years. Crucially, the MAVIS heart is designed to be fully implantable, powered by a subcutaneous component that receives energy wirelessly, thereby eliminating the driveline and its associated infection risk. The system is also controlled via a mobile application, representing a modern approach to the user interface for both clinicians and patients.

The success of the MAVIS project highlights a significant shift in the landscape of medical device innovation. Historically, MCS development was the domain of large, heavily funded government programs like the NIH's Artificial Heart Program or major corporations with vast R&D budgets. The ability of a university-based student team to produce an award-winning, functional TAH prototype that incorporates cutting-edge features like magnetic levitation and wireless power demonstrates a democratization of the innovation process. Accessible and powerful modern tools like CFD software and 3D printing have lowered the barriers to entry for high-concept medical device design, enabling agile, multidisciplinary academic teams to compete at the forefront of the field. This represents a new, more democratized model of innovation that can accelerate progress in parallel with traditional, capital-intensive corporate R&D.

The Distant Frontier: Speculative and Biological Solutions for Cardiac Support

While engineers work to perfect the mechanical heart, a parallel frontier of research is exploring solutions that move "beyond the machine." These speculative and biological approaches aim to solve the fundamental problem of biocompatibility not by improving the machine, but by merging it with living tissue or by regenerating the heart itself. This represents a paradigm shift from mechanical replacement to biological integration and restoration.

The Hybrid Heart: Merging Soft Robotics and Tissue Engineering

The most compelling vision in this domain is the "Hybrid Heart," a concept being pursued by European research consortia. This approach seeks to build a TAH that is part machine and part living organ. The external structure is a soft robotic shell made of flexible, compliant materials. Instead of a spinning rotor, this shell uses soft pneumatic actuators ("artificial muscles") that compress and twist, mimicking the natural, gentle, and efficient motion of the native myocardium [60]. This biomimetic motion is inherently less traumatic to blood cells than the high-speed shearing of rotary pumps.

The truly revolutionary aspect of the Hybrid Heart is its internal, blood-contacting surface. The plan is to line the soft robotic shell with a biodegradable scaffold that can be seeded with the patient's own cells. Over time, these cells would grow to form a living, confluent layer of endothelium, creating a perfectly biocompatible, non-thrombogenic surface. This strategy of in situ tissue engineering aims to solve the problem of blood clotting and immune reaction at its source. This concept has been demonstrated in other cardiac assist devices, such as the soft robotic sleeve developed at Harvard, which wraps around the failing heart and assists its contractions without ever touching blood, thereby avoiding the need for anticoagulation [61].

Rebuilding the Myocardium: Advances in Tissue-Engineered Cardiac Constructs

Moving even further along the biological spectrum is the field of cardiac tissue engineering, which aims not to assist or replace the heart, but to repair and regenerate damaged heart muscle directly. This approach is founded on three key pillars: biomaterial scaffolds, cell sources, and biofabrication techniques.

Biomaterial scaffolds, made from natural polymers like collagen or synthetic ones like polyglycolic acid (PGA), provide a three-dimensional structure that mimics the native extracellular matrix, giving cells a framework on which to grow and organize. The cell source of choice is increasingly human induced pluripotent stem cells (iPSCs), which can be generated from a patient's own skin or blood cells and then differentiated into beating cardiomyocytes. Advanced biofabrication techniques, particularly 3D bioprinting, allow researchers to precisely deposit layers of cells and scaffold materials to create complex, organized structures, such as prevascularized, beating cardiac patches [62].

The ultimate goal is to create functional cardiac tissue constructs that can be implanted onto an infarcted heart to remuscularize the scar tissue and restore contractile function. Significant challenges remain, including ensuring the long-term survival, vascularization, and electromechanical integration of the engineered tissue with the host myocardium [63]. However, this regenerative approach holds the promise of a true biological cure for heart failure, obviating the need for any mechanical device.

The Nanoscale Revolution: Nanomaterials and Nanotechnology in Cardiac Repair

The application of nanotechnology offers another speculative but powerful avenue for future cardiac support. At the device level, nanomaterials can be used to create novel surface topographies and coatings with enhanced biocompatibility, reducing protein adhesion and platelet activation to prevent thrombosis.

Beyond device enhancement, nanotechnology is a key tool for regenerative medicine. Biological nanocarriers, such as lipid nanoparticles or exosomes (tiny vesicles secreted by cells), can be engineered to deliver therapeutic payloads—such as growth factors, microRNAs, or drugs—directly to injured cardiac tissue. This targeted delivery could stimulate the heart's limited endogenous repair mechanisms, promote angiogenesis, and reduce harmful inflammation and fibrosis following a myocardial infarction [64]. While still largely in the preclinical phase, these nanoscale interventions represent a future where cardiac support may be delivered not by a macro-scale pump, but by billions of molecular-scale machines.

The trajectory from near-future engineering solutions to these distant-frontier concepts reveals a clear and profound trend: the future of cardiac support is integrative, not isolated. The most advanced concepts are not simply better pumps developed by mechanical engineers. They are fundamentally multidisciplinary, requiring the deep convergence of soft robotics, materials science, stem cell biology, tissue engineering, and even artificial intelligence. The Hybrid Heart explicitly merges robotics with living tissue. Tissue engineering itself is an amalgamation of cell biology, materials science, and advanced manufacturing. This convergence demonstrates that the community has recognized that the remaining challenges of long-term cardiac support are too complex for any single discipline to solve. The ultimate goal is no longer just to replicate the heart's pumping function, but to recapitulate its seamless biological integration.

Synthesis and Future Outlook

The journey of mechanical circulatory support is a remarkable narrative of medical and engineering perseverance. From its conceptual genesis in the early twentieth century and its practical birth as a consequence of the heart-lung machine, the field has progressed through distinct technological epochs. The initial era of large, external, and temporary pumps gave way to the ambitious but flawed first-generation TAHs and pulsatile VADs. The limitations of these early devices—mechanical failure and devastating thromboembolic complications—catalyzed the most significant paradigm shift in the field's history: the development of smaller, more durable, continuous-flow rotary pumps. These third-generation devices, exemplified by the HeartMate 3, have transformed MCS from a last-resort, short-term measure into a durable, life-extending therapy for thousands of patients with advanced heart failure.

Yet, despite this success, the field remains defined by a persistent set of clinical challenges. The fundamental bio-incompatibility of artificial materials with blood continues to impose a perilous balancing act between thrombosis and bleeding. The percutaneous driveline remains an Achilles' heel, serving as a constant source of debilitating and life-threatening infections. The reliance on external power supplies constrains patient quality of life, and the systemic physiological impact of non-pulsatile flow contributes to complications like right heart failure and neurological events.

The future of MCS is being shaped on multiple horizons, with each aiming to solve these enduring problems. In the near term, engineering-driven innovations promise an evolution of the current paradigm. The drive for miniaturization, coupled with less invasive surgical techniques, will reduce the initial morbidity of implantation. The development of robust transcutaneous energy transfer systems is on the cusp of creating a truly fully implantable VAD, a milestone that would eliminate driveline infections and dramatically improve patient freedom. Concurrently, advances in biomaterials, surface coatings, and intelligent, physiologically responsive control systems will continue to chip away at the problems of hemocompatibility and hemodynamic mismatch. The innovative work of researchers like UMF Iasi Artificial Heart group exemplifies this near-future vision, integrating miniaturization, wireless power, and advanced pump design into accessible, next-generation platforms.

On the more distant horizon, a revolutionary shift is underway, moving beyond purely mechanical solutions toward systems that are biologically integrated. The convergence of soft robotics and tissue engineering in concepts like the Hybrid Heart promises to create devices that are not only functionally biomimetic but also feature living, non-thrombogenic surfaces. Furthermore, the science of cardiac tissue engineering and the application of nanotechnology aim for the ultimate goal: the true regeneration of damaged heart muscle, rendering mechanical support obsolete.

The evolution of the field has demonstrated that progress is often a trade-off, where solving one problem may introduce another. The ultimate success of MCS, therefore, will not come from a single breakthrough but from the synthesis of these multi-horizon efforts. The future of durable cardiac support lies in creating systems that are fully implantable, intelligently adaptive to the body's needs, and, ultimately, indistinguishable from native tissue at the biological interface. This convergence of machine and organism is the final frontier in the long quest to provide a lasting solution for end-stage heart failure.

References

1. Khan S, Jehangir W. Evolution of artificial hearts: an overview and history. Cardiol Res. 2014;5(5):121–5. https://doi.org/10.14740/cr354w. Epub 2014 Oct 6. PMID: 28348709; PMCID: PMC5358116.
2. Helman DN, Rose EA. History of mechanical circulatory support. Prog Cardiovasc Dis. 2000;43(1):1–4. https://doi.org/10.1053/pcad.2000.7194. PMID: 10935552.
3. Nosé Y. The birth of the artificial heart programs in the world: a special tribute to Tetsuo Akutsu and Valerÿ Shumakov. Artif Organs. 2008;32(9):667–83. https://doi.org/10.1111/j.1525-1594.2008.00623.x. PMID: 18834376.
4. Liotta D, Crawford ES, Cooley DA, DeBakey ME, Urquia DE, M, Feldman L. Prolonged partial left ventricular bypass by means of an intrathoracic pump implanted in the left chest. Trans Am Soc Artif Intern Organs. 1962;8:90–9. https://doi.org/10.1097/00002480-196204000-00022. PMID: 14465672.
5. DeBakey ME. Left ventricular bypass pump for cardiac assistance. Clinical experience. Am J Cardiol. 1971;27(1):3–11. https://doi.org/10.1016/0002-9149(71)90076-2. PMID: 5538711.
6. Cooley DA, Liotta D, Hallman GL, Bloodwell RD, Leachman RD, Milam JD. Orthotopic cardiac prosthesis for two-staged cardiac replacement. Am J Cardiol. 1969;24(5):723–30. https://doi.org/10.1016/0002-9149(69)90460-3. PMID: 4899910.
7. Joyce LD, DeVries WC, Hastings WL, Olsen DB, Jarvik RK, Kolff WJ. Response of the human body to the first permanent implant of the Jarvik-7 Total Artificial Heart. Trans Am Soc Artif Intern Organs. 1983;29:81–7. PMID: 6673327.
8. Institute of Medicine (US) Committee on Technological Innovation in Medicine. In: Gelijns AC, Halm EA, editors. The changing economics of medical technology. Washington (DC): National Academies Press (US); 1991. (Medical Innovation at the Crossroads, No. 2.) 5, The Impact of Public Policy on Medical Device Innovation: a Case of Polyintervention. Available from: https://www.ncbi.nlm.nih.gov/books/NBK234317/.
9. Goldstein DJ, Oz MC, Rose EA. Implantable left ventricular assist devices. N Engl J Med. 1998;339(21):1522–33. https://doi.org/10.1056/NEJM199811193392107. PMID: 9819452.
10. Rose EA, Gelijns AC, Moskowitz AJ, Heitjan DF, Stevenson LW, Dembitsky W, Long JW, Ascheim DD, Tierney AR, Levitan RG, Watson JT, Meier P, Ronan NS, Shapiro PA, Lazar RM, Miller LW, Gupta L, Frazier OH, Desvigne-Nickens P, Oz MC, Poirier VL. Randomized evaluation of mechanical assistance for the treatment of Congestive Heart Failure (REMATCH) Study Group. Long-term use of a left ventricular assist device for end-stage heart failure. N Engl J Med. 2001;345(20):1435–43. https://doi.org/10.1056/NEJMoa012175. PMID: 11794191.
11. Patel SM, Throckmorton AL, Untaroiu A, Allaire PE, Wood HG, Olsen DB. The status of failure and reliability testing of artificial blood pumps. ASAIO J. 2005;51(4):440–51. https://doi.org/10.1097/01.mat.0000169083.90253.3c. PMID: 16156311.
12. Wampler RK, Moise JC, Frazier OH, Olsen DB. In vivo evaluation of a peripheral vascular access axial flow blood pump. ASAIO Trans. 1988;34(3):450–4. PMID: 3196544.
13. Burke DJ, Burke E, Parsaie F, Poirier V, Butler K, Thomas D, Taylor L, Maher T. The Heartmate II: design and development of a fully sealed axial flow left ventricular assist system. Artif Organs. 2001;25(5):380–5. https://doi.org/10.1046/j.1525-1594.2001.06770.x. PMID: 11403668.

14. Wampler R, Lancisi D, Indravudh V, Gauthier R, Fine R. A sealless centrifugal blood pump with passive magnetic and hydrodynamic bearings. Artif Organs. 1999;23(8):780–4. https://doi.org/10.1046/j.1525-1594.1999.06422.x. PMID: 10463507.
15. Loree HM, Bourque K, Gernes DB, Richardson JS, Poirier VL, Barletta N, Fleischli A, Foiera G, Gempp TM, Schoeb R, Litwak KN, Akimoto T, Kameneva M, Watach MJ, Litwak P. The Heartmate III: design and in vivo studies of a maglev centrifugal left ventricular assist device. Artif Organs. 2001;25(5):386–91. https://doi.org/10.1046/j.1525-1594.2001.025005386.x. PMID: 11403669.
16. Schmitto JD, Hanke JS, Rojas SV, Avsar M, Haverich A. First implantation in man of a new magnetically levitated left ventricular assist device (HeartMate III). J Heart Lung Transplant. 2015;34(6):858–60. https://doi.org/10.1016/j.healun.2015.03.001. Epub 2015 Mar 7. PMID: 25920932.
17. Heatley G, Sood P, Goldstein D, Uriel N, Cleveland J, Middlebrook D, Mehra MR. MOMENTUM 3 Investigators. Clinical trial design and rationale of the Multicenter Study of MagLev Technology in Patients Undergoing Mechanical Circulatory Support Therapy With HeartMate 3 (MOMENTUM 3) investigational device exemption clinical study protocol. J Heart Lung Transplant. 2016;35(4):528–36. https://doi.org/10.1016/j.healun.2016.01.021. Epub 2016 Jan 30. PMID: 27044532.
18. Pinney SP, Anyanwu AC, Lala A, Teuteberg JJ, Uriel N, Mehra MR. Left ventricular assist devices for lifelong support. J Am Coll Cardiol. 2017;69(23):2845–61. https://doi.org/10.1016/j.jacc.2017.04.031. Erratum in: J Am Coll Cardiol. 2017;70(10):1308. doi: 10.1016/j.jacc.2017.07.754. PMID: 28595702.
19. Frazier OH, et al. Use of the Flowmaker (Jarvik 2000) left ventricular assist device for destination therapy and bridging to transplantation. Cardiology. 2004;101(1-3):111–6. https://doi.org/10.1159/000075991.
20. Salerno CT, Hayward C, Hall S, Goldstein D, Saeed D, Schmitto J, et al. HVAD to HeartMate 3 left ventricular assist device exchange: best practices recommendations. J Thorac Cardiovasc Surg. 2022;163(6):2120–2127.e5. https://doi.org/10.1016/j.jtcvs.2021.11.085. PMID: 35065842.
21. Zein R, Patel C, Mercado-Alamo A, Schreiber T, Kaki A. A review of the Impella devices. Interv Cardiol. 2022;17:e05. https://doi.org/10.15420/icr.2021.11. PMID: 35474971; PMCID: PMC9026144.
22. Fraser CD Jr, Jaquiss RDB. The Berlin Heart EXCOR Pediatric ventricular assist device: history, North American experience, and future directions. Ann N Y Acad Sci. 2013;1291:96–105. https://doi.org/10.1111/nyas.12144.
23. Copeland J, et al. Total artificial heart update. Surg Technol Int. 2021;39:243–8. https://doi.org/10.52198/21.STI.38.CV1449.
24. Copeland JG. SynCardia Total Artificial Heart: update and future. Tex Heart Inst J. 2013;40(5):587–8. PMID: 24391330; PMCID: PMC3853833.
25. Kirklin JK, Naftel DC, Warner Stevenson L, Kormos RL, Pagani FD, Miller MA, Ulisney K, Young JB. INTERMACS database for durable devices for circulatory support: first annual report. J Heart Lung Transplant. 2008;27:1065–72.
26. Larose J, Timms D. Hemocompatibility in mechanical circulatory support. In: Kormos RL, Burkhoff D, editors. Mechanical circulatory support: a companion to Braunwald's heart disease. 2nd ed. Philadelphia: Elsevier; 2020. p. 83–9. https://doi.org/10.1016/B978-0-323-56699-5.00008-5.
27. Goh T, Ju LA, Waterhouse A. Thrombotic response to mechanical circulatory support devices. J Thromb Haemost. 2025;23(6):1743–57. https://doi.org/10.1016/j.jtha.2025.02.037.
28. Barnes GD. Combining antiplatelet and anticoagulant therapy in cardiovascular disease. Hematology Am Soc Hematol Educ Program. 2020;2020(1):642–8. https://doi.org/10.1182/hematology.2020000151. PMID: 33275740; PMCID: PMC7727581.
29. Tan MC, et al. Adverse events in total artificial heart for end-stage heart failure: insight from the Food and Drug Administration Manufacturer and User Facility Device Experience (MAUDE). Int J Heart Fail. 2023;6,2:76–81. https://doi.org/10.36628/ijhf.2023.0020.

30. Kranzl M, Stoiber M, Schaefer AK, Riebandt J, Wiedemann D, Marko C, Laufer G, Zimpfer D, Schima H, Schlöglhofer T. Driveline features as risk factor for infection in left ventricular assist devices: meta-analysis and experimental tests. Front Cardiovasc Med. 2021;8:784208. https://doi.org/10.3389/fcvm.2021.784208. PMID: 34977190; PMCID: PMC8716483.
31. Lumish HS, Cagliostro B, Braghieri L, Bohn B, Mondellini GM, Antler K, Feldman V, Kleet A, Murphy J, Tiburcio M, Fidlow K, Jennings D, Sayer GT, Takeda K, Naka Y, Demmer RT, Aaron JG, Uriel N, Colombo PC, Yuzefpolskaya M. Driveline infection in left ventricular assist device patients: effect of standardized protocols, pathogen type, and treatment strategy. ASAIO J. 2022;68(12):1450–8. https://doi.org/10.1097/MAT.0000000000001690. Epub 2022 Feb 27. PMID: 35239537; PMCID: PMC9469917.
32. Qu Y, McGiffin D, Kure C, Ozcelik B, Fraser J, Thissen H, Peleg AY. Biofilm formation and migration on ventricular assist device drivelines. J Thorac Cardiovasc Surg. 2020;159(2):491–502.e2. https://doi.org/10.1016/j.jtcvs.2019.02.088. PMID: 31056345.
33. Pereda D, Conte JV. Left ventricular assist device driveline infections. Cardiol Clin. 2011;29(4):515–27. https://doi.org/10.1016/j.ccl.2011.08.007. PMID: 22062325.
34. Mehra MR, Uriel N, Naka Y, Cleveland JC, Pinney M, Salerno CT, et al. A fully magnetically levitated left ventricular assist device — final report. N Engl J Med. 2019;380(17):1618–27.
35. Xie A, et al. Durability of continuous-flow left ventricular assist devices: a systematic review. Ann Cardiothor Surg. 2014;3(6):547–56. https://doi.org/10.3978/j.issn.2225-319X.2014.11.01.
36. Bravo CA, Navarro AG, Dhaliwal KK, Khorsandi M, Keenan JE, Mudigonda P, O'Brien KD, Mahr C. Right heart failure after left ventricular assist device: from mechanisms to treatments. Front Cardiovasc Med. 2022;9:1023549. https://doi.org/10.3389/fcvm.2022.1023549. PMID: 36337897; PMCID: PMC9626829.
37. Tinone G, Hoshino M, Lucato L, Comerlatti LR. Anticoagulation and stroke. Arq Neuropsiquiatr. 2022;80(5 Suppl 1):72–9. https://doi.org/10.1590/0004-282X-ANP-2022-S132. PMID: 35976322; PMCID: PMC9491440.
38. Dugal JK, Malhi AS, Singh Y, Razmi R, Vance J, Sharma D. Advances in Mechanical Circulatory Support (MCS): literature review. Biomedicine. 2025;13(7):1580. https://doi.org/10.3390/biomedicines13071580. PMID: 40722653; PMCID: PMC12292615.
39. Giridharan GA, Lee TJ, Ising M, Sobieski MA, Koenig SC, Gray LA, Slaughter MS. Miniaturization of mechanical circulatory support systems. Artif Organs. 2012;36(8):731–9. https://doi.org/10.1111/j.1525-1594.2012.01523.x. PMID: 22882443; PMCID: PMC3810069.
40. Dissanayake TD. An effective transcutaneous energy transfer (TET) system for artificial hearts [dissertation]. Auckland: University of Auckland; 2010.
41. Luu CH, Nguyen NT, Ta HT. Unravelling surface modification strategies for preventing medical device-induced thrombosis. Adv Healthc Mater. 2024;13(1):e2301039. https://doi.org/10.1002/adhm.202301039. PMID: 37725037; PMCID: PMC11468451.
42. Achneck HE, Serpe MJ, Jamiolkowski RM, Eibest LM, Craig SL, Lawson JH. Regenerating titanium ventricular assist device surfaces after gold/palladium coating for scanning electron microscopy. Microsc Res Tech. 2010;73(1):71–6. https://doi.org/10.1002/jemt.20757. PMID: 19642216; PMCID: PMC4062094.
43. Deveshkumar K, Hiren L, Nirav L. The impact of hydrophilic coatings on medical device performance: a comprehensive review. Int J Med Sci Clin Res Stud. 2025;5(11):1916–21. https://doi.org/10.47191/ijmscrs/v5-i11-20.
44. Vaidya Y, Riaz S, Dhamoon AS. Left ventricular assist devices. 2023 Aug 8. In: StatPearls [Internet]. Treasure Island: StatPearls Publishing; 2024. PMID: 29763004. Available at: https://www.ncbi.nlm.nih.gov/books/NBK499841/.
45. Mikhail J, Chivukula V, Khalili K. Advances in mechanical circulatory support (MCS): literature review. J Clin Med. 2025;14(13):3788. https://doi.org/10.3390/jcm14133788.
46. Kleinheyer M, Greatrex N, Nestler F, Timms DL. BiVACOR total artificial heart and future concepts. In: Mechanical circulatory support. Cham: Springer; 2025. p. 143–59. https://doi.org/10.1007/978-3-030-86172-8_14-1.

47. Perra E, Finocchiaro T, Jonasson D, Dual SA. Hemodynamic characterization of the Realheart® total artificial heart with a hybrid cardiovascular simulator. Artif Organs. 2022;46(8):1545–56. https://doi.org/10.1111/aor.14223.
48. Perra E, Jonasson D, Zaman SF, Ignell NB, Broomé M, Finocchiaro T, Perkins IL, Dual SA. Physiological control of Realheart total artificial heart. Artif Organs. 2025;49(10):1548–57. https://doi.org/10.1111/aor.15036.
49. Scandinavian Real Heart AB. Realheart® TAH receives Humanitarian Use Device designation by the U.S. Food and Drug Administration (FDA) [Internet]. Västerås: Scandinavian Real Heart AB; 2025. Available at: https://realheart.se/mfn_news/realheart-tah-receives-humanitarian-use-device-designation-by-the-u-s-food-and-drug-administration-fda/.
50. Carmat SA. The physiologic heart replacement therapy: Aeson® total artificial heart [Internet]. Vélizy-Villacoublay: Carmat SA; c2024. Available at: https://www.carmat-phrt.com/.
51. Jansen O, Finocchiaro T, Vandenberghe S, Van Meerbeeck G, Carrat F. Clinical experience with pressure sensor-based autoregulation of blood flow in an artificial heart. ASAIO J. 2019;65(8):779–86. https://doi.org/10.1097/MAT.0000000000001004. PMID: 31033621.
52. CARMAT. CARMAT delivers Q1 2025 results in line with its objectives [Internet]. Paris: CARMAT; 2025 Apr 9 Available at: https://www.carmatsa.com/carmat-content/uploads/2025/04/PR_CARMAT_Update_09-04-2025_EN_final-1.pdf.
53. Martin AC, Moussa MD, Panholzer B, Verde A, Guihaire J, et al. Initial experience with Aeson total artificial heart in cardiogenic shock patients on extracorporeal life support. JACC Heart Fail. 2025;13(6):1030–3. https://doi.org/10.1016/j.jchf.2025.01.023.
54. Fukamachi K, Karimov JH, Byram NA, Sunagawa G, Dessoffy R, Miyamoto T, Horvath DJ. Anatomical study of the Cleveland Clinic continuous-flow total artificial heart in adult and pediatric configurations. J Artif Organs. 2018;21(3):383–6. https://doi.org/10.1007/s10047-018-1039-0. PMID: 29616367.
55. Karimov JH, Horvath D, Byram N, Sunagawa G, Kuban B, Gao S, Dessoffy R, Fukamachi K. Abstract 16894: initial in vivo results of Cleveland Clinic pediatric continuous-flow total artificial heart implant. Circulation. 2017;136(Suppl_1):A16894. https://doi.org/10.1161/circ.136.suppl_1.16894.
56. Wang X, Zhou X, Chen H, Du J, Qing P, Zou L, Chen Y, Duan F, Yuan S, Shi J, Ji B, Wu R, Zhang Y, Jin Y, Hu S. Long-term outcomes of a novel fully magnetically levitated ventricular assist device for the treatment of advanced heart failure in China. J Heart Lung Transplant. 2024;43(11):1730–9. https://doi.org/10.1016/j.healun.2024.05.004.
57. CH Biomedical. MPA announcement | CH-VAD® approved for marketing in China: an implantable left ventricular assist device of CH Biomedical, opening a new era of heart failure treatment [Internet]. Suzhou: CH Biomedical; 2021. Available at: https://us.chbiomedical.com/news/detail-85.htm.
58. Lu Y, Zhao S, Han J, Lv Q, Du X, Hua Z, et al. Multicenter study for CH-VAD as a fully magnetically levitated left ventricular assist device. iScience. 2025;28(2):111764. https://doi.org/10.1016/j.isci.2025.111764.
59. Pleşoianu FA, Pleşoianu CE, Bararu Bojan I, Bojan A, Ţăruş A, Tinică G. Concept, design, and early prototyping of a low-cost, minimally invasive, fully implantable left ventricular assist device. Bioengineering (Basel). 2022;9(5):201. https://doi.org/10.3390/bioengineering9050201. PMID: 35621479; PMCID: PMC9137825.
60. Arfaee M, Vis A, Bartels PAA, van Laake LC, Lorenzon L, Ibrahim DM, et al. A soft robotic total artificial hybrid heart. Nat Commun. 2025;16(1):5146. https://doi.org/10.1038/s41467-025-5146-x.
61. Rogatinsky J, Recco D, Singh M, Yañez LZ, Matthews G, Ayers B, et al. A beating-heart procedure with soft robotic guidance. Adv Robot Res. 2025. [Epub ahead of print].; https://doi.org/10.1002/adrr.202400023.
62. Rayat Pisheh H, Nojabaei FS, Darvishi A, Rayat Pisheh A, Sani M. Cardiac tissue engineering: an emerging approach to the treatment of heart failure. Front Bioeng Biotechnol. 2024;12:1419972. https://doi.org/10.3389/fbioe.2024.1419972. PMID: 39021876; PMCID: PMC11252199.

63. Vunjak-Novakovic G, Tandon N, Godier A, Maidhof R, Marsano A, Martens TP, et al. Challenges in cardiac tissue engineering. Tissue Eng Part B Rev. 2010;16(2):169–87. https://doi.org/10.1089/ten.teb.2009.0352. PMID: 19712001; PMCID: PMC2846830.
64. Barani B, Rajasingh S, Rajasingh J. Exosomes: outlook for future cell-free cardiovascular disease therapy. Adv Exp Med Biol. 2017;998:285–307. https://doi.org/10.1007/978-981-10-4397-0_19. PMID: 28936747.

Managing Complications in Cardiac Interventions: Challenges and Solutions

16

Silviu Paul Stoleriu, Mihail Enache, Andrei Țăruș, Alberto Bacușcă, and Grigore Tinică

Classification of Interventions

Structural heart procedures can be categorized by access and technique.

- *Surgical interventions* include open approaches (median sternotomy or thoracotomy) with cardiopulmonary bypass (e.g., surgical valve replacement or repair, congenital defect closure, surgical maze or LAA ligation).
- *Minimally invasive procedures* use catheter-based or limited-incision approaches (e.g., TAVR, transcatheter mitral edge-to-edge repair (TEER, e.g., MitraClip), LAA occlusion devices, septal occluders, and endocardial ablation). These often avoid general cardiopulmonary bypass or full sternotomy.
- *Hybrid interventions* combine surgical and catheter techniques in a single setting (e.g., combined surgical LIMA-to-LAD plus PCI for multivessel disease, or a limited thoracotomy with percutaneous valve deployment). Hybrid methods aim to leverage the strengths of both approaches but can bring both sets of risks.
  - *Surgical AVR/MVR*: Full sternotomy with aortotomy or atriotomy. Risks include open-chest complications (e.g., mediastinitis).
  - *Minimally invasive surgery*: Limited incisions (mini-thoracotomy or hemisternotomy). These reduce trauma but may limit exposure; conversion to full sternotomy may be required [2, 3].

S. P. Stoleriu · M. Enache · A. Țăruș · A. Bacușcă (✉)
Faculty of Medicine, University of Medicine and Pharmacy "Grigore T Popa", Iasi, Romania

Institute of Cardiovascular Diseases "Prof. Dr. George I.M. Georgescu", Iasi, Romania

G. Tinică
Cardiovascular Surgery, Cardiovascular Diseases Institute, Iasi & Grigore T. Popa University of Medicine and Pharmacy, Iasi, Romania
e-mail: grigore.tinica@umfiasi.ro

G. Tinică, A. Burlacu (eds.), *Surgical, Hybrid and Minimally Invasive Structural Cardiac Interventions*, https://doi.org/10.1007/978-3-032-16676-0_16

- *TAVR and other transcatheter valves*: Percutaneous access (usually femoral artery for TAVR) or transapical, transseptal (for mitral) without CPB. Avoiding sternotomy reduces bleeding, but large sheaths can cause vascular injury and stroke.
- *TEER (MitraClip)*: Transseptal catheter-based mitral repair. Creates iatrogenic atrial septal defect and has device-specific risks (e.g., clip detachment).
- *LAA occlusion*: Endocardial devices (Watchman, Amulet, LAmbre, etc.) inserted via transseptal puncture to prevent stroke in AF. Acute risk of pericardial effusion is notable.
- *Septal defect closure*: Catheter closure of ASD/PFO/VSD with devices (Amplatzer, etc.). Requires transseptal or ventricular access; risk of device embolization or residual shunt.
- *Hybrid CABG/PCI*: Involves both surgical grafts and PCI in one procedure. Complications may include those of both CABG (sternotomy wound infection, bleeding) and PCI (contrast nephropathy, stent thrombosis).

Common Complications

Certain complications can occur with any structural intervention, though their incidence may vary by approach. Key common complications include (Table 16.1):

- *Bleeding*: All invasive procedures carry bleeding risk. Surgical cases often involve chest wall and mediastinal hemorrhage, while transcatheter cases risk access-site and retroperitoneal bleeding from large arterial or venous sheaths. Major bleeding (requiring transfusion or reoperation) occurs in both settings [1]. Antithrombotic regimens must balance thrombotic risk (e.g., stent thrombosis, device thrombosis) against hemorrhage.

Table 16.1 Complications associated with cardiac surgical procedures

Procedure	Common complications	Incidence	Management strategies
Coronary artery bypass grafting (CABG)	Postoperative bleeding, stroke, atrial fibrillation, renal failure, cognitive impairment	Bleeding: up to 20% require transfusion; stroke: 1.8%; atrial fibrillation: 30–40%; renal failure: Up to 18%	Bleeding: surgical hemostasis, transfusion; stroke: neuroimaging, anticoagulation; atrial fibrillation: rate/rhythm control, anticoagulation; renal failure: fluid management, dialysis if needed
Valve replacement	Paravalvular leak (PVL), prosthetic valve endocarditis, thromboembolism	PVL: 5–17%; endocarditis: 1–6%	PVL: percutaneous closure or reoperation; endocarditis: prolonged antibiotics, possible reoperation
Pacemaker implantation	Lead dislodgement, infection, pneumothorax	Lead dislodgement: 1–2%; infection: 1–2%	Lead dislodgement: lead repositioning; infection: device removal, antibiotics

- *Stroke/neurological events*: Embolic stroke is a feared complication, especially in TAVR and any procedure that manipulates the aorta or heart. Embolization of atheroma or debris during valve crossing can cause ischemic stroke. Rates of clinical stroke after TAVR or SAVR range ~1–5% [1]. Protocols include strict blood pressure control, intra-procedural anticoagulation, and embolic protection devices where available.
- *Infection*: This includes surgical site infection (superficial or deep sternal wound infections and mediastinitis after sternotomy), catheter-site infection (rare with sterility), and device-related endocarditis (infective endocarditis on prosthetic valves or devices). Prosthetic valve endocarditis (PVE) is a serious long-term risk, and guidelines emphasize antibiotic prophylaxis in high-risk scenarios. Rates of endocarditis are low (<1%/year for TAVR) but portend high mortality [4]. Prevention with sterile technique and perioperative antibiotics is critical.
- *Arrhythmias*: New-onset atrial fibrillation (AF) is common after open-heart surgery (seen in ~30% of AVR/MVR) and can complicate management with increased stroke risk. Postoperative AF usually peaks in the first few days and requires rate/rhythm control and anticoagulation per guidelines. TAVR and other transcatheter valves frequently cause conduction disturbances: new left bundle-branch block occurs in up to ~25%, and complete heart block requiring permanent pacemaker (PPM) occurs in ~5–20% (higher with certain valve types) [1]. Post-implant ECG monitoring and low threshold for PPM in persistent high-grade AV block are needed.
- *Vascular injury*: Large-bore arterial access (for TAVR, TEER, LAA devices) can cause arterial dissection, perforation, or pseudoaneurysm. Femoral artery or iliac artery injury may require endovascular stenting or open repair. Ultrasound guidance for access, careful sheath manipulation, and closure devices reduce these risks. Vessel tortuosity or calcification (common in elderly) increases risk of access trauma.
- *Renal injury*: Contrast-induced nephropathy and acute kidney injury (AKI) can occur with extensive imaging or angiography during transcatheter procedures or with cardiopulmonary bypass. Minimizing contrast volume, ensuring adequate hydration, and judicious use of nephrotoxic agents mitigate this. AKI is more common in surgical cases with CPB [1], but can occur in TAVR as well. Baseline chronic kidney disease is a major risk factor.
- *Pericardial effusion/tamponade*: Any intervention involving the heart or pericardium can cause bleeding into the pericardial space. Surgical cases often leave mild effusions, but aggressive bleeding (e.g., coronary or ventricular injury) can cause tamponade requiring urgent re-exploration. Transseptal puncture or device manipulation (e.g., LAA closure) can tear atrial or appendage walls, leading to effusion or tamponade [4, 5]. Pericardiocentesis or surgical drainage is required for tamponade. TEE is helpful intra-procedurally to detect pericardial fluid early.
- *Device failure or malposition*: Catheter-delivered devices (valves, clips, occluders) may malfunction. Examples include valve stent frame distortion, clip detachment, or device embolization. For instance, MitraClip single-leaflet detachment (SLDA) is a known issue [4], and LAA occluders can dislodge (embolic event) if not properly seated. Intra-procedural imaging (TEE, fluoroscopy) confirms device position. If a device embolizes, percutaneous snaring or urgent surgery may retrieve it.

Table 16.2 Summary of common complications, risk factors, prevention, and management

Complication	Incidence	Risk factors	Management strategies
Bleeding	Varies	Anticoagulation, vascular access site	Imaging, closure devices, hemostasis techniques
Stroke	Varies	Atherosclerosis, calcified valves	Cerebral protection, anticoagulation management
Infection	Varies	Prolonged procedures, immunosuppression	Aseptic technique, prophylactic antibiotics
Arrhythmias	Common	Atrial manipulation, ischemia	Monitoring, antiarrhythmic drugs, cardioversion
Acute kidney injury	Varies	Contrast use, pre-existing renal impairment	Hydration, renal function monitoring, medication adjustment

- *Paravalvular leak (PVL)*: In valve replacements (especially TAVR), incomplete seal between prosthesis and native annulus can cause PVL, leading to hemolysis or heart failure. Modern TAVR valves have lower PVL rates, but it remains more common than in surgical valves [1]. Moderate–severe PVL often requires intervention (post-dilation, plug, or re-do valve).
- *Procedural conversion*: A planned minimally invasive or transcatheter procedure may need to convert to open surgery. For example, a limited-thoracotomy AVR may be converted to full sternotomy for poor exposure or major bleeding [2, 3]. Similarly, TAVR may convert to emergent SAVR if catastrophic annular rupture or obstruction occurs (rare). Conversion rates in minimally invasive valve surgery range 1–4% [2, 3]. Teams should always be prepared to convert, with equipment (saw, sternal wires) ready.

For each complication, acute management is critical (e.g., controlling bleeding, treating arrhythmia, relieving tamponade). Equally important are prevention strategies: meticulous technique, appropriate patient selection, and protocolized care (Table 16.2).

Procedure-Specific Complications

Different interventions have characteristic risks in addition to the common ones above. Key examples include:

- *Surgical Valve Replacement/Repair (SAVR/S-MVR)*: In open surgery, bleeding from suture lines or graft sites can require re-exploration. Conduction tissue injury (e.g., from septal sutures in valve procedures) can cause AV block. Post-cardiotomy low cardiac output syndrome and coagulopathy are concerns. Sternotomy wounds may get infected (risk factors: diabetes, obesity). In a minimally invasive AVR (e.g., mini-thoracotomy), complications include limited field exposure (risk of inadvertent RV or mammary vessel injury) and need for groin cannulation (risk of infection or limb ischemia) [2]. Conversion to full sternotomy is usually safe but lengthens CPB time [2]. In minimally invasive mitral surgery (e.g., robotic or thoracoscopic), specific risks are phrenic nerve injury and aortic crossclamp management (balloon vs external clamp). Studies show conversion rates (e.g., to sternotomy) of ~2–3% with minimally invasive mitral approaches [3].

- *Transcatheter Aortic Valve Replacement (TAVR)*: Common complications include vascular injury (hematoma, dissection), conduction blocks (LBBB or heart block), and PVL [1]. Stroke (1–3%) occurs due to aortic arch manipulation; filter devices can reduce this risk. Rarely, TAVR may cause annulus rupture or coronary ostia obstruction, both catastrophic complications requiring immediate surgery or percutaneous bailout (e.g., chimney stent for coronary occlusion). Acute aortic dissection is another rare risk. Post-TAVR, many patients require PPM for persistent block. Preventive measures include careful sizing of the valve, rapid pacing during balloon inflation, and prophylactic pacemaker wires if high block is expected.
- *Mitral TEER (MitraClip)*: Unique complications include *single-leaflet device attachment* (SLDA) where the clip detaches from one leaflet, causing recurrent MR [4]. SLDA has decreased with newer device iterations but was historically seen in ~2–10% of cases. *Clip embolization* (detachment of entire clip) is rare (<1%) [4]. Iatrogenic atrial septal defect (iASD) from the transeptal puncture is universal; most are small and hemodynamically insignificant, but large defects can cause shunt that may require closure. Mitral stenosis (from too many clips) can occur if orifice is over-narrowed. Vascular complications are less common since venous access is used. Pericardial effusion can occur from transseptal or LA wall trauma [4]. Intra-procedure TEE is mandatory to guide clip placement and check for residual leak or clip stability. Overall, MitraClip is safe, with low in-hospital mortality (≈1–3%) [4].
- *Tricuspid TEER*: Emerging devices can cause heart block or leaflet injury. Data are evolving.
- *Left Atrial Appendage Closure*: Procedural tamponade is a leading acute risk. The LA appendage wall is thin and can perforate during device deployment. In a large series, tamponade occurred in ~3–6% of cases, usually within 7 days [5, 6]. Pericardial effusion, when it occurs, requires prompt drainage. Device embolization is a known complication (typically <1% if positioned correctly) [6]. *Peridevice leak (PDL)*—incomplete seal around the device—is not rare and portends higher stroke risk [7]. Even small leaks (<5 mm) may double stroke risk over time [7]. Management of PDL includes intensified anticoagulation or percutaneous plugging if significant. Device-related thrombosis (thrombus on the device) is another concern in the first months and requires antithrombotic therapy.
- *Atrial Septal/PFO Closure*: Embolization of the occluder is rare (<1%) but can cause stroke or require open retrieval. Residual shunt (left-to-right flow) may lead to paradoxical stroke if the patient has RA pressures > LA. Transient arrhythmias (atrial tachycardia) can occur after septal puncture. Device erosion (Atrium Septal) is very rare but catastrophic (aortic root erosion).

- *Valve-in-Valve and Other Advanced Transcatheter*: Implanting a transcatheter valve inside a failing bioprosthesis can risk coronary obstruction (if the prosthetic leaflets block a coronary ostium). This is assessed pre-procedure by CT ("virtual transcatheter heart valve-to-coronary ostium distance"). Management includes surgical conversion or snorkel stenting for acute obstruction. Valve embolization or malposition can occur if the landing zone is too large or calcified.
- *Congenital and Other Interventions*: Hybrid approaches in congenital heart disease (e.g., stage I palliation for HLHS) have unique risks, but are beyond this chapter's primary focus on acquired structural disease.

Diagnostic Tools

Effective diagnosis of complications relies on imaging and monitoring:

- *Echocardiography (TTE/TEE)* is indispensable. Intraoperative TEE is used in valve and clip procedures to guide repair and detect complications (air emboli, pericardial fluid, PVL, clip position). For example, TEE is mandated during minimally invasive surgery for safe cannula placement and deairing [1, 2]. Postoperatively, transthoracic echo at baseline (before discharge) and periodically (1 month, 1 year, then yearly) is recommended after valve implantation [1]. Echo assesses ventricular function, valvular gradients, paravalvular leak, pericardial effusion, and device position. Transesophageal echo or intracardiac echo can clarify uncertain findings.
- *Angiography/Fluoroscopy*: During TAVR or LAA closure, contrast angiography defines annular or LAA anatomy and confirms device occlusion. Vascular angiography can locate bleeding.
- *Computed Tomography (CT)*: Pre-procedural CT angiography is critical in TAVR planning (annulus sizing, access route, coronary height) and in transcatheter mitral planning (e.g., mitral annular calcification). Post-procedure, CT can evaluate valve position, coronary patency, or detect complications like pseudoaneurysm.
- *Electrocardiography/Monitoring*: Continuous ECG during and after procedures detects arrhythmias. Any new conduction block on ECG after TAVR warrants observation, as high-degree AV block can be delayed. Telemetry is used for at least 48–72 h post-intervention.
- *Laboratory Tests*: Hemoglobin/hematocrit monitor bleeding. Kidney function tests (Cr, BUN) gauge renal injury after contrast or bypass. Cardiac enzymes (troponin) might reflect infarction. Inflammatory markers and blood cultures are indicated if infection is suspected.
- *Neurologic Assessment*: Any new neurologic deficit triggers immediate neurologic evaluation and brain imaging (CT/MRI) to distinguish stroke vs hemorrhage. Stroke protocols (NIHSS scoring, neuro-imaging, possible thrombolysis or thrombectomy) should be ready in cath lab settings.

Management Protocols

Management of complications must be prompt and evidence-based, often guided by contemporary society guidelines and studies. Key strategies include:

- *Bleeding*: For surgical bleeding, return to OR for exploration and hemostasis is often required. Transfusion protocols (e.g., maintaining hemoglobin >7–8 g/dL unless ongoing ischemia) follow institutional guidelines. Antifibrinolytics (tranexamic acid) are given in cardiac surgery to reduce bleeding. For catheter-access bleeding, apply manual or device-assisted compression; severe cases may need covered stents or surgical repair of vessels. If anticoagulation has been given (heparin, bivalirudin), reversal agents (protamine sulfate for heparin) should be used. In massive hemorrhage, activate massive transfusion protocol. (Guidance: manage according to "Society of Thoracic Surgeons" or local transfusion guidelines.)
- *Stroke*: Ischemic stroke management follows stroke protocol. If identified immediately during TAVR, possible options include intravenous thrombolysis (risky post-procedure) or mechanical thrombectomy (if large vessel occlusion). In practice, most centers do supportive care and early rehabilitation. Prevention includes dual antiplatelet therapy or anticoagulation post-TAVR as per trials (recent evidence supports single vs dual antiplatelet based on bleeding risk) [1, 8]. Rigorous control of risk factors (AF anticoagulation, atherosclerosis) is mandatory.
- *Infection*: Prophylactic antibiotics are administered perioperatively. For confirmed infection (e.g., mediastinitis or endocarditis), broad-spectrum IV antibiotics are started, and imaging (TEE) is done to assess for abscess or dehiscence. In prosthetic valve endocarditis, early surgical intervention is often indicated (valve excision and replacement) per endocarditis guidelines [9]. Mediastinitis requires surgical debridement and vacuum-assisted closure. All indwelling lines/catheters should be removed. Negative-pressure wound therapy can help salvage sternal wounds.
- *Arrhythmias*: New-onset AF post-surgery is treated per guidelines (rate control with β-blockers or calcium-channel blockers; rhythm control if unstable; anticoagulation if stroke risk is high). Amiodarone may be used for prophylaxis or treatment in the immediate post-op setting. Conduction blocks from TAVR: PPM implantation is indicated if complete heart block persists >48–72 h [1], or if new high-grade AV block occurs. Temporary pacing wires placed during surgery or TAVR allow monitoring and bridging if needed. Ventricular arrhythmias are rare but require ACLS protocols; underlying causes (electrolyte imbalance, ischemia) should be corrected.
- *Vascular injury*: Access vessel dissection or perforation during catheter insertion may be managed by endovascular stenting (covered stent for perforation) or balloon tamponade. If endovascular measures fail, surgical cut-down and repair are done. Retroperitoneal bleed signs prompt immediate reversal of anticoagulation

and hemodynamic support. Limb ischemia from cannulation requires urgent angiography and possible embolectomy.

- *Renal injury*: For contrast nephropathy, aggressive IV hydration (isotonic saline) is given peri-procedure. Avoid nephrotoxins (NSAIDs) postoperatively. Use low-contrast protocols and iso-osmolar agents if possible. If AKI progresses to >2× baseline creatinine or oliguria, nephrology consultation and renal replacement therapy (dialysis) are considered. In CPB-associated AKI, maintain perfusion pressure and consider ultrafiltration.
- *Pericardial effusion/tamponade*: Any hypotension with rising central venous pressure and echo evidence of effusion mandates urgent drainage. TEE/echo-guided pericardiocentesis is first-line. If drainage is inadequate or effusion is loculated, surgical sternotomy or thoracoscopic drainage is required. Avoid excessive positive pressure ventilation. Intravenous fluids and inotropes may stabilize hemodynamics while arranging drainage.
- *Device malfunction*: If a MitraClip detaches, options include adding another clip, surgical repair, or replacement if MR is severe [4]. Late leaflet detachment may be managed with re-intervention if feasible. Embolized devices (valve or occluder) should be retrieved percutaneously if stable, or surgically extracted if hemodynamic compromise. Paravalvular leak is treated with additional transcatheter occluders or surgical patch closure, guided by imaging. Failed bioprostheses (high gradients or stenosis) may be addressed with valve-in-valve replacement or reoperation, depending on patient risk and anatomy.
- *Paravalvular leak*: Mild PVL can be observed; moderate–severe PVL causing hemolysis or CHF usually requires intervention. Transcatheter PVL plugs (Amplatzer Vascular Plugs) can seal leaks in suitable anatomy. If PVL is refractory, surgical re-replacement of the valve is indicated.
- *Conversion*: When conversion to open surgery is needed (e.g., for uncontrollable bleeding or anatomy issues), hemodynamic support (inotropes, bypass) is initiated quickly. Communicating early within the team is vital: even in minimally invasive AVR, having the sternal saw ready is a recommendation [2]. Extending an incision or performing full sternotomy should be done calmly but decisively, as conversion is reported to be safe if done under controlled conditions [2, 3]. After conversion, expect longer bypass times; closely watch for low-output syndrome.

Standardized protocols (e.g., "code bleed", "code stroke") can expedite multidisciplinary response. Figures/flowcharts may illustrate management algorithms (e.g., a flowchart for "post-TAVR hypotension" evaluating tamponade vs MI vs vascular bleed). Early consultation with specialists (cardiac surgeons, neuro, vascular, nephrology) improves outcomes.

Post-Intervention Surveillance

Vigilant follow-up is essential to detect late complications. Surveillance strategies include:

- *Echocardiographic follow-up*: Both surgical and transcatheter prosthetic valves require echocardiography at 30 days (to establish a new baseline), at 1 year, and annually thereafter [1]. Imaging assesses for prosthetic dysfunction (degeneration, thrombosis, PVL) and ventricular function. For MitraClip and surgical repairs, echo evaluates residual or recurrent regurgitation and device stability. New or progressing shunts (ASD/PFO, valve paravalvular leak) are monitored by color Doppler.
- *Clinical monitoring*: Patients should have regular clinical exams (initially within 1–3 months post-op, then yearly). Monitor for new murmurs, heart failure symptoms, arrhythmias, or signs of infection. Check blood pressure and heart rhythm at each visit; 12-lead ECG to screen for late conduction issues. Palpate pulses and inspect access sites for late pseudoaneurysm formation.
- *Laboratory tests*: For valve patients on anticoagulants, check INR (if warfarin) and adjust dose. Monitor renal function periodically in patients who had AKI. Check complete blood count (hemoglobin) for delayed bleeding or hemolysis from PVL. For.
- LAAO patients, periodic imaging (TEE or CT) at 45 days and 6–12 months is often done per device protocols to confirm endothelialization and rule out device thrombus or leak.
- *Antithrombotic therapy and prophylaxis*: Follow guidelines for post-procedure anticoagulation. For example, after TAVR, many experts use short-term dual antiplatelet therapy or warfarin for 3 months if bleeding risk is low [1]. After MitraClip, antiplatelets or anticoagulants are used per atrial fibrillation status. Prophylaxis for infective endocarditis should follow current guidelines (e.g., antibiotic prophylaxis only for highest-risk patients undergoing dental or invasive GI/GU procedures).
- *Surveillance for specific issues*: Screen for late-onset complications like structural valve degeneration (SVD) of bioprostheses (annual echo gradients rising over time). Check for signs of device erosion or endocarditis (e.g., repeat blood cultures if fever). Periodically assess LV function and size by echo or MRI, especially if before intervention function was reduced. For hybrid CABG/PCI, perform routine angiographic or noninvasive stress testing to ensure graft and stent patency (Table 16.3).

Table 16.3 Outlined surveillance schedule (clinical, echo, ECG, labs) at discharge, 1 month, 6–12 months, and annually

Time point	Clinical evaluation	Investigations	Patient education topics
At discharge	Review surgical course Assess wound & vitals	Baseline ECG Echocardiogram (if indicated) Basic labs (CBC, renal fx, INR if on warfarin)	Signs of infection (fever, redness) Stroke/tia symptoms dvt/pe signs Anticoagulation adherence Smoking cessation, diet, activity guidance
1 month	Symptom review (dyspnea, chest pain, fatigue) Wound healing Medication compliance	ECG Echocardiogram (if valve repair/replacement or pericardial effusion risk) INR (if applicable) Renal function & CBC	Activity levels and cardiac rehab Monitoring for late complications (e.g., arrhythmias) Lifestyle adherence
6–12 months	Physical exam Review symptoms Risk factor optimization	ECG Repeat echo if structural concern or persistent symptoms Lipid panel, glucose/HbA1c	Reinforcement of stroke and infection warning signs Emphasize long-term lifestyle change
Annually thereafter	General cardiac review Evaluate functional status Update medications	Annual ECG Echo every 1–2 years (earlier if symptoms or prosthetic valve) Labs: renal, INR, lipids	Vaccinations (e.g., influenza, pneumococcus) Lifelong endocarditis prophylaxis if indicated

Conclusion

Advances in surgical, hybrid, and minimally invasive structural heart interventions have greatly expanded treatment options for valvular and structural disease. However, these complex procedures bring a spectrum of potential complications. Multidisciplinary care (surgery, interventional cardiology, anesthesiology, imaging, and intensive care) is vital for prevention, early detection, and management of complications. Evidence-based guidelines (ESC/EACTS, ACC/AHA) and recent studies emphasize individualized risk stratification (e.g., for TAVR vs SAVR) and tailored management of adverse events [1, 5]. By understanding the patterns of complications—from bleeding and stroke to device-specific failures—clinicians can optimize perioperative protocols and surveillance. Future improvements in device technology and procedural technique should further reduce these risks. Ultimately, diligent prevention (such as embolic protection in high-risk TAVR patients), vigilant monitoring (routine echo surveillance), and prompt, protocol-driven interventions (e.g., standardized stroke pathways) will improve outcomes in structural heart patients.

Key Points

- TAVR vs. SAVR have different complication profiles (TAVR: vascular, conduction, PVL; SAVR: bleeding, AKI, AF) [1].
- MitraClip most common failure is single-leaflet detachment; manage with clip repositioning or surgery [4].
- LAA closure's major acute risk is tamponade; peridevice leaks increase stroke risk [5, 7].
- Protocol-driven response (bleeding, stroke, infection) and planned conversion strategies improve safety [4].
- Regular follow-up with echo (30-day, 1-year, yearly) is essential for surveillance [1].

Postoperative Complications in Cardiac Surgery

Postoperative Bleeding

Postoperative bleeding is a major complication following cardiac surgery, contributing to increased morbidity, re-exploration rates (2–6%), transfusion requirements, prolonged ventilation, and mortality (up to 20%) [10, 11]. It may result from surgical bleeding (technical causes) or coagulopathy (acquired platelet dysfunction, hypothermia, CPB-related hemodilution, anticoagulant effects, hyperfibrinolysis) (Table 16.4) [10, 12].

Incidence

- Mild to moderate bleeding requiring transfusion: ~20–50% [10].
- Re-exploration for bleeding/tamponade: 2–6% [2].
- Mortality after re-exploration: up to 20% [10].

Hemostatic Agents

- *Tranexamic acid (antifibrinolytic)*: IV 10–30 mg/kg bolus at incision, often followed by 1–10 mg/kg/h infusion during surgery [13]. (Example: 1 g IV bolus then 1 g over 4 h). No routine titration; stop after surgery. Use cautiously (renal impairment, seizure risk at high dose) and monitor for thrombosis.

Table 16.4 Risk factors for postoperative bleeding

Category	Risk factors
Patient factors	Age, low body weight, preoperative antiplatelets (clopidogrel within 5 days), anticoagulation, liver dysfunction, renal dysfunction
Surgical factors	Prolonged CPB time (>120 min), complex surgery, redo surgery, emergency surgery
Postoperative factors	Hypothermia, metabolic acidosis, residual heparin, platelet dysfunction, hypofibrinogenemia

- *Epsilon-aminocaproic acid (antifibrinolytic)*: Alternative to tranexamic acid, e.g., 100 mg/kg IV at the start of surgery. (Less commonly used in Europe.)
- *Protamine sulfate (heparin antagonist)*: Administer to reverse heparin: ~1 mg protamine per 100 units remaining heparin, titrated to ACT normalization. Use cautiously (allergy risk, hypotension).
- *Prothrombin complex concentrate (PCC, clotting factors II/VII/IX/X concentrate)*: For refractory bleeding or urgent reversal of vitamin-K antagonists. Dose 25–50 IU/kg IV based on INR; give with IV vitamin K. Monitor INR. Contraindications: DIC.
- *Recombinant Factor VIIa (Novoseven, factor VIIa)*: Rescue therapy if bleeding persists despite conventional measures. Dose ~90 μg/kg IV bolus (may repeat once); no titration protocol. Duration: single dose or very short course. *Note:* High thrombotic risk; use only when bleeding life-threatening and after informed decision. Monitor for thrombosis.
- *Blood products*: Platelets, FFP, cryoprecipitate as needed per bleeding indices and coagulation studies; not drugs per se.

Management of Postoperative Bleeding

Step 1: Assessment

Quantify chest tube output:

200 mL/h × 2 h or >300 mL in 1 h → consider active bleeding.

Check hemodynamic status (tachycardia, hypotension, low urine output).

Evaluate coagulation:

- INR, APTT, fibrinogen, platelet count.
- Thromboelastography (TEG) or ROTEM for functional assessment [10].

Bedside echocardiography to exclude tamponade.

Step 2: Initial medical management

- Maintain *normothermia (≥36 °C)* [12].
- Correct *metabolic acidosis (target pH >7.3).*
- Reverse residual heparin with *protamine (1 mg per 100 IU heparin, adjust based on ACT)* [11].
- *Transfusion thresholds*:
  - Hb <7–8 g/dL → transfuse PRBCs.
  - Platelet count <50,000/μL → transfuse platelets (1 apheresis unit or 4–6 pooled units).
  - Fibrinogen <1.5–2 g/L → Cryoprecipitate (2–4 pools) or fibrinogen concentrate (2–4 g IV) [10].
  - Prolonged INR/APTT → consider FFP 15 mL/kg.
- *Tranexamic acid 10–15 mg/kg IV over 20 min, then 1 mg/kg/h infusion* if hyperfibrinolysis suspected, guided by ROTEM (APTEM vs EXTEM) [12].

Table 16.5 Postoperative bleeding—summary

Aspect	Details
Incidence	20–50% require transfusion; 2–6% re-exploration
Risk factors	CPB >120 min, platelet inhibitors, redo surgery, hypothermia
Management	Stepwise: (1) assess, (2) correct coagulopathy, (3) re-explore if needed
Preventive measures	Normothermia, antifibrinolytics, preoperative planning

Step 3: Re-Exploration

Indications:

- Ongoing bleeding (>300 mL/h) unresponsive to correction.
- Hemodynamic instability despite resuscitation.
- Cardiac tamponade.

Surgical re-exploration should *not be delayed* in active surgical bleeding [10].

Preventive Measures

- Preoperative cessation of clopidogrel ≥5 days before elective surgery.
- Maintain normothermia during CPB [12].
- Use cell savers intraoperatively.
- Careful surgical hemostasis before chest closure.
- Prophylactic tranexamic acid (10–15 mg/kg IV at induction + infusion 1 mg/kg/h) in high-risk bleeding cases per EACTS guidelines [12].
- Use of point-of-care coagulation monitoring to guide targeted transfusion and avoid dilutional coagulopathy (Table 16.5) [10].

Flowchart: Postoperative Bleeding Management

1. Chest tube output monitoring
   - If >200 mL/h for 2 consecutive hours.
   - OR >300 mL in 1 h
     Investigate active bleeding.
2. Assess hemodynamics and laboratory values
   - Blood pressure, heart rate, urine output.
   - Laboratory evaluation:
     - Hemoglobin (Hb).
     - Platelet count.
     - INR, APTT.
     - Fibrinogen.
   - TEG/ROTEM if available.

3. Correction measures
   - Maintain normothermia (≥36 °C).
   - Correct acidosis (target pH >7.3).
   - Reverse residual heparin with protamine.
   - Transfusion as needed:
     - PRBCs if Hb <7–8 g/dL.
     - Platelets if <50,000/μL.
     - Cryoprecipitate or fibrinogen concentrate if fibrinogen <1.5–2 g/L.
     - FFP for coagulopathy.
   - Administer tranexamic acid (TXA) if hyperfibrinolysis is suspected.
4. Perform bedside echocardiography
   - Assess for cardiac tamponade.
5. Decision point
   If bleeding decreases and patient is stable: Continue monitoring.
   If bleeding persists or instability is present: Proceed to surgical re-exploration.

Neurologic Complications

Cardiac surgery with cardiopulmonary bypass (CPB) can cause various neurological issues. Common complications include stroke (intra- or postoperative), delirium, prolonged cognitive dysfunction, seizures, visual deficits, phrenic nerve palsy, etc. The overall stroke rate is ~1–5% (higher after valve/DHCA surgery), and delirium occurs in 10–50% of patients (elderly and high-risk patients are most susceptible. Seizures occur in ~1–8%, often linked to high-dose tranexamic acid. Risk factors include advanced age, atherosclerosis, valve operations, prolonged CPB/DHCA, anemia or renal failure, and high systemic inflammation [14, 15].

- *Stroke*: Incidence ~1–17% early (during or within 48 h) and ~1% late [14]. Risk: severe atherosclerosis, valve surgery, emboli. *Management:* Rapid neurologic evaluation (CT/MRI), avoid CPB if possible, postpone anticoagulation if hemorrhage, and follow stroke guidelines (Table 16.6).
- *Postoperative delirium*: Occurs immediately in 10–50% (peaks post-op day 1–2). Risk: age >65, prior cognitive impairment, polypharmacy, transfusions. *Prevention:* Reorientation, avoid sedatives, optimize pain control. *Treatment:* Nonpharmacologic measures; consider antipsychotics only if severe agitation [14].
- *Cognitive dysfunction*: Long-term cognitive decline (1–42%). Risk: vascular disease, frailty. Manage expectantly and arrange neurocognitive testing, but no proven therapy [14].
- *Seizures*: Immediate seizures (1–8%) often due to TXA or electrolyte imbalance. Treat with IV benzodiazepines or antiepileptics (e.g., levetiracetam 1 g IV) [14].

Table 16.6 Postoperative stroke—incidence, risk factors, and management

Aspect	Details
Incidence	Incidence varies among different types of surgery and is considerably higher in cardiac surgeries.
Risk factors	Advanced age, atherosclerosis, atrial fibrillation, prolonged aortic cross-clamp time, manipulation of the aorta.
Management	Immediate neuroimaging, supportive care, and, in select cases, thrombolytic therapy.
Preventive measures	Preoperative carotid screening, minimizing aortic manipulation, maintaining optimal perfusion pressures during surgery.

Key Points Maintain normal perfusion/oxygenation, avoid cerebral ischemia (keep hematocrit >25–30%). Monitor neuro exam. There are no specific drug "doses" aside from stroke/ICU care (e.g., maintain MAP >65 mmHg, avoid hyperglycemia). Early neurologic consultation is advised.

- *Stroke (Ischemic & Hemorrhagic)*
  Etiology:
  - Embolic (air, thrombus).
  - Aortic manipulation.
  - Hypoperfusion.

- *Ischemic stroke (thrombotic/embolic)*: If within window, IV alteplase (tPA, fibrinolytic): 0.9 mg/kg IV (max 90 mg), with 10% as bolus and reminder over 60 min.
- *Titration:* none; single infusion. Duration: one dose.
- *Contraindications:* recent major surgery (within ~14 days), active bleeding, uncontrolled hypertension.
- After treatment: *Aspirin* 75–100 mg daily started >24 h after tPA (if no hemorrhage) or immediately if no tPA.
- If noncardioembolic minor stroke or TIA: dual antiplatelet (aspirin 75–100 mg + clopidogrel 75 mg daily) for 21–90 days. If cardioembolic (e.g., postop AF): start *anticoagulation* (e.g., heparin IV infusion then vitamin K antagonist or DOAC) after bleeding risk subsides (often 1–2 weeks post-stroke).

- *Hemorrhagic stroke*: Lower blood pressure to prevent expansion: IV labetalol (β-blocker) 10–20 mg IV push (may repeat) or infusion (2–8 mg/min) and/or nicardipine (CCB) infusion (5 mg/h, titrate up to 15 mg/h) to target SBP ~140–160 mmHg. Administer osmotherapy for intracranial hypertension: Mannitol 0.25–1 g/kg IV bolus or hypertonic saline (e.g., 23.4% 30 mL IV) if signs of herniation; may repeat if needed. Duration: titrate BP agents to maintain goals until acute phase resolves. Reverse anticoagulants (PCC or idarucizumab) if needed.

Table 16.7 Acute ischemic stroke management

Medication	Dose	Notes
Alteplase (IV tPA)	0.9 mg/kg IV (max 90 mg); 10% bolus, rest over 60 min	Avoid within 14 days of major surgery [5]
Aspirin	75–100 mg/day	Start 24–48 h after tPA if no bleeding
DOAC (e.g., Apixaban)	5 mg BID (adjusted by renal function/age)	Start 1–2 weeks post-stroke depending on infarct size

No ESC/EACTS guideline specifically covers postoperative stroke; management follows general stroke guidelines. Thrombolysis after recent surgery is typically contraindicated. Blood pressure control in ICH is guided by European Stroke Society recommendations (aim SBP <140–160), and neurosurgical consultation is required [16] (Table 16.7).

Hemorrhagic Stroke

- *BP control*:
  - *Labetalol*: 10–20 mg IV, repeat q10min; or infusion 2–8 mg/min.
  - *Nicardipine*: Start 5 mg/h IV; titrate to 15 mg/h.
- *ICP management*:
  - *Mannitol*: 0.25–1 g/kg IV 4–6 h.
  - *Hypertonic saline*: 23.4% 30 mL IV over 10 min.

Flowchart: Postoperative Stroke Management

1. Identify Sudden Neurological Deficit
   - Observe for weakness, speech disturbances, facial droop.
2. Perform Immediate Neurological Exam + NIHSS Scoring.
3. Obtain Urgent Non-Contrast Brain CT
   - If hemorrhage ➔ Neurosurgical consult.
   - If no hemorrhage ➔ Ischemic stroke.
4. Evaluate Treatment Options
   - Consider mechanical thrombectomy (if LVO, within window).
   - Systemic thrombolysis rare post-op due to bleeding risk.
5. Provide Supportive Care
   - Blood pressure control (<185/110 unless poor perfusion).
   - Maintain oxygenation and normoglycemia.
   - Early rehabilitation, transfer to stroke unit as indicated.

Flowchart: Postoperative Delirium Management

1. Identify Agitation or Confusion
   - Acute changes in attention, awareness, or cognition.
2. Check for Reversible Causes
   - Hypoxia, hypoglycemia, infection.
   - Pain, urinary retention, medication effects.

Table 16.8 Infections—incidence, risk factors, and management

Aspect	Details
Incidence	Surgical site infections occur in 3–27% of cases.
Risk factors	Obesity, diabetes, prolonged surgery, re-exploration, poor glycemic control.
Management	Antibiotic therapy, surgical debridement for deep infections, wound care.
Preventive measures	Preoperative skin antisepsis, perioperative antibiotic prophylaxis, glycemic control.

3. Initiate Non-Pharmacological Management
   - Reorient the patient regularly.
   - Reduce noise and ensure a day-night cycle.
   - Encourage family presence if feasible.
4. Pharmacological Management (If Severe)
   - Low-dose haloperidol (0.5–1 mg PO/IV every 8 h).
   - Avoid benzodiazepines unless managing alcohol withdrawal.
5. Monitor Hydration and Electrolyte Balance.

Postoperative Infections

Surgical Site Infections (SSI) are a major concern. Overall SSI rates after cardiac surgery range ~3–27%. The chest (sternotomy) wound is at highest risk, particularly mediastinitis (deep SSI) which has ~3–20% mortality (Table 16.8) [17]. Common pathogens: *Staphylococcus aureus* (incl. MRSA), coagulase-negative staphylococci.

Risk Factors Obesity, diabetes, COPD, malnutrition, renal failure, re-operation, prolonged surgery or CPB time, blood transfusions, and *S. aureus* nasal carriage [17].

Prevention
- *Decolonization*: Preop nasal mupirocin (2% ointment, 2× daily ×5 days) and chlorhexidine baths for *S. aureus* carriers.
- *Antibiotic prophylaxis*: Give IV cefazolin 2 g (3 g if weight >120 kg) within 60 min of incision; redose every 4 h intra-op. In beta-lactam allergy or MRSA risk, use vancomycin 15 mg/kg IV (maximum 2 g).
- *Glucose control*: Maintain blood glucose <180 mg/dL perioperatively.
- *Aseptic technique*: Strict sterile prep, minimize OR traffic, and careful sternal closure [17].

Diagnosis Superficial SSI (skin only) vs deep (fascia/mediastinum). Look for fever, drainage, sternal instability, leukocytosis; confirm with culture and imaging (CT/MRI).

Table 16.9 Treatment postoperative infections [17]

Infection Type	Timing	Prevention	Treatment
Superficial SSI	≤30 days	Preop decolonization, IV cefazolin 2 g	Wound care, targeted antibiotics
Deep SSI / mediastinitis	≤90 days	Above + strict sterility	Debridement + prolonged antibiotics (e.g., vancomycin 15 mg/kg IV)
Pneumonia (postop)	Post-ICU	Early extubation, pulmonary toileting	IV antibiotics (e.g., ceftriaxone 1–2 g + azithromycin 500 mg)

Treatment

- Superficial SSI: Local care, antibiotics based on cultures (Table 16.9).
- Deep SSI (mediastinitis): Urgent surgical debridement/irrigation. Consider vacuum-assisted closure (VAC) therapy. Broad antibiotics (e.g., vancomycin 15 mg/kg IV + piperacillin–tazobactam 4.5 g IV q6h) guided by cultures. Wean drains only when output minimal.
- Graft site infections: Also suspect saphenous or internal mammary harvest site infection. Manage similarly (drain + antibiotics).

Flowchart: SSI Detection & Management

1. Identify Fever or Wound Changes
   - Fever, drainage, or new wound symptoms.
2. Examine the incision Site
   - Look for redness, warmth, discharge.
   - Assess for sternal instability.
3. If superficial SSI Suspected
   - Initiate local wound care.
   - Start oral or IV antibiotics as indicated.
4. Deep SSI/Mediastinitis Suspected
   - Order CT chest for evaluation.
   - Obtain surgical consult for debridement.
   - Start IV antibiotics (e.g., vancomycin + piperacillin-tazobactam).
5. Consider VAC (Negative Pressure) Therapy
   - If appropriate for wound management post-debridement.

Postoperative Atrial Fibrillation (POAF)

New-onset AF is the most common arrhythmia after cardiac surgery (25–65% incidence) [18]. It typically occurs on postop days 2–4. Risk factors include older age, prior AF, COPD, valvular surgery, LA enlargement, withdrawal of β-blockers, and high inflammatory/adrenergic state [19].

Table 16.10 Management of POAF

Strategy	ESC class (Level)	Key point
Continue β-blocker peri-op	I (B)	Reduces POAF incidence
Peri-op amiodarone prophylaxis	IIa (A)	Consider in high-risk (e.g., CHF, prior AF)
Rate control (BB/CCB)	I (B)	Target HR <100 bpm (stable patients)
Rhythm control (amiodarone/ cardioversion)	IIa–IIb	No proven mortality benefit; use if unstable or recurrent
Anticoagulation (≥48 h AF)	IIa (C)	Based on stroke risk vs. bleeding
Sotalol prophylaxis	IIb (C)	Not routine; consider if recurrent despite BB

Guidelines: Welker/Ramakrishna 2023 commentary [18]; POAF review [19]

Prevention

- *β-Blockers*: Class I (ESC) recommendation to continue or start peri-op (e.g., metoprolol 50–100 mg PO daily or esmolol 50–200 mcg/kg/min IV).
- *Amiodarone*: Class IIa for prophylaxis (e.g., loading 600 mg PO daily 3 days before or IV 5–10 mg/kg bolus then 1 mg/min for 6 h).
- *Posterior pericardiotomy (surgical technique)*: Class IIa in high-risk patients [19].

Management of POAF Focus on rate control, anticoagulation, and deciding rhythm control (Table 16.10):

- *Rate control*: First-line for stable patients. Give IV β-blockers (metoprolol 2.5–5 mg IV q5min up to 15 mg) or non-dihydropyridine CCB (diltiazem 5–10 mg IV). Target HR <100–110 bpm in ICU setting (some recommend <80 in LV dysfunction) [18].
- *Rhythm control*: Consider if hemodynamic instability or symptomatic. IV amiodarone (150 mg IV over 10 min, then 1 mg/min × 6 h, then 0.5 mg/min), or cardioversion if unstable.
- *Antico*agulation: If AF >48 h or high stroke risk (CHA_2DS_2-VASc ≥2), start heparin/LMWH bridging to warfarin (INR target 2.0–3.0) for valve patients. [18] For brief (<48 h) AF with low risk, may hold anticoagulation initially (practice varies).

Algorithm: POAF Management

1. Detect New-Onset Atrial Fibrillation
   - Confirm with ECG.
2. Assess Hemodynamic Stability
   - Unstable (hypotension, ischemia)? ➔ Immediate electrical cardioversion.
   - Stable ➔ Proceed to rate control.
3. Rate Control (if stable):
   - IV metoprolol 2.5–5 mg IV every 5 min up to 15 mg.
   - OR diltiazem 0.25 mg/kg IV over 2 min.

Table 16.11 AKI—incidence, risk factors, and management

Aspect	Details
Incidence	AKI occurs in 20% to 40% of cardiac surgery patients.
Risk factors	Pre-existing renal impairment, diabetes, prolonged cardiopulmonary bypass, low cardiac output.
Management	Optimization of hemodynamics, avoidance of nephrotoxic agents, initiation of renal replacement therapy if indicated.
Preventive measures	Adequate hydration, minimizing use of contrast agents, careful monitoring of renal function.

Risk factors and prevention summarized from Brown 2013 [20]

4. If AF Persists:
   - Rhythm control: IV amiodarone 150 mg over 10 min, then 1 mg/min infusion.
5. Anticoagulation:
   - CHA_2DS_2-VASc assessment.
   - If AF >48 h ➔ LMWH/heparin bridging ➔ warfarin per protocol.
6. Monitor:
   - Electrolytes (K^+, Mg^{2+}), volume status, and oxygenation.

Acute Kidney Failure (AKI)

AKI occurs in 20–40% of cardiac surgery patients (KDIGO criteria: ↑SCr ≥0.3 mg/dL or ↑50% within 48 h) and predicts higher morbidity [20]. About 2–5% require renal replacement therapy. Common risk factors are chronic kidney disease, age, diabetes, CHF, low EF, COPD, perioperative hypotension, long CPB duration, intra-aortic balloon pump use, anemia/transfusion, and vasopressor use (Table 16.11) [15, 20].

Prevention Optimize renal perfusion and avoid nephrotoxins:

- Maintain MAP >60–65 mmHg; use vasopressors (norepinephrine 0.01–0.5 μg/kg/min) as needed to sustain perfusion.
- Avoid hypotension during/after CPB.
- Use balanced fluids, avoid excessive crystalloids or colloids.
- Minimize CPB time and transfusions if possible.
- Continue ACE-inhibitors/ARBs with caution (hold if pre-renal risks).
- No proven drug prevents AKI: diuretics (furosemide 20–40 mg IV) *do not* improve outcomes unless volume overloaded. Fenoldopam and natriuretic peptides have not shown benefit.
- KDIGO "bundle": tight glucose control (target 110–140 mg/dL), discontinue nephrotoxins, consider KDIGO protocols (e.g., Zarbock et al. study).

Monitoring Strictly follow urine output and creatinine. If oliguria (<0.5 mL/kg/h) or rising creatinine, correct reversible factors (fluids, pressors).

Treatment Supportive. Give IV fluids (target CVP ~8–10 mmHg) if prerenal; start vasopressors if needed. Start diuretics *only* for fluid overload once pressure is OK (furosemide 40–80 mg IV). For severe AKI (oliguria, metabolic acidosis, hyperkalemia), initiate RRT (CRRT or hemodialysis) in ICU.

Flowchart: AKI Management

1. Identify AKI:
   - Rising creatinine.
   - Urine output <0.5 mL/kg/h for >6 h.
2. Assess:
   - Volume status (clinical, CVP).
   - Hemodynamics (MAP >65 mmHg).
   - Review nephrotoxic medications.
3. Initial measures:
   - Optimize intravascular volume (crystalloids).
   - MAP support with norepinephrine if needed.
   - Avoid nephrotoxic agents.
4. If Volume overload:
   - IV furosemide 40 mg, titrate as needed.
5. Persistent AKI:
   - Consider renal replacement therapy (RRT) if:
     - Hyperkalemia >6.5 mmol/L.
     - pH <7.1 (refractory acidosis),
     - Fluid overload with hypoxia.
6. Low Cardiac Output Syndrome (LCOS)

   LCOS (postcardiotomy shock) is a state of inadequate cardiac output causing organ hypoperfusion (Table 16.12). It occurs in ~10–20% of complex adult cardiac surgeries (higher in pediatrics). Definition varies (e.g., cardiac index <2.0 L/min/m^2 plus signs of shock) [21].

Risk Factors Preop LV dysfunction, reoperation, long CPB or cross-clamp time, prolonged ischemia, bleeding, acidosis, and residual mechanical issues.

Table 16.12 LCOS—incidence, risk factors, and management

Aspect	Details
Incidence	10–12% in adult cardiac surgery
Risk factors	Preop LV dysfunction, reoperation, long CPB or cross-clamp time, prolonged ischemia, bleeding, acidosis, and residual mechanical issues
Management	Inotropes, vasopressors, mechanical support
Preventive measures	Optimize myocardial protection, minimize CPB time

Management Algorithm

1. *Optimize Preload*: Give IV fluids (crystalloids) cautiously to maintain adequate filling (target CVP ~10–12 mmHg or PAWP ~12–15 mmHg).
2. *Maintain Perfusion*: If hypotensive (SBP <90), start vasopressor support: *norepinephrine* infusion (titrate 0.02–0.5 µg/kg/min) to raise MAP. Add *vasopressin* (0.01–0.04 U/min) if needed to reduce catecholamines.
3. *Inotropes*: If CI remains low despite adequate filling:
   - *Dobutamine*: 2–10 µg/kg/min IV (start at 2.5 µg/kg/min, titrate up) (*European adult dose*).
   - *Milrinone*: 0.375–0.75 µg/kg/min IV without load (or 50 µg/kg bolus + infusion 0.5 µg/kg/min)—especially if pulmonary hypertension or RV dysfunction. Adjust in renal impairment.
   - *Epinephrine*: 0.02–0.1 µg/kg/min IV if severe shock.
   - *Levosimendan* (not available in all countries): 0.05–0.2 µg/kg/min IV for 24 h infusion. (Loading dose rarely used in adults on CPB due to hypotension risk.)
   - *Dopamine*: generally avoid in adults (ineffective for renal or CO improvement).
4. *Afterload reduction*: If high SVR, consider vasodilators (nitroprusside 0.1–2 µg/kg/min or nitroglycerin 5–20 µg/min) once BP permits. This can improve cardiac output.
5. *Mechanical support*: If refractory: insert intra-aortic balloon pump (IABP) or ECMO/VAD. Early consultation with cardiac surgery/ICU for mechanical support is critical.

Adjuncts Correct anemia (transfuse to Hgb ~8–10), keep normothermia, correct electrolytes (e.g., Ca^{2+}). Inotropic support also serves to correct lactic acidosis and improve urine output [21].

Algorithm: LCOS Management

1. Identify:
   - Hypotension, high lactate, low urine output, low cardiac index.
2. Assess Preload:
   - Cautious IV fluids.
   - Target CVP 10–12 mmHg.
3. If Hypotensive:
   - Norepinephrine 0.02–0.5 µg/kg/min to maintain MAP >65 mmHg.
4. Add Inotropes if Low Cardiac Index:
   - Dobutamine 2–10 µg/kg/min.
   - OR milrinone 0.375–0.75 µg/kg/min.
5. If Refractory:
   - Consider IABP or ECMO for mechanical support.
6. Correct Secondary Factors:
   - Anemia, acidosis, and electrolyte disturbances.

Table 16.13 Cardiac tamponade—incidence, risk factors, and management [22]

Feature	Tamponade (Post-cardiac surgery)
Incidence	~0.5–6% (4.3% after valve surgery)
Timing	Early (<48 h): hemorrhagic; Late (days): serous effusion
Signs	Hypotension, ↑CVP, pulsus paradoxus, oliguria
Diagnosis	Echocardiography (RV/RA collapse); CXR (enlarged silhouette)
Treatment	Urgent pericardial drainage (surgical or percutaneous)

Cardiac Tamponade

Postoperative tamponade (pericardial effusion causing compression) can occur *early* (<48 h, usually bleeding) or *late* (>48 h, usually serous inflammation). Incidence is ~0.3–6%; one valve surgery series reported 4.3% (other studies: CABG ~0.2%, valve ±CABG ~0.6%) (Table 16.13) [22].

Risk Factors valve operations, redo surgery, incomplete hemostasis, postoperative anticoagulation, and infective endocarditis [22].

Presentation Hypotension, tachycardia, elevated JVP, pulsus paradoxus, low cardiac output. Beck's triad (muffled heart sounds) may appear. If on TEE/echo immediately post-op, look for increasing pericardial collection.

Management

- *Early tamponade (hours after surgery)*: Suspect if hemodynamic collapse or sudden chest tube output. Most often requires *return to OR* for sternotomy and evacuation of hematoma.
- *Late tamponade*: If subacute (days later) present with subtle hypotension, echo is diagnostic (RA/RV diastolic collapse). Management often percutaneous drainage under echo/fluoroscopy guidance, or subxiphoid pericardial window. If effusion loculated or re-accumulates, may need surgical pericardial window or re-sternotomy.
- *Medical measures*: Temporize with IV fluids and inotropes to maintain perfusion (but this is usually ineffective long-term). Avoid positive-pressure ventilation if possible (it can worsen venous return).

Flowchart: Tamponade Management

1. Identify Clinical Signs:
   - Hypotension.
   - Elevated CVP.
   - Pulsus paradoxus.

Table 16.14 PVL—incidence, risk factors, and management

Aspect	Details
Incidence	PVL occurs in 7% to 17% of mitral valve replacements, with 1% to 5% being clinically significant.
Risk factors	Infective endocarditis, annular calcification, technical issues during surgery.
Management	Percutaneous closure using devices like Amplatzer vascular plug, or surgical re-intervention.
Preventive measures	Meticulous surgical technique, thorough debridement of infected tissue, appropriate sizing of prosthetic valves.

Guidelines: 2021 ESC/EACTS Valvular Disease [1]

2. Confirm Diagnosis:
   - Bedside echocardiography.
3. Management:
   - Early postoperative tamponade ➔ Urgent surgical re-exploration.
   - Late tamponade ➔ Pericardiocentesis or surgical window.
4. Supportive Measures:
   - IV fluids for preload.
   - Inotropes as needed for hemodynamic support.

Paravalvular Leak (PVL)

A PVL is regurgitation around a prosthetic valve sewing ring. Incidence after valve replacement: Mitral PVL ~7–17%, aortic PVL ~3–10% (most are small and asymptomatic; only ~1–5% require intervention) (Table 16.14) [1].

Causes Endocarditis, annular calcification, suture dehiscence, excessive valve oversizing, or tissue friability.

Symptoms New CHF (murmur of regurgitation), hemolytic anemia (jaundice, ↑LDH, schistocytes), or low output. Evaluate with TEE (best test) or TTE. Check hemolysis labs (LDH, haptoglobin).

Management

- *Asymptomatic/minor leak*: Conservative. Treat anemia (iron 100–200 mg IV daily, folate, erythropoietin 40,000 IU weekly) and heart failure (diuretics). Beta-blockers may reduce regurgitant flow energy.
- *Symptomatic PVL (HF or hemolysis)*: If leak is due to endocarditis or causes severe hemolysis/CHF, *reoperation* for surgical repair/replacement is Class I (ESC. Otherwise, evaluate for percutaneous closure:
  - If patient high-risk for surgery and leak anatomy suitable, *transcatheter device closure* is Class IIa recommendation. Devices (Amplatzer occluders) can be placed via transseptal or transapical approach. This requires TEE guidance.

  - Otherwise, plan reoperation with patch or new prosthesis.
- *Medical therapy*: Manage volume and anemia supportively. ESC notes use of iron, β-blockers, and epoetin in those who cannot undergo closure.

Algorithm: PVL Management

1. Suspect PVL:
   - New murmur, heart failure symptoms, or hemolytic anemia post valve surgery.
2. Confirm Diagnosis:
   - Transesophageal echocardiography (TEE).
3. If Mild/Asymptomatic:
   - Conservative medical management.
   - Regular monitoring.
4. If Symptomatic (Heart Failure, Hemolysis):
   - Evaluate for:
     - Surgical repair or valve re-replacement.
     - OR Percutaneous closure with vascular plug devices.
5. Supportive Care:
   - Manage anemia and volume overload.

Gastrointestinal (GI) Complications

GI issues are less common but often severe. The gut is vulnerable to hypoperfusion after CPB. The most frequent GI complications are paralytic ileus, upper GI bleeding (stress ulcers), and mesenteric ischemia (Table 16.15). Less common are acute cholecystitis and pancreatitis. Overall GI complications occur in ~3–5% of cases, but have high mortality (especially mesenteric ischemia ~50–100%) [15].

Table 16.15 GI complications—incidence, risk factors, and management

Complication	Incidence (estimate)	Risk factors	Prevention/treatment
Paralytic ileus	1–3%	Opioids, electrolyte imbalance, hypoperfusion	Bowel rest, NG tube decompression; metoclopramide 10 mg IV q6h; correct electrolytes. Early mobilization.
GI bleeding (ulcer)	0.2–2%	Stress ulcers, coagulopathy, steroids	PPI prophylaxis (pantoprazole 40 mg IV q24h), H2 blockers; stop NSAIDs; transfuse PRBCs; endoscopic eval & therapy as needed.
Mesenteric ischemia	<0.1% (<1%)	Low CO, arrhythmias, atherosclerosis	High suspicion (acidosis, pain out of proportion). Early CT angiogram; urgent laparotomy/embolectomy.
Pancreatitis	Rare (<0.5%)	Low perfusion, transfusion-related	Supportive care (fluids, NG tube); avoid propofol infusion (some cases).
Hepatic dysfunction	Variable	Shock, transfusions	Support: maintain perfusion, consider N-acetylcysteine (no proven benefit).

Key Measures Maintain gut perfusion and avoid stress: keep BP stable, limit vasopressors if possible. Use GI prophylaxis (PPI). Early enteral nutrition when feasible. Monitor abdominal exam/ileus (no flatus or stool by day 4 is ileus), and hematocrit for occult bleeding. High lactate or sudden ileus should prompt CT scan for ischemia [15].

Flowchart: GI Complications Management

1. Identify:
   - Abdominal pain, distension, GI bleeding.
2. Evaluate:
   - Laboratory tests (lactate, hemoglobin).
   - Physical abdominal examination.
3. Paralytic Ileus:
   - Nasogastric decompression.
   - Correct electrolytes (K^+, Mg^{2+}).
4. GI Bleeding:
   - IV proton pump inhibitor (pantoprazole 40 mg IV).
   - Transfusion if needed.
5. Suspected Mesenteric Ischemia
   - CT angiography.
   - Surgical consultation for possible intervention.

Respiratory Complications

Pulmonary issues are very common and contribute to morbidity. The most frequent are atelectasis and pleural effusion. Others include pneumonia, ARDS, pulmonary edema, pneumothorax, and phrenic nerve injury (hemidiaphragm paralysis). Nearly 20–30% of patients develop some pulmonary complication (Table 16.16) [23].

- *Atelectasis*: Caused by pain, shallow breathing, CPB inflammation. Prevent with incentive spirometry, chest physiotherapy, and adequate analgesia (paracetamol or NSAIDs; use opioids judiciously).
- *Pleural effusion*: Often small; tap if large and causing dyspnea. Frequent after mammary artery harvest.
- *Pneumonia*: Risk with prolonged ventilation. Prevention: early extubation (<6 h), oral care, mobilization. Treat with IV antibiotics (e.g., ceftriaxone 2 g IV q24h + azithromycin 500 mg IV daily).
- *Pulmonary edema/ARDS*: Aggressive capillary leak or LV failure. Use lung-protective ventilation (Vt 6 mL/kg ideal body weight, PEEP as needed) and diuretics for volume overload.
- *Phrenic nerve palsy*: Cold injury from internal mammary graft harvest; leads to dyspnea/atelectasis on ipsilateral side. Supportive; usually recovers.

Table 16.16 Respiratory complications—incidence, risk factors, and management

Complication	Prevention	Treatment
Atelectasis	Deep breathing, early extubation, analgesia	Incentive spirometry, CPAP, physiotherapy
Pleural effusion	Gentle fluid management	Thoracentesis or chest tube if large
Pneumonia	Ventilator bundles, mobilization	IV antibiotics (e.g., vancomycin + pip/tazo if MRSA/aspiration risk)
ARDS	Low-tidal ventilation, conservative fluids	Ventilator with PEEP, prone if needed, diuresis
Pulmonary embolism	DVT prophylaxis (LMWH 40 mg SC daily), early ambulation	IV heparin, IVC filter if contraindications
Bronchospasm	Minimize histamine/restrict propofol	Bronchodilators (salbutamol nebs), steroids
Phrenic nerve palsy	Cautious cooling during IMA harvest	Noninvasive ventilation, usually resolves

Respiratory PPCs cited from CORONARY trial/VENICE cohort [23]

Monitoring Pulse oximetry/ABG, chest X-ray. Keep PaO_2 >80 mmHg (FiO_2 as needed), $PaCO_2$ ~35–45 mmHg. Mobilize early and use CPAP/EBPOD as indicated.

Summary Early recognition and protocolized care (ventilator bundles, aggressive pulmonary toilet, fluid balance) help mitigate these complications. Implement pre-operative rehabilitation (incentive spirometry) and postoperative physiotherapy, as evidence shows these measures significantly reduce pulmonary events [23].

Algorithm: Postoperative Respiratory Management

1. Monitor:
   - SpO_2, respiratory rate, ABG as needed.
2. Atelectasis:
   - Incentive spirometry.
   - Early mobilization.
3. Pleural Effusion:
   - Therapeutic thoracentesis if symptomatic.
4. Pneumonia:
   - IV antibiotics per hospital protocol.
5. ARDS:
   - Low tidal volume ventilation (6 mL/kg IBW).
   - Appropriate PEEP for oxygenation.
6. Phrenic Nerve Palsy:
   - Supportive care.
   - Monitor respiratory function and recovery.

Complications in Hybrid Structural Cardiac Interventions

Hybrid structural procedures involve close collaboration between interventional cardiologists, cardiac surgeons, anesthesiologists, and imaging specialists. Coordination failures in this multidisciplinary "heart team" can cause serious complications. In one series, video analysis of hybrid cath-lab procedures found that even routine sequences (e.g., controlled apnea for imaging) had communication breakdowns in ~11% of steps [24]. Such breakdowns (missed requests, unclear commands) can delay critical actions or lead to errors. Contemporary practice mandates a formal *heart team* approach: guidelines stress that "multidisciplinary dialogue between different specialists is required to deliver optimal, patient-centred care" [25]. In practice, this means structured protocols, checklists, and closed-loop communication (e.g., read-backs) to ensure everyone hears critical information. Simulation training has been shown to improve team readiness and patient safety: a systematic review found that high-fidelity simulation effectively transfers procedural skills and is recommended as an adjunct to traditional training to reduce trainee errors [26]. Regular simulation of emergencies (e.g., TAVI arrest, device embolization) can practice coordinated management. Proactive strategies include assigning a case coordinator, standard handoff protocols, and immediate "time-outs" if miscommunication is detected. When breakdowns occur, "conversational repairs" (confirmation queries) are needed [24]. Overall, strong communication protocols and team training mitigate coordination failures and improve outcomes [25].

Intraoperative Conversion to Open Surgery

Emergent conversion to open surgery is a feared outcome of hybrid cases. In large TAVI registries, ~0.7–0.8% of procedures required immediate surgical bailout. The most common triggers were guidewire perforation of the left ventricle (causing tamponade) and annular/root rupture [27]. For example, in a 27,760-patient TAVI registry, emergent cardiac surgery was needed in 212 cases (0.76%), most often for LV perforation by a stiff wire (28%) or annular rupture (21%) [27]. Other triggers include valve embolization or malposition, aortic dissection, or uncontrollable paravalvular leak. Cardiac tamponade from any cause (wire or catheter perforation) is also a recognized complication. One single-center study found tamponade in 4.3% of TAVI cases (often due to temporary pacemaker lead perforation), with 23.5% mortality when caused by left-sided structural injury [28].

Current guidelines and expert consensus uniformly recommend that all complex structural procedures be done in a hybrid OR with on-site cardiac surgery and perfusion ready [25, 29]. This ensures rapid sternotomy, cardiopulmonary bypass, or vessel repair if needed. Teams should pre-brief conversion protocols (who clamps where, conversion drill, instrument availability). Simulation of "conversion" scenarios (rapid switch from cath-lab to open) can shorten response times.

Emergency surgery carries high risk, patients undergoing bailout had 34.6% immediate procedural mortality and 46% in-hospital mortality. Annular rupture had the worst prognosis (~62% in-hospital mortality) [27]. Survival at 1 year post-bailout was only ~40% for initial survivors. These sobering outcomes underscore the need for prevention (careful technique, imaging guidance) and swift surgical support when complications occur.

Device-Specific Complications

- *TAVI devices*:
  - *Valve embolization/migration*: Rare (approximately 1–2% of TAVI cases) but serious. Often seen with bulky calcifications or severe LV outflow-angulation. A displaced valve may be retrieved by snare or crushed against the aortic wall and a second valve deployed; uncorrected embolization may mandate surgery. In one series, 54 embolizations occurred in 3757 TAVIs (~1.4%), with most patients managed percutaneously. Risk factors include horizontal aorta, use of self-expanding valves, and low LVEF [30].
  - *Annular or root rupture*: Uncommon (~1% of cases) but life-threatening. Rupture typically results from oversizing or heavily calcified annulus. Management requires emergent surgery and aortic root repair. Historically, ~1% of TAVIs had annular rupture [31]. Nearly all cases are clinically evident (tamponade), but subclinical micro-rupture may go undetected. Mortality is very high (~60% if rupture occurs).
  - *Coronary artery obstruction*: Extremely rare (<1%) but catastrophic. Nationwide studies report <0.5–1% incidence. It occurs when native or bio-prosthetic leaflets (or TAVI frame) block a coronary ostium, usually the left main. Pre-procedure CT is *essential* to assess valve-to-coronary distance and leaflet height. One review emphasized that "accurate pre-procedural planning, mainly based on cardiac CT, is crucial to determining…risk of coronary obstruction". Intra-procedurally, TEE Doppler of coronary flow and selective angiography should be ready to detect obstruction [29]. If obstruction occurs, strategies include placing "chimney" stents or the BASILICA leaflet-laceration technique; in dire cases urgent surgery is needed [32]. Even with prompt management, 30-day mortality of coronary obstruction is ~50% [29].
- *MitraClip (transcatheter mitral repair)*:
  - *Leaflet detachment (SLDA)*: Incomplete capture of a leaflet by the clip can cause sudden single-leaflet device attachment. Large registries report SLDA in ~1–5% of cases. In the EXPAND study, adjudicated leaflet adverse events (mostly SLDA) occurred in ~2.0% of patient [33]. Earlier trials (ACCESS-EU) reported ~4.8% SLDA. Risk factors include thin or calcified leaflets, wide flail gaps, or leaflet injury during grasping.
  - *Residual mitral regurgitation*: A suboptimal reduction (≥2+ MR post-clip) is not uncommon, especially with complex anatomy. While not a "device failure" per se, significant residual MR may necessitate additional clips or surgical referral. Studies show that residual ≥2+ MR at discharge is associated with worse long-term outcomes [34].

- *Device embolization*: Extremely rare. There are virtually no reported cases of a complete MitraClip detachment (embolizing freely) in modern practice [28]. Most detachments manifest as SLDA rather than full embolization.
- *Management*: If SLDA occurs, often the operator will reposition or implant an additional clip to grasp the freed leaflet. If regurgitation is severe or anatomy unsuitable, surgical repair may be required. Post-procedure echocardiography and careful imaging of leaflet attachments are mandatory.

- *ASD/VSD occluders (e.g., Amplatzer devices)*:
  - *Device embolization/migration*: Uncommon (<1–3%) but critical; usually occurs early if device is undersized or malpositioned. Devices can embolize to the left ventricle or aorta. Early embolizations are usually captured percutaneously with snares or forceps. Late embolizations (days to weeks) are rarer. To prevent this, careful sizing and ensuring adequate septal rims are key.
  - *Cardiac erosion*: A rare but serious complication, typically seen with deficient aortic rim (<2 mm) and oversized devices. Incidence is very low (<0.5%). Erosion usually presents late (months to years) as pericardial effusion. Risk factors include an absent anterior (aortic) rim and oversized occluder.
  - *Device-related thrombus*: Occurs in ~1–2% of ASD/PFO closures [35]. Thrombi usually form early (within 4 weeks) on the device. This can lead to embolic stroke. Most thromboses are managed by intensifying anticoagulation (e.g., temporary warfarin) until resolution.
  - *Management*: Migrated devices are often retrieved percutaneously if discovered early; otherwise, surgical removal is indicated. Erosions necessitate surgical correction (device removal and patch). Thrombi on occluders are treated with anticoagulation (heparin/warfarin) and sometimes thrombolysis. Appropriate antithrombotic prophylaxis (see below) is crucial for prevention.
- *Left Atrial Appendage (LAA) occluders (e.g., Watchman, Amulet)*:
  - *Device migration*: Uncommon with good initial seating, but can occur if an undersized device is used. Most embolizations happen during the procedure and can be immediately retrieved; late migration is rare.
  - *Device-related thrombus*: Reported in ~2–4% of patients. For example, a multi-center study of the Amplatzer Cardiac Plug found 3.2% incidence of device thrombus and 12.5% incidence of any peri-device leak [36]. Thrombus may form if the device isn't fully endothelialized or if post-procedure anticoagulation is inadequate.
  - *Peri-device leak*: Small residual flow (gap) around the occluder is common (seen in ~10–15% for mild leaks) [36]. Clinically significant leaks (>5 mm) are rare (<1%). Any leak warrants continued anticoagulation or repeat closure.
  - *Management*: Thrombus on LAA occluders is usually managed by resuming or intensifying anticoagulation (heparin bridged to warfarin/DOAC) until resolution. Significant leaks may prompt adding antiplatelet therapy or even placing a second device. Ensuring optimal device positioning at implant and proper post-procedure anticoagulation prevents many of these issues (Table 16.17).

Table 16.17 Key device-related complications and management strategies

Procedure/ device	Complication	Incidence	Prevention/management
TAVI	Valve embolization	~1–2%	Secure valve with correct depth; snare or deploy second valve if occurs; surgery if unstable [37].
	Annular/root rupture	~1%	Careful sizing; surgical repair if occurs. (high mortality.) [31]
	Coronary obstruction	<1%	Pre-procedure CT risk assessment; prophylactic stenting or BASILICA; urgent revascularization or surgery [29].
MitraClip (TEER)	Single-leaflet detachment (SLDA)	~2% (4–5% in early registries)	Use transesophageal guidance to ensure leaflet capture; add another clip or refer for surgery if SLDA [33].
	Residual MR (≥2+)	Common (varies)	Aim for ≤1+ MR; implant additional clips if needed; surgical evaluation for severe residual leak.
	Device embolization	~0%–very rare [38]	Rare; ensure clip locks properly.
ASD/VSD Occluder	Device embolization	<1–3%	Correct sizing and rim evaluation; percutaneous snare removal if embolized.
	Cardiac erosion	<0.5%	Avoid oversized devices, ensure aortic rim; surgical removal if erosion.
	Device-associated thrombus	~1–2% [35]	DAPT post-procedure; treat thrombus with anticoagulation; continue ASA for 6 mo.
LAA Occluder	Device embolization	~1% (early cases)	Proper sizing; surgical retrieval or percutaneous capture if embolized.
	Device-associated thrombus	~3–4% [36]	Warfarin/NOAC for 45 days post-implant (see below); treat thrombus with anticoagulation.
	Peri-device leak	~12% any leak (mostly mild) [36]	Verify seal on imaging; continue anticoagulation or consider re-closure for significant leak.

Imaging for Prevention and Diagnosis of Complications

Multimodality imaging is integral to both preventing and promptly diagnosing hybrid procedure complications. Transesophageal echocardiography (TEE) is used in most procedures (TAVI, MitraClip, ASD closure) to visualize device placement and function in real time. For example, TEE can quickly detect a new pericardial effusion (tamponade) during TAVI, ensure complete leaflet capture during MitraClip, or confirm device expansion in ASD closure. Intracardiac echocardiography (ICE) is increasingly used for LAA closures and select mitral/tricuspid interventions: ICE avoids general anesthesia, allows the operator to manipulate the probe directly, and can provide 3D guidance for septal puncture and device deployment. One review notes that ICE's advantages (no general anesthesia, single-operator) have enabled its routine use in LAA closure, transseptal puncture, and tricuspid interventions [39].

Computed Tomography (CT) is critical *pre-procedurally*. In TAVI, contrast CT of the aortic root measures annulus size, leaflet calcification, and coronary heights. This directly predicts risk of annular rupture and coronary obstruction. In fact, one state-of-art review on ViV-TAVR emphasizes that CT-based planning is "crucial to determining…risk of coronary obstruction" [29]. CT is also used for LAA morphology to choose device size and detect accessory lobes that could leave leaks. In cases of suspected complication (e.g., unexplained hypotension post-TAVI), urgent CT can diagnose aortic dissection or valve malposition.

Fluoroscopy is the workhorse for device deployment. It shows the position and expansion of catheters and implants. Fluoro "cusp overlap" views can minimize conduction block during TAVI, and continuous fluoroscopic monitoring can reveal sudden device shifts. However, fluoroscopy alone can miss soft-tissue issues (like pericardial effusion), so it is always complemented by echo or angiography. Fusion imaging (overlaying CT or 3D echo onto fluoroscopy) is an emerging technique to improve accuracy of device delivery, though it is still investigational.

In summary, an imaging-supported approach is mandatory: TEE/ICE guidance during implantation can prevent maldeployment, while real-time monitoring (echo and fluoroscopy) allows immediate recognition of complications (e.g., pericardial effusion, severe regurgitation). Follow-up imaging is also crucial (see below).

Antithrombotic Protocols and Medical Management

Procedure Anticoagulation During structural procedures, unfractionated heparin is usually given to maintain activated clotting time (ACT) >250–300 s (or per protocol). Immediate reversal (protamine) is on hand if life-threatening bleeding occurs. Temporary pacemaker leads (in TAVI) should be managed carefully to avoid RV perforation, as pacing leads caused >50% of tamponades in one series [28].

Post-procedure Antithrombotics Regimens vary by device and patient risk:

- *TAVI*: For patients without other indications, current practice is aspirin lifelong plus a short course of clopidogrel. Most heart-team protocols use clopidogrel 75 mg daily for 1–3 months post-TAVI, then single aspirin [40]. If the patient requires chronic anticoagulation (e.g., atrial fibrillation), guidelines suggest continuing OAC and possibly adding a single antiplatelet agent. These recommendations come from expert consensus (e.g., recent trials found single antiplatelet to be as effective as DAPT in TAVI without increasing stroke, but guidelines still vary).
- *MitraClip*: There are no firm evidence-based guidelines. Many centers give dual antiplatelet therapy for ~1 month if there is no other indication. If the patient has atrial fibrillation, standard anticoagulation (warfarin or DOAC) is continued per AF protocol. A single-center report noted no consensus, but recommended at least aspirin and often add clopidogrel for 4–6 weeks in patients in sinus rhythm [41]. It is reasonable to treat MitraClip as a bioprosthetic valve: aspirin plus

30 days of clopidogrel, then aspirin alone, unless systemic anticoagulation is indicated.
- *ASD/VSD occluders*: Current guidance is aspirin 75–100 mg daily plus clopidogrel 75 mg for 3 months, then aspirin alone up to 6 months [42]. This covers the period of endothelialization of the device. In patients at high thrombosis risk, some operators extend DAPT or use temporary anticoagulation, but this is individualized. Warfarin for 6 months is recommended only for exceptionally high-risk cases (e.g., large ASD with very low flow).
- *LAA occluders (Watchman/Amulet)*: The classic protocol (PROTECT-AF/PREVAIL trials) is warfarin + aspirin for 45 days post-implant; if the 45-day TEE confirms good seal (<5 mm leak) and no thrombus, discontinue warfarin and use dual antiplatelet (aspirin + clopidogrel) for 6 months, then aspirin indefinitely [43]. In patients who cannot take warfarin, alternative regimens (e.g., DOAC for 45 days, or dual antiplatelet only) are used based on physician judgment and institutional protocol.

If bleeding occurs, reversal agents are available: vitamin K and prothrombin complex for warfarin, protamine for heparin, idarucizumab for dabigatran, orexanet alfa for Xa inhibitors (if applicable). Platelet transfusion can be considered if on antiplatelets. The antithrombotic strategy should balance embolic vs bleeding risk, especially in elderly TAVI patients.

Follow-Up and Prevention

Long-term follow-up is crucial for detecting late complications and ensuring device success. Follow-up schedules often include:

- *Echocardiography*:
  - *TAVI:* Transthoracic echo before discharge and at 30 days to assess valve function (gradient, leaks) and left ventricular function. Subsequent echocardiograms (e.g., at 1 year annually) monitor for valve degeneration or new regurgitation.
  - *MitraClip:* Echo at 1 month to quantify residual MR and mitral gradient. Lifelong annual checks as for surgical mitral repair.
  - *ASD/VSD occluders:* Echo at 1–3 months and 6–12 months to ensure complete closure, exclude pericardial effusion, and check device position. After 6–12 months, annual or biannual echo is reasonable to detect erosion or late leaks.
  - *LAA occluders:* TEE at ~45 days to confirm complete LAA seal and absence of thrombus (per trial protocols) [43]. A further TEE at 6 months is often done if concerns remain. Transthoracic echo is also used in follow-up to screen for pericardial effusion or device position.
- *Electrocardiography*: All TAVI patients should have EKG monitoring and a 12-lead EKG before discharge to detect new conduction blocks; ambulatory monitoring can detect transient heart block. Pacemaker implantation should be

Table 16.18 Key complications of common transcatheter structural procedures, with reported incidence and management strategies

Procedure/device	Complication	Approximate incidence	Management/prevention
TAVI	Valve embolization	~1–2%	Ensure proper valve positioning; snare or deploy second valve if embolized; surgical retrieval if unstable [30]
	Annular/root rupture	~1%	Avoid excessive oversizing; emergent surgical repair if rupture detected. (high mortality.) [31]
	Coronary obstruction	<1%	Pre-procedure CT planning; prophylactic coronary wiring/stenting or BASILICA if high-risk; urgent PCI or surgery if occurs [29].
MitraClip	Single-leaflet detachment	~2%	Use TEE guidance to verify leaflet capture; implant additional clip or refer for surgery if detachment causes severe MR [33].
	Residual ≥2+ MR	Common (variable)	Aim for ≤1+ MR; add clips if needed; surgical evaluation if severe.
	Complete device embolization	Very rare	None reported in modern series; ensure clip locks completely.
ASD/PFO Occluder	Device migration/embolization	<1–3%	Confirm device release position before detachment; retrieve embolized device percutaneously or surgically.
	Cardiac erosion	<0.5%	Avoid oversized device with deficient rims; surgical removal and repair if erosion occurs.
	Device thrombosis	~1–2%	DAPT for 3 mo then ASA (6 mo); treat any thrombus with anticoagulation [42].
LAA Occluder	Device embolization	~1% (procedural)	Careful sizing; emergency percutaneous or surgical retrieval if occurs.
	Device thrombosis	~3–4%	Warfarin/NOAC for 45 days post-implant; treat thrombus with anticoagulation.
	Peri-device leak	~12% (mostly mild)	Check seal by imaging; continue anticoagulation or re-close if leak >5 mm.

done before discharge if high-grade AV block persists. MitraClip and occluder procedures rarely affect conduction, but a baseline EKG is still advisable.

- *Medical follow-up*: Manage hypertension and diabetes aggressively to protect implants. Continue recommended antithrombotics (e.g., antiplatelets). Antibiotic prophylaxis for endocarditis (if indicated by guidelines, e.g., first 6 months post-implant for prosthetic material) should be considered, especially for septal occluders or prosthetic valves.
- *Prevention*: Before any hybrid procedure, careful planning reduces complications. This includes high-quality 3D imaging, patient selection by heart team, and discussion of bailout strategies. Avoiding overly aggressive device oversizing (to prevent rupture or erosion) and ensuring backup equipment and personnel are on hand (e.g., perfusionist for bypass) are key preventive measures (Table 16.18).

Key Points

- Hybrid structural cardiac interventions require structured team coordination and imaging guidance to prevent complications.
- Emergent surgical conversion during TAVI or hybrid procedures is rare (~0.7–0.8%) but high-risk, requiring preparedness and immediate surgical availability.
- Device-specific complications:
  - TAVI: Valve embolization, annular rupture, coronary obstruction.
  - MitraClip: Single-leaflet detachment, residual MR.
  - ASD/VSD occluders: Device embolization, erosion, thrombosis.
  - LAA occluders: Device migration, thrombosis, peri-device leaks.
- Multimodality imaging (TEE, ICE, CT) is critical for prevention, detection, and follow-up of complications.
- Post-procedural antithrombotic strategies:
  - TAVI: Aspirin lifelong + short-term clopidogrel.
  - MitraClip: Short-term DAPT or anticoagulation if AF.
  - ASD/VSD: DAPT for 3 months.
  - LAA occluders: Warfarin + aspirin 45 days, then DAPT, then aspirin lifelong.
- Routine follow-up (echo, ECG, clinical) is essential to detect late complications and optimize outcomes.

Complications in Minimally Invasive Structural Cardiac Interventions

Device Failure or Malposition

Percutaneous devices can embolize or sit improperly. For example, ASD/PFO closure devices embolize in roughly 0.01–0.55% of cases (up to 1.4% in some series) [44], LAA occluders in ≈0.01% (e.g., Watchman FLX) [45], and transcatheter valves migrate in ≈1% of TAVI procedures [46]. Management centers on immediate percutaneous correction: deploy a snare or catheter-based device to retrieve or reposition the displaced implant. In ASD/PFO device embolization, gooseneck snares usually succeed, reserving surgery only if retrieval fails [44]. Embolized TAVI valves to the aorta can sometimes be snared or a second valve implanted; valves embolized into the left ventricle generally require emergency surgery. LAA occluders are typically retrieved percutaneously by snaring the device knob [45]. After any retrieval/redeployment, repeat imaging (TTE/TEE and angiography) confirms correct placement and excludes injury.

Imaging TEE or fluoroscopy is used throughout retrieval. After reposition, routine TEE at 24–48 h ensures no new shunt or complication.

Antithrombotic Therapy After a corrected implantation, resume standard post-procedure therapy. For ASD/PFO closure this means dual antiplatelet therapy (aspi-

Table 16.19 Antithrombotic therapy management in minimally invasive cardiac interventions

Device	Incidence	Acute management	Follow-up/ imaging	Post-procedure antithrombotics
ASD/PFO occluder	~0.01–0.55% embolization	Percutaneous snare retrieval; surgery if unsuccessful	TEE immediately and at 3 mo to check for residual shunt	DAPT (aspirin+clopidogrel) ~3 months, then aspirin
TAVI prosthesis	~1% migration/ embolization	Snare if in aorta or implant another valve; surgery if LV embolus	TEE/ angiography intra-procedure; echo at 1 mo to assess valve and PVL	DAPT 3–6 months then aspirin
LAA occluder	~0.01% embolization	Percutaneous snare (usually successful)	TEE at 45 days and 6 mo (per protocol)	DAPT (aspirin+clopidogrel) ~1–3 months, then single antiplatelet

rin 75–100 mg plus clopidogrel) for ~3 months then aspirin alone. After TAVI, ESC guidelines recommend aspirin+clopidogrel for 3–6 months (Class IIa) followed by aspirin [47]. After LAA closure, a brief course of DAPT (e.g., aspirin + clopidogrel for 1–3 months) followed by single antiplatelet is typical [45] (Table 16.19).

Vascular Access Complications

Large-bore access (e.g., transfemoral TAVI) poses risks of bleeding, hematoma, pseudoaneurysm, AV fistula, and retroperitoneal hemorrhage. Incidence is substantial: registry series report any vascular injury in up to 25% of TAVI patients (most minor), with major complications in ~7–10% [48].

- *Bleeding/Hematoma*: Control with firm pressure or closure devices (e.g., Proglide sutures). Transfusion and reversal of anticoagulation may be needed for major bleeds.
- *Pseudoaneurysm*: Diagnose by Doppler ultrasound. Many can be treated nonsurgically with ultrasound-guided thrombin injection; large or expanding pseudoaneurysms may require surgical or endovascular repair.
- *AV Fistula*: Diagnose on Doppler; symptomatic or large fistulae often need endovascular coil/plug closure or surgery.
- *Retroperitoneal Hemorrhage*: Suspect with flank pain or hypotension after femoral puncture. Confirm by CT. Manage with blood products, reversal of anticoagulation, and urgent endovascular stent-graft or surgical repair.
- *Dissection/Occlusion*: Often managed by percutaneous angioplasty/stenting; surgery if limb threatened.

Imaging Early vascular ultrasound or CT angiography is indicated whenever bleeding or ischemia is suspected. Duplex ultrasound is used to confirm pseudoaneurysm or AV fistula. Follow-up Doppler is done after pseudoaneurysm treatment.

Antithrombotic Therapy In bleeding complications, hold all antiplatelet/anticoagulant drugs and reverse them (e.g., protamine for heparin) until hemostasis. Once stabilized, restart single antiplatelet (usually aspirin) unless bleeding risk remains high. There are no specific ESC guideline prescriptions for these scenarios, but minimizing sheath size and using closure devices are recommended to prevent complications [47].

Residual Shunts (Post-ASD/PFO Closure)

Residual interatrial shunt (trivial flow through or around a device) is common immediately post-closure but usually small. In early series, a moderate/large residual ASD shunt was seen in ~8% immediately and ~ 2% at 1 year, with small shunts in ~26% at 1 year. Modern devices achieve >90% complete closure by 6–12 months. Residual shunts after PFO closure are typically <10% [49].

Management Small, asymptomatic residual shunts are usually observed. Significant shunts (e.g., large flow, bidirectional flow, or causing RV volume load) may be closed by a second device or surgery. After PFO closure for stroke, persistent shunting with recurrent events may prompt re-intervention or lifelong antiplatelets.

Imaging TTE (with contrast) at 3–6 months is standard to detect residual flow. If TTE is equivocal or the patient has symptoms, TEE is indicated. Thereafter, annual clinical and echo follow-up ensures no late complications (device erosion is rare).

Antithrombotic Therapy Post-closure antithrombotic regimens apply whether or not a shunt remains. Typically, dual antiplatelet therapy (aspirin + clopidogrel) is given for 3–6 months and then aspirin alone. ESC guidelines endorse antiplatelets in PFO/ASD closure (Class I for indications) [47]. If atrial fibrillation or other indication arises, manage per standard (e.g., anticoagulation if AF). No additional lifelong anticoagulation is required for a small residual shunt alone.

Paravalvular Leak (Post-TAVI)

Paravalvular leak (PVL) occurs when blood flows around the implanted valve. Mild PVL is common; moderate/severe PVL occurs in only a minority. In one large study, ≥mild PVL was seen in 29.3% of patients (moderate in 5.9%, severe 0.8%) [50]. Newer valves and sizing have reduced these rates, but mild PVL still occurs in a quarter of cases.

Management Most mild PVLs are managed conservatively. Significant PVL (≥moderate) causing heart failure or hemolysis should be addressed.

Treatment options include:

1. *Percutaneous PVL closure*: transcatheter plug placement via transseptal or trans-aortic approach, under TEE guidance.
2. *Valve reintervention*: implanting an additional TAVI valve ("valve-in-valve") if anatomy allows.
3. *Surgical repair*: for severe leaks, especially if concomitant surgery is indicated. ESC/EACTS guidelines advise considering closure for PVL causing hemolysis or heart failure [51].

Imaging After TAVI, systematic TTE assesses PVL grade. If PVL is suspected (new murmur or hemolysis), TEE is recommended. Three-dimensional TEE or CT angiography can localize leak sites for planning. Repeat echo is done post-closure intervention to confirm success [51].

Antithrombotic Therapy Patients continue standard post-TAVI therapy (often single antiplatelet per current practice [47]. For PVL with hemolysis, manage anemia (folate, transfusion). Some experts use oral anticoagulation (warfarin) if hemolysis is significant, though evidence is limited. Heart-failure therapy (ACE inhibitors, diuretics) is given as needed. Guidelines do not mandate special drugs for PVL beyond general TAVI recommendations; management focuses on leak closure if indicated.

Key Points These complications are uncommon but serious following structural cardiac interventions.

- Early recognition (often via imaging) is critical to reduce morbidity and mortality.
- A Heart Team approach ensures appropriate decision-making between percutaneous and surgical repair.
- Follow-up protocols should include:
  - Routine echocardiography after closure procedures to check for leaks or residual shunts.
  - Clinical monitoring for vascular complications and rhythm disturbances.
  - Medication regimens should align with current ESC guidance:
  - Dual antiplatelet therapy (DAPT) for 3–6 months after TAVI or septal device placement (tctmd.com; cdt.amegroups.org).
  - Short-term DAPT following LAA occlusion as per device protocol and patient risk profile (openaccess.sgul.ac.uk).
  - Anticoagulation strategies tailored to rhythm, valve type, and bleeding risk.
- Education on signs of complications (dyspnea, stroke symptoms, leg pain, wound changes) and lifestyle modification (rehabilitation, medication adherence) is essential in long-term follow-up.
- Using structured protocols and team-based surveillance improves outcomes in patients undergoing structural cardiac interventions.

References

1. Vahanian A, Beyersdorf F, Praz F, Milojevic M, Baldus S, Bauersachs J, et al. 2021 ESC/EACTS guidelines for the management of valvular heart disease. EuroIntervention. 2022;17(14):e1126–e96.
2. Moscoso Luduena M, Rastan AJ. Complications and conversions in minimally invasive aortic valve surgery. Ann Cardiothorac Surg. 2015;4:94.
3. van der Merwe J, Van Praet F, Vermeulen Y, Casselman F. Complications and pitfalls in minimally invasive atrioventricular valve surgery utilizing endo-aortic balloon occlusion technology. J Vis Surg. 2018;4:248.
4. Schnitzler K, Hell M, Geyer M, Kreidel F, Münzel T, von Bardeleben RS. Complications following MitraClip implantation. Curr Cardiol Rep. 2021;23(9)
5. Zou Q, Jiang C, Lin P, Yu Y, Li J, Zhao F, et al. Management of complications associated with percutaneous left atrial appendage closure with or without ablation: experience from 512 cases over a 4-year period. Front Cardiovasc Med. 2024;11:11.
6. Yu Y, Chu H, Wang B, He B, Fu G. Pericardial effusion following percutaneous left atrial appendage closure using the LAmbre device. Front Cardiovasc Med. 2023;10:1188322.
7. Alkhouli M, De Backer O, Ellis CR, Nielsen-Kudsk JE, Sievert H, Natale A, et al. Peridevice leak after left atrial appendage occlusion: incidence, mechanisms, clinical impact, and management. JACC Cardiovasc Interv. 2023;16(6):627–42.
8. Walther T, Arsalan M, Hecker F. Managing stroke during transcatheter aortic valve replacement. Interv Cardiol Rev. 2017;12(01):25.
9. Delgado V, Ajmone Marsan N, de Waha S, Bonaros N, Brida M, Burri H, et al. 2023 ESC guidelines for the management of endocarditis. Eur Heart J. 2023;44(39):3948–4042.
10. Raphael J, Mazer CD, Subramani S, Schroeder A, Abdalla M, Ferreira R, et al. Society of Cardiovascular Anesthesiologists Clinical Practice Improvement Advisory for Management of Perioperative Bleeding and Hemostasis in Cardiac Surgery Patients. Anesth Analg. 2019;129(5):1209–21.
11. Pagano D, Milojevic M, Meesters MI, Benedetto U, Bolliger D, von Heymann C, et al. 2017 EACTS/EACTA guidelines on patient blood management for adult cardiac surgery. Eur J Cardiothorac Surg 2017;53(1):79–111.
12. Kozek-Langenecker SA, Afshari A, Albaladejo P, Santullano CA, De Robertis E, Filipescu DC, et al. Management of severe perioperative bleeding: guidelines from the European Society of Anaesthesiology. Eur J Anaesthesiol. 2013;30(6):270–382.
13. Myles PS, Smith JA, Kasza J, Silbert B, Jayarajah M, Painter T, et al. Tranexamic acid in coronary artery surgery: one-year results of the Aspirin and Tranexamic Acid for Coronary Artery Surgery (ATACAS) trial. J Thorac Cardiovasc Surg. 2019;157(2):644–52.e9.
14. Gilbey T, Milne B, de Somer F, Kunst G. Neurologic complications after cardiopulmonary bypass—a narrative review. Perfusion. 2022;38(8):1545–59.
15. Viana FF, Chen Y, Almeida AA, Baxter HD, Cochrane AD, Smith JA. Gastrointestinal complications after cardiac surgery: 10-year experience of a single Australian centre. ANZ J Surg. 2013;83(9):651–6.
16. Steiner T, Purrucker JC, Aguiar de Sousa D, Apostolaki-Hansson T, Beck J, Christensen H, et al. European Stroke Organisation (ESO) and European Association of Neurosurgical Societies (EANS) guideline on stroke due to spontaneous intracerebral haemorrhage. Eur Stroke J. 2025:23969873251340815.
17. Zukowska A, Zukowski M. Surgical site infection in cardiac surgery. J Clin Med. 2022;11(23)
18. Welker CC, Ramakrishna H. Postoperative atrial fibrillation: guidelines revisited. J Cardiothorac Vasc Anesth. 2023;37(12):2413–5.
19. Suero OR, Ali AK, Barron LR, Segar MW, Moon MR, Chatterjee S. Postoperative atrial fibrillation (POAF) after cardiac surgery: clinical practice review. J Thorac Dis. 2024;16(2):1503–20.
20. Cheruku SR, Raphael J, Neyra JA, Fox AA. Acute kidney injury after cardiac surgery: prediction, prevention, and management. Anesthesiology. 2023;139(6):880–98.

21. Aslan N, Yildizdas D. Low cardiac output syndrome after cardiac surgery: a life-threatening condition from the perspective of pediatric intensivists. Turk Kardiyol Dern Ars. 2022;50(4):284–92.
22. Cavarretta E, You SC, Shim CY, Hong G-R, Kim D, Cho IJ, et al. Incidence, predictors, and clinical outcomes of postoperative cardiac tamponade in patients undergoing heart valve surgery. PLoS One. 2016;11(11)
23. Fischer MO, Brotons F, Briant AR, Suehiro K, Gozdzik W, Sponholz C, et al. Postoperative pulmonary complications after cardiac surgery: the VENICE international cohort study. J Cardiothorac Vasc Anesth. 2022;36(8 Pt A):2344–51.
24. Ivarsson J, Åberg M. Role of requests and communication breakdowns in the coordination of teamwork: a video-based observational study of hybrid operating rooms. BMJ Open. 2020;10(5):e035194.
25. Leonardi S, Capodanno D, Sousa-Uva M, Vrints C, Rex S, Guarracino F, et al. Composition, structure, and function of heart teams: a joint position paper of the ACVC, EAPCI, EACTS, and EACTA focused on the management of patients with complex coronary artery disease requiring myocardial revascularization. Eur J Cardiothorac Surg. 2021;59(3):522–31.
26. Kweki AG, Sarwar Khan Tharin M, Baptista V, Kenneth E, Rohin F, Scoote M, et al. The impact of simulation-based training in cardiovascular medicine: a systematic review. Cureus. 2023;
27. Eggebrecht H, Vaquerizo B, Moris C, Bossone E, Lämmer J, Czerny M, et al. Incidence and outcomes of emergent cardiac surgery during transfemoral transcatheter aortic valve implantation (TAVI): insights from the European Registry on Emergent Cardiac Surgery during TAVI (EuRECS-TAVI). Eur Heart J. 2018;39(8):676–84.
28. Rezq A, Basavarajaiah S, Latib A, Takagi K, Hasegawa T, Figini F, et al. Incidence, management, and outcomes of cardiac tamponade during transcatheter aortic valve implantation: a single-center study. JACC Cardiovasc Interv. 2012;5(12):1264–72.
29. Prandi FR, Niv Granot Y, Margonato D, Belli M, Illuminato F, Vinayak M, et al. Coronary obstruction during valve-in-valve Transcatheter aortic valve replacement: pre-procedural risk evaluation, intra-procedural monitoring, and follow-up. J Cardiovasc Dev Dis. 2023;10(5)
30. Frumkin D, Pietron M, Kind A, Brand A, Knebel F, Laule M, et al. Valve embolization during transcatheter aortic valve implantation: incidence, risk factors and follow-up by computed tomography. Front Cardiovasc Med. 2022;9:9.
31. Cutchins VCA, Goldstein JC. Taking a new path: Intracardiac shunt calculation to aid in decision-making with annular rupture after transcatheter aortic valve replacement deployment. J Cardiothorac Vasc Anesth. 2018;32(5):2444–8.
32. Lederman RJ, Babaliaros VC, Rogers T, Khan JM, Kamioka N, Dvir D, et al. Preventing coronary obstruction during transcatheter aortic valve replacement. JACC Cardiovasc Interv. 2019;12(13):1197–216.
33. Asch FM, Little SH, Mackensen GB, Grayburn PA, Sorajja P, Rinaldi MJ, et al. Incidence and standardised definitions of mitral valve leaflet adverse events after transcatheter mitral valve repair: the EXPAND study. EuroIntervention. 2021;17(11):e932–e41.
34. Buzzatti N, De Bonis M, Denti P, Barili F, Schiavi D, Di Giannuario G, et al. What is a "good" result after transcatheter mitral repair? Impact of 2+ residual mitral regurgitation. J Thorac Cardiovasc Surg. 2016;151(1):88–96.
35. Olasinska-Wisniewska A, Grygier M. Antithrombotic/antiplatelet treatment in transcatheter structural cardiac interventions—PFO/ASD/LAA Occluder and interatrial shunt devices. Front Cardiovasc Med. 2019;6:6.
36. Saw J, Tzikas A, Shakir S, Gafoor S, Omran H, Nielsen-Kudsk JE, et al. Incidence and clinical impact of device-associated thrombus and peri-device leak following left atrial appendage closure with the Amplatzer cardiac plug. JACC Cardiovasc Interv. 2017;10(4):391–9.
37. Frumkin D, Pietron M, Kind A, Brand A, Knebel F, Laule M, et al. Valve embolization during transcatheter aortic valve implantation: incidence, risk factors and follow-up by computed tomography. Front Cardiovasc Med. 2022;9:928740.
38. Bilge M, Alsancak Y, Ali S, Duran M, Biçer H. An extremely rare but possible complication of MitraClip: embolization of clip during follow-up. Anatol J Cardiol. 2016;16(8):636–8.

39. Agricola E, Meucci F, Ancona F, Pardo Sanz A, Zamorano JL. Echocardiographic guidance in transcatheter structural cardiac interventions. EuroIntervention. 2022;17(15):1205–26.
40. Vavuranakis M, Kalogeras K, Kolokathis AM, Vrachatis D, Magkoutis N, Siasos G, et al. Antithrombotic therapy in TAVI. J Geriatr Cardiol. 2018;15(1):66–75.
41. Calabrò P, Gragnano F, Niccoli G, Marcucci R, Zimarino M, Spaccarotella C, et al. Antithrombotic therapy in patients undergoing transcatheter interventions for structural heart disease. Circulation. 2021;144(16):1323–43.
42. Olasinska-Wisniewska A, Grygier M. Antithrombotic/antiplatelet treatment in transcatheter structural cardiac interventions-PFO/ASD/LAA occluder and interatrial shunt devices. Front Cardiovasc Med. 2019;6:75.
43. Magdi M, Renjithal SLM, Mubasher M, Mostafa MR, Lathwal Y, Mukuntharaj P, et al. The WATCHMAN device and post-implantation anticoagulation management. A review of key studies and the risk of device-related thrombosis. Am J Cardiovasc Dis. 2021;11(6):714–22.
44. Cho JY, Kim KH, Yoon HJ, Seon HJ, Ahn Y, Jeong MH, et al. Percutaneous retrieval of embolized amplatzer septal Occluder after treatment of double atrial septal defect: a case report. J Korean Med Sci. 2015;30(9):1361–6.
45. Potpara T, Grygier M, Hausler KG, Nielsen-Kudsk JE, Berti S, Genovesi S, et al. Practical guide on left atrial appendage closure for the non-implanting physician: an international consensus paper. Europace. 2024;26(4)
46. Kim WK, Schafer U, Tchetche D, Nef H, Arnold M, Avanzas P, et al. Incidence and outcome of peri-procedural transcatheter heart valve embolization and migration: the TRAVEL registry (TranscatheteR HeArt Valve EmboLization and Migration). Eur Heart J. 2019;40(38):3156–65.
47. Nusca A, Bressi E, Colaiori I, Miglionico M, Di Sciascio G. Antiplatelet therapy in valvular and structural heart disease interventions. Cardiovasc Diagn Therapy. 2018;8(5):678–93.
48. Sumii Y, Morisaki A, Okai T, Taniuchi S, Shintani A, Kawase T, et al. Vascular access site complications after transfemoral transcatheter aortic valve implantation: a comparison of open and percutaneous puncture approaches. J Thorac Dis. 2023;15(11):5901–12.
49. Sievert H, Babic UU, Hausdorf G, Schneider M, Höpp HW, Pfeiffer D, et al. Transcatheter closure of atrial septal defect and patent foramen ovale with ASDOS device (a multi-institutional European trial). Am J Cardiol. 1998;82(11):1405–13.
50. Hagar A, Li Y, Wei X, Peng Y, Xu Y, Ou Y, et al. Incidence, predictors, and outcome of paravalvular leak after transcatheter aortic valve implantation. J Interv Cardiol. 2020;2020:8249497.
51. disease SECWGftEEgftmovh, Committee SECG. Comments on the 2021 ESC/EACTS guidelines for the management of valvular heart disease. Rev Esp Cardiol (Engl Ed). 2022;75(6):466–471.

Ethical and Legal Considerations in Cardiac Surgery

17

Beatrice Gabriela Ioan

Introduction

Cardiac surgery is an advanced medical specialty that involves technical procedures with notable risks of morbidity and mortality. Cardiac surgery is performed within the general ethical framework applicable in medical practice. This medical field, however, has particularities that generate specific ethical challenges and dilemmas. Particularities derive from surgical specialties and also from the technological progress and innovation, which generate specific clinical circumstances and risks [1]. Minimally invasive cardiac surgery (MICS) allows interventions on and inside the structures of the heart and the great vessels without completely opening the chest wall. The main goal of minimally invasive techniques is to reduce collateral tissue damage and, therefore, morbidity—while ensuring the complete surgical repair. MICS has the following advantages: faster and better postoperative mobilization, reduced chest wall trauma, fewer postoperative complications- such as infections, hemorrhage requiring blood transfusion, cardiac arrhythmias, and reduced number of functional re-explorations. The spectrum of MICS approaches ranges from partial chest opening to keyhole surgery performed with endoscopic and robotic manipulation and hybrid techniques [2, 3].

The demographic and medical profile of the patients has been changing as well. For instance, the percutaneous coronary intervention (angioplasty) has changed both the volume and the clinical presentation of coronary artery bypass grafting [4], with patients now older, having more comorbidities, and having undergone more prior procedures. In the field of valve surgery, transcatheter aortic valve replacement (TAVR) has led to a dramatic decrease in "surgical" aortic valve replacements

B. G. Ioan (✉)
Grigore T. Popa University of Medicine and Pharmacy, Iasi, Romania
e-mail: beatrice.ioan@umfiasi.ro

G. Tinică, A. Burlacu (eds.), *Surgical, Hybrid and Minimally Invasive Structural Cardiac Interventions*, https://doi.org/10.1007/978-3-032-16676-0_17

(SAVR), and the technology of minimally invasive mitral valve surgery is advancing rapidly [1].

Minimally invasive techniques derived from adult cardiac surgery are gradually finding applications in congenital cardiac surgery. Currently, an increasing number of procedures in the pediatric population are performed using a minimally invasive approach, i.e., from the correction of simple defects such as atrial septal defects (DSA) and ventricular septal defects (DSV), to Fallot tetralogy, mitral valve repair, etc. [5]. However, while MICS is now a well-established intervention for adults, minimally invasive congenital cardiac surgery (MICCS) still faces limitations due to the complexity of the cases, the wide range of ages and body weights of patients, the need to often address multiple anatomical segments in one operating field, limited access to peripheral cannulation for cardiopulmonary bypass (CPB), and the lack of appropriately sized instruments. Because infants and children do not experience major additional morbidity from the thoracic opening itself, aesthetics have remained secondary to the completion of the surgical procedure [5, 6]. However, MICCS in the pediatric population has the potential to ameliorate the psychological impact of scars from sternotomy incisions. MICCS in the pediatric population also minimizes surgical trauma and pain, reduces blood product consumption, and shortens the recovery period [5].

In this chapter, the author analyzes the ethical issues raised by the conventional cardiac surgery and the minimally invasive cardiac surgery using the principles of bioethics formulated by Beauchamp and Childress: autonomy, beneficence, non-maleficence, and justice [7]. By virtue of the four moral principles formulated by Beauchamp and Childress, physicians must use their knowledge and skills for the benefit of patients (beneficence), while minimizing risks (non-maleficence). Physicians also have the obligation to intervene on patients only with their informed consent (by virtue of the principle of autonomy) and, at the same time, to treat all patients with respect and dignity (justice). These four principles form a duty-based ethical framework, which must be applied and interpreted in the particular context of each medical specialty, considering the fact that in there are medical circumstances in which moral theories based on duties cannot be applied and it becomes necessary to apply alternative theories, such as the utilitarianist theory that becomes relevant in solving ethical dilemmas generated by scarce resource allocation [1].

Autonomy and Informed Consent

The principle of autonomy is fundamental for the proper conduct of medical activity and, implicitly, cardiovascular surgery and clinics. By virtue of the principle of autonomy, patients have the right to make informed and voluntary decisions (i.e., in the absence of any coercion) regarding their medical treatment. Respect for the autonomy of the competent patient is mandatory both in the case of the patient accepting the proposed medical care and in the case of the patient deciding to forgo medical care [1].

Informed consent and an appropriate patient framework approach are essential for building trust. Cardiac surgical procedures often involve significant risks and aim to achieve significant outcomes, making obtaining the patient's informed consent particularly relevant, by ensuring the integration of evidence-based data with the patient's clearly expressed preferences. However, patients may have difficulty fully understanding cardiac surgery procedures and their implications, especially if they are not medically trained or have certain cognitive impairments, which are common in elderly or frail patients [8].

Physicians are responsible for translating complex medical language into information that can be understood by patients, providing them with a so-called "reasonable certainty" regarding the benefit of the medical interventions [9].

It is important that the clinical reasoning made by surgeons considers the patient's best interests and wishes. In the case of elective surgery, a voluntary agreement must be established between the patient and the surgeon, in which neither the patient nor the surgeon is obliged to accept the other's opinions. In cardiac surgery, patient information goes beyond risks, and information that allows the patient to fully understand the treatment options, the long-term effects, and the impact of the surgery on their quality of life is essential. Ultimately, the patient is the one who makes the decision, and the surgeon may or may not accept it. If the surgeon does not agree with the patient's decision, they may or may not agree to perform the surgery and allow the patient to consult another doctor. An exception to this approach is in emergency situations, in which the medical intervention is absolutely necessary to save the patient's life [1].

Ethical dilemmas may arise when a surgeon is asked to perform a surgery that is considered unnecessary or when there are better alternatives for the patient. In such situations, the surgeon may refuse to perform the operation because it cannot be forced to provide an inappropriate procedure. Moreover, the surgeon has an obligation to use their best clinical judgment for the benefit of the patient. In practice, however, there are also less clear situations—for example, a patient with aortic dissection and unclear neurological status. It is currently recognized that the results of the aortic dissection repair in patients with severely altered neurological status are very weak, and it may be inappropriate to offer such an operation in such settings. However, the patient's neurological status may be unclear due to the administration of sedative medication, which makes it more appropriate to offer the patient the surgical intervention under the principle of beneficence [1].

In the case of an incompetent patient, who lacks the mental capacity to make decisions for themselves, family members or legal representatives have the right to make decisions regarding the patient's medical care, according to the doctrine of *substitute judgment*, i.e., what the patient would have decided if they had the capacity to make the decision themselves [7]. In general, if the patient is unable to decide, the surgeon must respect the decision made by the family or the patient's designated legal representative, including the waiver of medical treatment [1].

Consensus between the patient and physician is sometimes constrained by the patient's wishes and cultural values, which may require adaptations of the surgical technique to accommodate them. An example of this is "bloodless" heart surgery for Jehovah's Witnesses, who refuse blood transfusions because of their religious beliefs. This situation requires the multidisciplinary heart team to respect patient's autonomy by applying specific methods that reduce blood loss and achieve good outcomes, such as preoperative correction of anemia, careful intraoperative techniques like myocardial salvage, and careful postoperative monitoring [10].

Patient Information in Cardiac Surgery

Conventional cardiac surgery has undergone extensive changes in the last decade, which means that it is currently competing with other intervention options, such as MICS, which is a field in continuous development. Thus, patients can choose between conventional cardiac surgery techniques and minimally invasive ones. Studies show that the perception of patients is often that a smaller incision or percutaneous cannulation of the inguinal vessels is associated with lower risk or gentler procedures. This perception is also observed among physicians, but it is often not supported by concrete evidence, with mortality being identical in hospital or at 30 days, regardless of whether the procedure was interventional aortic valve implantation versus surgical replacement or cardiopulmonary bypass procedure versus a percutaneous intervention. However, patients treated with minimally invasive techniques can be extubated early postoperatively, wound infections usually have a milder course, and they are not at risk of permanent sternal instability. It should be noted, however, that these potential advantages are often offset by longer periods of cardiopulmonary bypass and longer times of aortic clamping. Given that short- and long-term outcomes are relatively similar, patients should be adequately informed to make an informed choice of preferred technique [6].

When informing patients, surgeons must balance providing sufficient and coherent information and avoiding technical overload that could hinder patient decision-making. In cardiac surgery, patient information should include, in addition to risks, details of available treatment alternatives, as well as long-term and quality-of-life effects [8].

To prevent unauthorized transfer of medical information or violation of patient autonomy, it is essential that during the admission phase, the individuals involved in the communication process, any advance directives (such as blood transfusion preferences), and the patient's legal representatives are identified [11].

Communication in Cardiac Surgery

Effective physician-patient communication promotes adherence throughout the care process and improves the overall quality of medical care. Preoperative consultations—which involve the direct participation of the doctor or medical team and the patient—can be supplemented with various additional tools such as information brochures, possibly containing QR codes to explanatory videos [11].

Physician-patient communication is an important modifiable factor in patient mortality. Improving teamwork and communication has the potential to ensure the safety and quality of patient care in cardiac surgery. A study conducted in Australia that aimed to explore communication problems in a cohort of patients who died after cardiothoracic surgery identified poor communication in 10% of the deaths. Communication problems occurred throughout the patients' hospitalizations, especially pre- and postoperatively. The majority of cases involved surgeons, both in terms of communication received from other medical professionals (doctors from other medical departments, such as ICU or junior doctors) and that transmitted to other parties (ICU doctors, doctors from other surgical departments, patients). The main problems identified by this study concerned the communication between members of the medical team, such as failure of the shared decision making, lack of notification of the patient's deterioration, or erroneous reporting of the patient's condition. Poor communication between the cardiac surgeon and the patient was also identified, reflected in deficiencies in obtaining informed consent, for example, failure to communicate the degree of risk of surgical procedures. Poor communication between the cardiac surgeon and the patient may also be due to language barriers or the urgency of the medical situation, which does not allow for adequate communication. There are also situations in which the extent of the surgical intervention is greater than that established during the preoperative discussion between the surgeon and the patient [12].

Inadequate communication and communication failures can have serious consequences for patients. Rabøl et al. found that more than 50% of serious patient incidents or near misses in hospital involved communication errors [13]. However, in the operating room, surgeons tend to rate the quality of teamwork and communication more favorably than nurses and anesthesiologists [14].

Beneficence and Non-maleficence

Medical practice is associated with dilemmas and controversies generated by the desire of medical professionals to do what is right and good for their patients. These dilemmas are accentuated by new techniques and practices that, in turn, supplement the so-called "classic" dilemmas or controversies, making it difficult to decide what is right and good for patients in the new medical environment.

Minimally invasive cardiac surgery procedures have the potential to reduce the surgical trauma caused by sternotomy, characteristic of conventional cardiac surgery. A good clinical outcome after MICS is demonstrated by the lower morbidity and mortality rates in certain procedures. MICS also involves reduced use of blood products, less pain, and faster recovery [5, 15].

Median sternotomy, performed in conventional cardiac surgery, can cause major complications, such as mediastinitis (in 0.3–5% of patients, with a mortality rate of 14–47%), or sternal instability, which is the leading cause of postoperative morbidity and mortality. These complications can lead to prolonged hospitalization and, subsequently, higher healthcare costs [15]. In addition, conventional cardiac surgery causes aesthetic damage through the long midline scar of the anterior chest wall and a risk of chronic post-sternotomy pain, both of which have the potential to negatively affect the patient's life in the long term [16].

The quality of the patient's recovery is also important. Quality of recovery is a complex concept that includes several dimensions of physical, psychological, and social health, and is a subjective experience of the patient [15]. Myles and colleagues found that the quality of life of patients who underwent cardiac surgery in the first three months postoperatively depends on the quality of recovery during the hospital stay, which suggests the need for effective support strategies initiated during the hospital stay, such as counseling, home care, local physician notification, and cardiac rehabilitation [17].

A literature review, which included articles published after 1999 and which followed the quality of recovery (QoR) after minimally invasive cardiac surgery, assessed with quality of life assessment tools, indicated that patients benefit from both minimally invasive and conventional cardiac surgery, but patients recover faster and to a greater extent after MICS. However, the authors showed that a firm conclusion could not be drawn due to the limited studies available, and randomized controlled clinical trials are needed in this respect. Both patients who underwent conventional cardiac surgery and those with MICS experienced benefits in terms of quality of life (QoL). Overall, general health status, as well as the energetic score, improved in both groups after surgery. However, patients with MICS reported a more rapid improvement in their general health and indicated that they had significantly more energy than patients with conventional cardiac surgery [15].

Standard of Care

The current standard of care for minimally invasive cardiac surgery involves referral by cardiologists to cardiac surgery clinics, where patients are scheduled for cardiac surgery. They are usually admitted to the hospital the day before surgery and are given information about anesthesia and surgery on the day of surgery. After surgery, patients are intubated and transferred to the intensive care unit, where they stay overnight before being transferred to the cardiac surgery unit, if they have not experienced a complication. In the cardiac surgery unit, patients receive physiotherapy sessions, and they continue rehabilitation after discharge, when available [18].

The current standard of care in cardiac surgery is set to be dramatically modified by the introduction of the *ERAS (enhanced recovery after surgery) protocol*, a comprehensive perioperative management protocol applied in minimally invasive cardiac surgery, which has the potential to improve the prognosis of patients by streamlining treatment and patient involvement.

This care protocol aims to optimize and shorten the recovery process after surgery by reducing stress and supporting physiological functions. The ERAS protocol allows patients to regain independence and return to work at an earlier stage, as well as reduce healthcare costs by reducing the length of hospital stay by up to 50% and postoperative complications [17].

The implementation of the ERAS protocol is possible with the help of a multidisciplinary team that includes a cardiac surgeon, anesthesiologist, physiotherapist, perfusionist, psychologist, rehabilitation team, nutritionist, nurses, and with the patient being at the center of the process and actively participating in their own care. For the effective implementation of the ERAS protocol and patient involvement, an ERAS coordinator (often a nurse) is designated, who has the role of supervising and ensuring the connection between all relevant parties [18, 19].

Implementation of the ERAS protocol begins in the preoperative period with prehabilitation (to prevent postoperative atelectasis and pneumonia), i.e., preoperative physiotherapy with functional/respiratory exercises and nutritional support, continues intraoperatively with the use of short-acting anesthetics with extubation on the operating table and early postoperative mobilization and functional training [18].

Schmid et al. showed that the ERAS protocol has multiple benefits perceived by patients. Effective and seamless communication was identified as a critical factor in patient satisfaction. Comprehensive preoperative education including information sessions 2–4 weeks prior to surgery and adequate communication throughout the perioperative care were essential for patient satisfaction and to optimize the care process. Interprofessional preoperative discussions allowed patients to more effectively manage anxiety related to surgery, increased their confidence, and gave them sufficient time to mentally prepare for surgery. Preoperative education allowed patients to have realistic expectations and appropriate behavior regarding their treatment. Physical activity, nutrition, and mental health were considered significant in preoperative preparation. Involvement and active participation of patients and their families in the treatment process allowed for superior postoperative care, intensive physiotherapy, psychological support, and faster recovery. The functional flow of information throughout the care process was perceived as vital by patients. Patients were involved in all stages of their care through preoperative discussions, which allowed them to understand what the disease was, to be fully informed and therefore to take responsibility for their own care, all decisions being made with their consultation. In the event of complications, patients understood the reasons and were supported by the medical team. The involvement of family members, which was encouraged by the medical team, was perceived as beneficial by patients and by their family members who were able to cope better with the circumstances and provide the necessary support to the patients [18]. Education and comprehensive involvement of patients require personnel and time resources, but the initial investment of time can generate long-term benefits, as well as responsible management of patients and the care process, a more efficient and appropriate allocation of resources, thus contributing to a robust and cost-effective health system [20]. More favorable patient appreciation for all medical professionals involved in treatment has the potential to strengthen a positive workplace climate and staff satisfaction [21].

Risk Assessment in Cardiac Surgery

Therapeutic decisions in cardiac surgery involve balancing potential benefits against the risk of harm, taking into account the immediate and long-term results and the patient's quality of life, as well as their cultural values [22].

A correct and well-documented assessment of the risk-benefit ratio is essential, especially for certain complex diagnostic and treatment procedures, as it takes into account both preoperative risks and subsequent results [11]. Given the complexity of the cases, it is beneficial to evaluate patients by multidisciplinary teams and to refer to guidelines or the best available evidence in the field [11, 23].

Comparative assessment of the risks and benefits of cardiac surgery becomes particularly problematic when it comes to the elderly, frail patients who suffer from multiple comorbidities. In such cases, short-term risks must be considered such as complications or mortality, as well as long-term risks, such as pulmonary disease or prolonged suffering. An honest discussion with the patient is needed regarding the influence of comorbidities and reduced psychological reserve on intra- and postoperative results. In this way, patients have realistic expectations from the medical act, and informed consent can be expressed in knowledge [24].

In the specific context of cardiovascular surgery, fundamental concepts of risk prevention and outcome standardization are inconsistently applied, often due to high staff turnover. Basic concepts such as following safety recommendations to prevent compress retention or misidentification of patients are widely recognized, but their implementation varies significantly across medical facilities, indicating the need for their systematic review and reinforcement through ongoing staff training. Risk management methods also require regular updating to adapt to the changing contexts. Audits of cases of death or serious adverse events are important for the objective reconstructing of the events, reviewing surgical indications, and evaluating patient management and team communication. Poor socioeconomic and family conditions can also have a significant impact on health outcomes through patient non-adherence to treatment, unhealthy lifestyle, and limited access to care [11].

Justice

The principle of justice in cardiac surgery includes the fair distribution of medical resources, equitable access to new treatments and technologies, and taking social factors into account in medical decision-making.

Cardiac surgery uses advanced procedures and technologies, which are both costly and limited, requiring careful allocation based on medical need and potential benefit, so as to avoid discrimination or basing clinical judgment on the patient's social worth and financial status [25].

The use of advanced technologies, such as extracorporeal life support (ECLS), although with increased potential to provide benefits to surgical patients, requires an analysis and balancing of the potential benefits against the use of resources at the societal level [22].

An important issue is the role of the cardiac surgical in the public politicies and in the allocation of scarce resources, such as organs for transplantation, financial resources for ventricular assist devices, or ICU bed allocation. Surgeons clearly have a duty to support their patients, but the needs of society at large should also be considered, which creates ethical dilemmas regarding balancing the needs of the patient with those of society, the hospital, or the patients of other physicians. The allocation of resources at the individual level must consider the short-term benefits to the patient versus the comorbidities the patient suffers from and that dramatically limit life expectancy even when receiving a modern device to support cardiac function. One such example is a patient with severe heart failure who might benefit in the short term from a left ventricular assist device (LVAD), but whose long-term benefit is severely limited by the important comorbidities it suffers from [1].

A problematic aspect is the fixed hospital budget within which those providing medical and surgical care, including cardiac surgeons, must fit. This situation becomes more problematic if the patient does not have additional medical insurance that can cover the considerable costs of the new devices used in cardiac surgery [1].

In cardiac surgery, it is particularly important to consider actions that could have been taken earlier to prevent and manage chronic diseases. It is also important to understand the shortcomings in patients' compliance with general health care recommendations, as many patients focus exclusively on the curative aspects of surgery, without adapting their lifestyle, nutrition, rehabilitation, medical compliance, smoking habits, or routine check-ups [11].

Cardiac surgeons may experience pressure from the management of the medical institution to increase the number of cases assisted or prioritize low-risk patients to optimize outcome reporting, which leads to overtreatment or non-provision of cardiovascular care to patients in high-risk groups. This approach clearly contradicts the principles of medical ethics that impose the placement of patient benefit above any financial or reputational gains [26].

Health policies should consider the geographical distribution of medical facilities and the access of persons in need to these facilities. Medical facilities intended for cardiac surgery must meet minimum organizational, structural, technological, volumetric, and staffing requirements to ensure safe, high-quality, and appropriate care [11].

For example, the development of an effective and sustainable MICS program for patients with congenital heart disease must consider the technical challenges and the specific training for the medical team members, as well as the appropriate selection of initial cases. Such a program involves a coordinated team approach, together with meticulous preoperative planning. In the initial stages, avoiding patients who are at high risk, have multiple comorbidities, or require highly complex procedures ensures patient safety and minimizes complication and conversion rates to conventional techniques. At the same time, the cardiac surgeons should be aware of the fact that complication rates tend to be higher in the early stages [5].

The efficiency of regionalization of cardiac surgery care and the better outcomes obtained in high-volume centers have been recognized [27]. Chang and colleagues reported a 24% reduction in mortality that, theoretically, could have occurred if patients had been transferred from low-volume hospitals to high-volume hospitals [28]. Austin et al. showed that an overall 26% reduction in deaths could theoretically have been prevented if high-risk operations in patients with coronary artery disease had been performed in hospitals with high patient volumes [29].

The development and evaluation of new cardiovascular surgical technologies involve financial transactions, which can lead to conflicts of interest that could influence clinical decisions and the integrity of scientific research. In cardiovascular surgery, self-regulation requires transparent disclosure of financial resources and careful consideration of how industry-pharmaceutical partnerships may affect clinical practice. It is important to foster beneficial collaborations that improve cardiovascular patient care while preventing conflicts that could undermine professional judgment or patient trust [9].

Medical Liability in Cardiac Surgery and MICS

Responsibility for one's work and decisions concerning the patients is a key asset for a cardiac surgeon. Surgical talent, medical education, and professional responsibility must go together and complement each other. Rapid progress in medicine, on the one hand, and the expectations of patients, their families, and society toward medical activity impose increased legal responsibility on healthcare professionals [30].

Risk prevention and liability assessment are typically based on the usual diligence of the average practitioner, taking into account their specific experience and training and the context of patient care. At the same time, it must be kept in mind that the central factor in determining the right to health and the risk-benefit ratio is the patient and not the surgeon [11].

In recent decades, medical liability has become a challenge in medical practice. This phenomenon has reached the scale and severity of a pandemic in the medical world globally [31]. Malpractice claims have a significant impact on patient outcomes and healthcare costs [11]. The main consequences are new economic pressures, loss of physician autonomy, and the practice of defensive medicine, with increased unnecessary diagnostic testing, referrals, and treatment of low-risk patients [31], for the purpose of medical protection and not necessarily for the benefit of the patient.

Given the prevalence of cardiovascular diseases in the population, healthcare planning and organizational needs, as well as the effects and costs of adverse events and litigation in this area, an integrated and multidisciplinary perspective of analysis is needed, allowing for the identification of risks and the prevention of adverse events [32].

The feelings of harm experienced by patients or their family members usually lead to malpractice complaints on their part. The significant emotional impact of severe adverse events on families hinders the settlement of claims for compensation and may lead to criminal proceedings against healthcare professionals. The massive exposure of healthcare services in the media and the emotional and professional burden on healthcare providers must also be considered [11].

Patients may have unrealistic expectations regarding recovery from minimally invasive cardiac surgical (MICS) procedures, leading to a mismatch between expectations and outcomes and, consequently, reduced patient satisfaction. Improving and individualizing preoperative patient communication and education as part of the informed consent process could help better manage individual expectations, especially in populations at high medical risk [33].

According to the literature, the procedures most frequently involved in complaints are: management of acute coronary syndrome and differential diagnosis, especially differentiation of myocardial infarction from acute aortic dissection; coronary angiography and cardiac catheterization; pacemaker-defibrillator implantation; valvular surgery and treatment of congenital heart disease. The main causes identified in the perioperative phase include inadequate fitting or securing of prosthetic valves, local infections (at the surgical site), perfusion-related complications, failure to diagnose or treat complications in a timely and appropriate manner, and vascular perforation, dissection, or thrombosis. In the postoperative phase, complaints include bleeding or tamponade, infective endocarditis, and sepsis, as well as information and communication issues. These findings should be contextualized within broader demographic trends, such as increased preoperative risk. Other factors contributing to medical liability in cardiac surgery include a higher prevalence of intravascular implants, increased use of advanced technology, increased patient expectations, increased life expectancy, and the more frequent use of minimally invasive surgical approaches for complex cases. In addition, one must consider the notable deficit, both in the number and appropriate qualification of healthcare professionals, as well as the financing of healthcare and medical facilities [11].

Written informed consent obtained from patients before surgery often falls short of the goal of patient engagement, partly because it is part of a broader communication process aimed at reducing legal claims. In the instance of a patient's death as a result of an adverse event, the legal representative initiates the claim, while the medical information is provided to the patient who consented for the surgery. However, adequate information and communication provided to the patient and family members, documented in the medical record, promotes trust and may demonstrate diligent and collaborative professional behavior on the part of the surgeon and medical team [11].

Communication with the patient and their family is crucial in the event of surgical complications and, more generally, in the event of adverse events occurring during hospitalization. At the same time, honest and clear communication, within the team, in a secure environment, about both the surgical indication and potential intra-procedural complications can strengthen the personal medical relationship with the patient and his family. This approach allows for careful management of information, explanation of errors when necessary, and reduces the likelihood of misinterpretation of events or blame seeking, especially in cases of serious complications or death [34].

The Professionalism of Cardiac Surgeons

The surgeon has clear duties to their patient, i.e., to provide good quality care and to act in the best interests of the patient. The surgeon also has duties to their employer. Principles of professionalism, however, tend to prioritize duties to the patient concerning professional performance and clinical judgment. Medical professionals should have some freedom to exercise discretionary judgment, even if it is not in the best interests of the employer. Friedson has identified four characteristics of a successful employer-patient-professional relationship: adequate resources for the professional to perform well; an organizational structure that allows the professional some independence in the activities they perform; recognition of the professional's specialized knowledge; and an element of performance measurement that is recognized by the professional community [1].

Cardiac surgery requires extraordinary professional skills, manual talent enriched by relentless hard work of self-development and, often, exceeding one's own limits. A surgeon must face physical fatigue, overcome its weaknesses, and acquire the ability to practice a special way of thinking, that of a "lifesaver" [30].

Patient perceptions and expectations have changed. Patients are increasingly demanding a minimally invasive approach that leaves the sternum intact. Therefore, physicians who wish to meet this new challenge must understand that minimal incisions in cardiac surgery require increased technical skills that can be acquired through specific training [6].

In the context of over-specialization, healthcare professionals must be aware of the limits of their expertise and the challenges they may create. It is therefore important that practitioners are informed about the consequences of exceeding the limits of their clinical competence and assuming risks beyond these limits. Practitioners may be held liable for performing procedures without the necessary equipment specified in the guidelines, both in case management and in the event of complications. To avoid such situations, healthcare institutions are required to implement clinical guidelines that standardize medical practices based on current scientific evidence, and staff should be trained to comply with them [11].

Cardiac surgeons should collaborate with interventional cardiologists as part of the so-called *cardiac team*. The goal is for patients to benefit from the care of a skilled team of physicians and to achieve better outcomes at lower costs. Teamwork requires trust between professionals and a fair distribution of gains and losses. Such an approach minimizes duplication or overlap of services, allows for prioritization of patient outcomes, while the professionals' work is evaluated based on overall outcomes rather than individual productivity [1].

A study conducted in Australia, which analyzed the communication problems in the case of patients who died after cardiac surgery interventions, drew attention to the deficiencies of communication between members of the interdisciplinary medical teams that treated the patients. Communication errors led to failure in decision-making within the team and the lack of notification of the deterioration of the patients' condition. The failure to make shared decisions within the multidisciplinary team was determined by insufficient information of the medical team members either because of the erroneous reporting of the patient's condition or because of the lack of informing the surgeon about the patient's deterioration. The lack of notification of the deterioration of the patient's condition, or erroneous reporting, most often between the surgical team and the ICU team, did not allow the surgical team to intervene in a timely manner to save the patient's life. In other cases, it was a matter concerning the lack of appropriate and timely reaction of the cardiac surgeon to alarm signals transmitted by the ICU doctor. The absence of consensus between cardiac surgeons and ICU doctors on the treatment administered to the patients, especially fluids and inotropic/vasopressor substances, also proved to be problematic [12].

Conclusion

Ethical approaches in cardiac surgery have evolved from being an implicit part of clinical practice to key elements of contemporary cardiovascular care, involving complex, high-stakes decisions that impact the lives of patients. Healthcare professionals continue to ask fundamental ethical questions that balance autonomy, beneficence, non-maleficence, justice, and also professional responsibility in order to adapt to the latest technological advances and evolving healthcare environments. Making such decisions requires high technical skills and a commitment to ethical principles in the context of patient-centered care.

Future ethical advances in cardiovascular surgery and interventional cardiology depend on continued collaboration within cardiovascular surgery teams, namely surgeons, cardiologists, ethicists, patients, and society, ensuring that technological innovations support the well-being of all patients and align with the principles and values of medical ethics.

References

1. Whyte RI, Wood DE. Ethical issues in cardiothoracic surgery. In: Ferreres A, editor. Surgical ethics. Cham: Springer; 2019.
2. Kiraly L, Aye WMM, Subbian SK, Kofidis T, Al Hakami A. Minimal incision and less invasive techniques in congenital cardiac surgery: a narrative review. Pediatr Med. 2024;7:14.
3. Dieberg G, Smart NA, King N. Minimally invasive cardiac surgery: a systematic review and meta-analysis. Int J Cardiol. 2016;223:554–60.
4. Cornwell LD, Omer S, Rosengart T, Holman WL, et al. Changes over time in risk profiles of patients who undergo coronary artery bypass graft surgery: the veterans affairs surgical quality improvement program (VASQIP). JAMA Surg. 2015;150(4):308–15.
5. Karangelis D, Androutsopoulou V, Tzifa A, Chalikias G, et al. Minimally invasive cardiac surgery: in the pursuit to treat more and hurt less. J Thorac Dis. 2021;13(11):6209.
6. Doenst T, Diab M, Sponholz C, Bauer M, Färber G. The opportunities and limitations of minimally invasive cardiac surgery. Dtsch Arztebl Int. 2017;114(46):777.
7. Beauchamp TL, Childress JF. Principles of biomedical ethics. 7th ed. New York: Oxford University Press; 2013.

8. Wleklik M, Uchmanowicz I, Sobański P, Pasierski T. Ethical issues concerning cardiac surgery in elderly patients- the nurse's role as a patient advocate: a case report. Med Res J. 2020;5(2):120–5.
9. Kavarana MN, Sade RM. Ethical issues in cardiac surgery. Futur Cardiol. 2012;8(3):451–65.
10. Maheta DK, Frishman WH, Aronow WS. Bloodless cardiac surgery in Jehovah's witness: a comprehensive review. Cardiol Rev. 2024. https://doi.org/10.1097/CRD.0000000000000725.
11. Bolcato V, Speziale G, Savini C, Mikus E, et al. Litigation in cardiovascular surgery: risk management considerations in the Italian context. Surgeries. 2024;5(4):1072–83.
12. Chan JC, Gupta AK, Stewart S, Babidge W, et al. "Nobody told me": communication issues affecting Australian cardiothoracic surgery patients. Ann Thorac Surg. 2019;108(6):1801–6.
13. Rabøl LI, Andersen ML, Østergaard D, Bjørn B, et al. Descriptions of verbal communication errors between staff. An analysis of 84 root cause analysis-reports from Danish hospitals. BMJ Qual Saf. 2011;20:268–74.
14. Mills P, Neily J, Dunn E. Teamwork and communication in surgical teams: implications for patient safety. J Am Coll Surg. 2008;206:107–12.
15. Claessens J, Rottiers R, Vandenbrande J, Gruyters I, et al. Quality of life in patients undergoing minimally invasive cardiac surgery: a systematic review. Indian J Thorac Cardiovasc Surg. 2023;39(4):367–80.
16. Piarulli A, Chiariello GA, Bruno P, Cammertoni F, et al. Psychological effects of skin incision size in minimally invasive valve surgery patients. Innovations. 2020;15:532–40.
17. Myles PS, Hunt JO, Fletcher H, Solly R, Woodward D, Kelly S. Relation between quality of recovery in hospital and quality of life at 3 months after cardiac surgery. Anesthesiology. 2001;95(4):862–7.
18. Schmid ME, Stumm J, Stock S, Girdauskas E. Patient perspectives on health care models in cardiac surgery: a qualitative evaluation. BMC Health Serv Res. 2024;24(1):1309.
19. Kubitz JC, Schulte-Uentrop L, Zoellner C, Lemke M, et al. Establishment of an enhanced recovery after surgery protocol in minimally invasive heart valve surgery. PLoS One. 2020;15(4):e0231378.
20. Burgess LC, Arundel J, Wainwright TW. The effect of preoperative education on psychological, clinical and economic outcomes in elective spinal surgery: a systematic review. Healthcare (Basel). 2019;7(1):48.
21. Krogstad U, Hofoss D, Veenstra M, Hjortdahl P. Predictors of job satisfaction among doctors, nurses and auxiliaries in Norwegian hospitals: relevance for micro unit culture. Hum Resour Health. 2006;4:3.
22. Hull SC, Mullen JB, Kirkpatrick JN. The case for Cardioethics. JACC Adv. 2023;2(2):100273.
23. Mazza A, Iafrancesco M, Bruno P, Chiariello GA, et al. The multidisciplinary heart team approach for patients with cardiovascular disease: a step towards personalized medicine. J Cardiovasc Med. 2023;24:906–13.
24. Boulin M. Ethical considerations in cardiovascular research and treatment. J Interv Gen Cardiol. 2024;8(4):1–2.
25. Canver CC, Carpenter AJ, Ceppa DP, Chen EP, et al. Global health initiatives in cardiothoracic surgery: ethical considerations and guidelines. J Thorac Cardiovasc Surg. 2021;161(6):2114–8.
26. Lin PJ. Some ethical legal issues in heart disease surgery. Acta Cardiol Sin. 2014;30(6):529–37.
27. Backer CL, Pasquali SK, Dearani JA. Improving national outcomes in congenital heart surgery: the time has come for regionalization of care. Circulation. 2020;141:943–5.
28. Chang RK, Klitzner TS. Can regionalization decrease the number of deaths for children who undergo cardiac surgery? A theoretical analysis. Pediatrics. 2002;109:173–81.
29. Austin JM, Derk JM, Pronovost PJ. An analysis of publicly reported pediatric heart surgery data and patient mortality implications. J Hosp Manag Health Policy. 2018;2:50.
30. Skalski JH. Ethics in cardiac surgery, the new times. Philosophy in the background. Folia Med Cracov. 2024;LXIV(3):47–53.
31. Montisci R, Licciardi M, Cecchi R, Kondo T, et al. Malpratice claims in cardiology and cardiac surgery: a medico-legal issue. Legal Med. 2023;65:102319.

32. Leape L, Berwick D, Clancy C, Conway J, et al. Transforming healthcare: a safety imperative. Qual Saf Health Care. 2009;18:424–8.
33. Catalano MA, Hemli JM, Yu PJ, Scheinerman SJ, et al. Patient satisfaction scores after cardiac surgery: should they be risk-adjusted? Semin Thorac Cardiovasc Surg. 2023;35(4):696–704.
34. Mostafapour M, Fortier JH, Garber G. Exploring the dynamics of physician-patient relationships: factors affecting patient satisfaction and complaints. J Healthc Risk Manag. 2024;43:16–25.

Artificial Intelligence in Cardiac Surgery and Educational Tools: Current Applications and Future Directions

18

Alexandru Burlacu, Crischentian Brinza, and Adrian Covic

Introduction

Artificial intelligence (AI) became increasingly relevant in medicine, offering practical tools to support diagnosis, clinical decision-making, as well as surgical training. The application of AI in surgical fields has evolved at a slower pace compared to other clinical specialties, due to the complexity of intraoperative dynamics and the variability in surgical workflows [1, 2].

Cardiac surgery presents both challenges and opportunities for implementing AI tools. The procedures are often complex, the patient population tends to have multiple comorbidities, and the timing of interventions is critical. These characteristics make it a suitable field for integrating systems that can process large volumes of clinical data quickly and help guide decisions in real time [3, 4].

The demand for greater accuracy in perioperative decision-making has grown substantially in recent years, particularly in cardiac surgery. Cardiovascular disease remains the primary cause of mortality globally, with ischemic heart disease and heart failure contributing significantly to the overall burden [5]. Also, the patients

A. Burlacu (✉)
Interventional Cardiology, Cardiovascular Diseases Institute, Iasi & Grigore T. Popa University of Medicine and Pharmacy, Iasi, Romania
e-mail: alexandru.burlacu@umfiasi.ro

C. Brinza
Faculty of Medicine, University of Medicine and Pharmacy "Grigore T Popa", Iasi, Romania
e-mail: crischentian.brinza@d.umfiasi.ro

A. Covic
Faculty of Medicine, University of Medicine and Pharmacy "Grigore T Popa", Iasi, Romania

Nephrology Clinic, Dialysis, and Renal Transplant Center – "C.I. Parhon" University Hospital, Iasi, Romania
e-mail: adrian.covic@umfiasi.ro

G. Tinică, A. Burlacu (eds.), *Surgical, Hybrid and Minimally Invasive Structural Cardiac Interventions*, https://doi.org/10.1007/978-3-032-16676-0_18

undergoing cardiac procedures have changed considerably. Patients are often older and present with multiple comorbidities such as chronic kidney disease (CKD), diabetes, and pulmonary dysfunction, factors that complicate both the surgical procedure and the recovery process [6, 7]. These changes have made it increasingly important to refine existing methods for evaluating operative risk, anticipating complications, and ensuring favorable outcomes [7].

Machine learning techniques could be applied in case of patients requiring cardiac surgery. In the preoperative phase, algorithms have been developed to assist with interpreting advanced imaging modalities such as CT angiography and 3D echocardiography, enabling more precise anatomical assessments and supporting procedural planning [3, 8]. Also, AI models can generate individualized risk predictions, offering improved accuracy compared to traditional scoring systems, particularly in patients with complex profiles [9, 10]. Intraoperatively, AI integration into robotic surgical systems could enhance real-time decision-making, including vessel identification, tissue tracking, and prediction of technical complications [3, 11]. These applications suggest that AI may improve consistency in care delivery and enable earlier interventions in critical phases of the surgical process [3].

AI is also changing the way surgeons are trained. Simulation platforms can now provide structured feedback, assess technical performance, and adjust training based on individual learning pace. These tools offer more consistent and measurable forms of education, which are especially valuable in cardiac surgery [12, 13].

However, several challenges remain, including the accuracy of AI systems in diverse patient populations, potential bias in the data used to train algorithms, and the need to maintain transparency in clinical decisions. Surgeons should work closely with data scientists and engineers to ensure that new tools improve clinical workflows without replacing the essential judgment of the surgical team [3, 14].

This chapter reviews current applications of AI in cardiac surgery and in surgical education, with a focus on practical tools that have been supported by research. Also, it explores how these tools might evolve in the coming years, and what considerations must be addressed to ensure their responsible and effective use.

AI in Cardiac Surgery: Clinical Applications

The adoption of machine learning and data-driven tools is reshaping many aspects of cardiac surgery. These tools could outperform traditional risk models, such as EuroSCORE II or STS score, for predicting mortality and postoperative complications. Also, these innovations could be useful from preoperative planning and intraoperative guidance to postoperative monitoring and outcome prediction [3, 15].

Preoperative Planning

Machine learning has shown significant value in pre-surgical evaluation. A recent study proposed a fully automated method for analyzing coronary artery morphology and calcium burden using coronary computed tomography angiography (CCTA). The system was designed to perform both segmentation of coronary arteries and objective quantification of coronary artery calcium (CAC) and tortuosity. The segmentation process relied on a two-stage neural network architecture. For model development, 281 CCTA scans with manual annotations were used, and the final segmentation achieved a Dice coefficient of 0.896. Notably, coronary segments with stenosis were correctly identified. These results suggest that the proposed approach can provide reproducible and time-efficient assessment of coronary anatomy and disease markers, with potential utility in both clinical and research settings [16].

Another study evaluated the performance of an automated deep learning model for the segmentation of multiple cardiovascular structures using CCTA images. The dataset included 206 patients and encompassed over five billion imaging pixels. Eight anatomical regions were manually annotated as reference, including the proximal ascending aorta, descending aorta, superior and inferior vena cavae, pulmonary artery, coronary sinus, right ventricular wall, and left atrial wall. A deep learning architecture, based on a U-Net-derived framework, was trained and tested. The overall segmentation accuracy was favorable, with a median Dice score of 0.820. Among individual structures, the highest median Dice scores were observed for the ascending aorta (0.969), descending aorta (0.953), and superior vena cava (0.937). These results demonstrated that deep learning methods can achieve reproducible and anatomically detailed segmentation of multiple cardiac and vascular structures in CCTA imaging, potentially refining preoperative evaluation and structural analysis [17].

In a retrospective analysis, Allyn et al. evaluated the ability of different models to predict in-hospital mortality following elective cardiac surgery. The study included 6520 patients who underwent cardiac surgery in 2005 and 2012, with an observed in-hospital mortality rate of 6.3%. When comparing predictive performance for mortality, the machine learning model achieved a significantly higher area under the receiver operating characteristic (AUC) curve (AUC 0.795, 95% CI: 0.755–0.834) than both the EuroSCORE II (AUC 0.737, 95% CI: 0.691–0.783) and a traditional logistic regression model (AUC 0.742, 95% CI: 0.698–0.785), $P < 0.0001$. These findings support the potential of machine learning algorithms to offer improved predictive accuracy in risk assessment prior to cardiac surgery, especially when compared to established scoring systems like EuroSCORE II. These methods could assist surgeons in selecting candidates, planning surgical approaches, and preparing patients more effectively [15].

A retrospective study assessed the performance of several machine learning models in predicting postoperative mortality among adults undergoing cardiac surgery. The dataset included 5443 patients treated between 2008 and 2017. Using preoperative and intraoperative variables, the investigators developed four different models: random forest, neural network, support vector machine, and gradient boosting machine. These models were compared against traditional scoring systems, including EuroSCORE I, EuroSCORE II, the STS risk model, and logistic regression. Among all models tested, random forest achieved the highest predictive power (AUC of 0.87), followed by gradient boosting (AUC of 0.82). In contrast, the AUCs for EuroSCORE II and the STS model were 0.73 and 0.71, respectively. Therefore, machine learning approaches could offer improved accuracy and greater adaptability in mortality prediction when compared to widely used clinical risk scores [18].

Machine learning techniques demonstrated substantial potential in enhancing preoperative assessment in cardiac surgery. Automated image segmentation tools have shown reliable anatomical delineation across diverse cardiovascular structures, supporting efficient and reproducible pre-surgical evaluation. Moreover, multiple comparative studies have indicated that machine learning models could outperform traditional risk scores, such as EuroSCORE II and STS, in predicting perioperative mortality, offering more individualized and accurate risk stratification. These developments underscore the growing role of data-driven approaches in refining surgical planning and patient selection [3].

Intraoperative Support

Advances in computational analysis during surgery are beginning to assist the surgical team in real time, offering potentially enhanced navigation, perfusion management, and resource use [3].

(a) Robotic and Image Guidance

The combination of advanced imaging systems and robotic-assisted surgical techniques has already contributed to improved outcomes in various surgical specialties. However, the complexity of interpreting high-resolution imaging in real time and the cognitive load associated with managing robotic interfaces continue to pose practical challenges for surgeons. To address these limitations, recent developments have focused on integrating computational tools with robotic platforms to enhance intraoperative decision-making. These tools can process large volumes of data derived from preoperative imaging and assist in overlaying critical anatomical information onto the surgical field during procedures. This integration has the potential to improve surgical accuracy by marking anatomical boundaries, highlighting areas of concern, and supporting intraoperative navigation. While most clinical systems remain under development or in early stages of use, the concept of combining algorithm-based guidance with robotic control is gaining attention as a means of refining operative workflow and improving patient-specific planning [19].

(b) Intraoperative Decision Support

A recent study investigated the potential of machine learning to anticipate critical decisions made during cardiopulmonary bypass in the context of cardiac surgery. Using data from 148 high-fidelity simulations replicating intraoperative events, the research team developed predictive models capable of identifying appropriate responses to evolving clinical scenarios. The model achieved a prediction accuracy of 78.2% (95% CI: 77.8–78.6%) when tested across 30-fold cross-validation using different random seeds. These findings suggest that such data-driven tools may eventually support intraoperative decision-making during bypass, offering early warnings in complex situations and potentially enhancing safety during the most critical phases of cardiac procedures [20].

(c) Intraoperative Transfusion Risk Prediction

A retrospective study evaluated the performance of statistical learning models to predict the need for red blood cell (RBC) transfusion in patients undergoing mitral valve surgery. The analysis included 698 cases, with approximately one-quarter of patients requiring intraoperative transfusion. Thirteen modeling techniques were tested, and among them, the CatBoost algorithm demonstrated the highest predictive performance, achieving an AUC of 0.88 (95% CI: 0.845–0.909) in the test cohort. The model identified several key variables associated with transfusion risk, including low hematocrit, older age, lower body weight and BMI, reduced hemoglobin and red blood cell count, female sex, and specific surgical. In the validation subset, the model correctly classified transfusion status in 86.8% of patients. These findings suggest that such tools may assist surgical teams in anticipating transfusion needs and optimizing intraoperative preparation [21].

Wang and collaborators developed a predictive approach to estimate intraoperative RBC transfusion requirements in cardiothoracic surgery using detailed perioperative data from over 2400 procedures. The study applied a hybrid modeling framework, combining Gaussian Process regression and classification algorithms. The regression model showed strong accuracy for patients receiving no transfusion or limited transfusion (1–3 units). For cases involving ≥4 units of RBCs, the classification component achieved an AUC of 0.826. These results suggest that locally trained data-driven tools can provide useful estimates of intraoperative transfusion requirements, which may support individualized preparation and more efficient blood product allocation in cardiothoracic procedures [22].

These findings underscore the clinical value of machine learning models in predicting transfusion needs during cardiac surgery. By incorporating a wide array of preoperative and intraoperative variables, such models can offer more accurate and individualized assessments than traditional empirical methods. Their ability to identify high-risk patients before and during surgery may improve operative planning, reduce unnecessary blood product use, and support more efficient inventory management. As these models continue to be validated and integrated into clinical workflows, they may become essential components of perioperative care strategies in cardiac surgery [22].

Postoperative Monitoring and Outcomes Prediction

Effective postoperative surveillance in the intensive care unit (ICU) after cardiac surgery is essential for identifying early signs of critical complications and enabling timely intervention. Recent efforts have focused on creating predictive models that use real-time patient data to anticipate issues such as sepsis, atrial arrhythmias, and acute kidney injury [23–25].

(a) ICU Surveillance for Early Complications

One study explored the use of data-driven models to predict postoperative complications and short-term mortality in critically ill patients who had undergone open-heart surgery. The analysis was based on data extracted from the MIMIC-III database and included 6844 patients who underwent procedures such as coronary artery bypass grafting and valve replacements. The authors aimed to predict four clinically relevant outcomes: 30-day mortality, septic shock, thrombocytopenia, and liver dysfunction. Several modeling techniques were tested, including random forest, logistic regression, artificial neural networks, and extreme gradient boosting (XGBoost). Among these, the XGBoost model achieved the best performance across all outcomes. Specifically, it yielded an AUC of 0.88 for 30-day mortality, 0.98 for septic shock, 0.88 for thrombocytopenia, and 0.89 for liver dysfunction. These results highlighted that learning models based on routinely collected ICU data may help identify patients at increased risk for adverse postoperative events [26].

(b) Atrial Fibrillation Prediction

Postoperative atrial fibrillation remains a major concern. A recent study investigated the occurrence of new-onset postoperative atrial fibrillation (POAF) in patients undergoing mitral valve surgery and evaluated the ability of machine learning models to predict this complication. The study examined data from 27,856 mitral valve procedures performed across 910 centers in the United States between 2017 and 2020, using the Society of Thoracic Surgeons National Adult Cardiac Database. All patients included had no prior history of atrial fibrillation or permanent pacemaker implantation. The overall incidence of POAF was 35.4%. Patients who developed POAF were generally older and more likely to have comorbidities. The authors applied several modeling strategies, including gradient boosting, random forest, decision trees, and penalized logistic regression, and found that the machine learning approaches modestly outperformed conventional logistic regression in terms of sensitivity, specificity, and precision. Despite these improvements, the models achieved only moderate predictive performance, underlining the complexity of identifying patients at risk for POAF using structured clinical data alone [27].

A scoping review assessed current evidence on the use of data-driven predictive models for POAF following cardiac surgery. The incidence of POAF reported in the studies included varied between 21.5% and 37.1%. The predictive performance of the models showed considerable variability, with sensitivity values ranging from 0.22 to 0.91 and AUC scores between 0.67 and 0.94. Across studies, patient age, sex, left atrial dimension, kidney function, and ventilation duration were among the key factors influencing POAF risk. While the reviewed models demonstrated potential for individualized risk stratification, the authors noted significant heterogeneity in study designs and a lack of external validation, both of which limit their immediate applicability in clinical settings [28].

(c) Prediction of Acute Kidney Injury

A systematic review and meta-analysis evaluated the performance of various predictive models for anticipating acute kidney injury (AKI) following cardiac surgery. The analysis included 38 studies comprising over 255,000 patients and assessed 60 distinct modeling approaches. Among these, logistic regression was the most frequently used method, although other models, such as neural networks, support vector machines, random forests, and extreme gradient boosting, were also examined. Across the pooled data, the overall discrimination for predicting cardiac surgery-associated AKI (CSA-AKI) was moderate, with a C-index of 0.76 in training sets and 0.79 in validation cohorts. The findings underscore the growing role of computational models in the early identification of CSA-AKI and call for further development of tools that use noninvasive factors to enhance prognostic utility in the perioperative setting [29].

Another study explored a dynamic approach to anticipate AKI in patients undergoing cardiac surgery by developing a model that integrated a wide range of perioperative and intensive care data. The study included 4267 patients treated at a tertiary center, and the model was trained to issue hourly predictions of AKI risk within a 48-hour window following surgery. The model demonstrated strong performance, with an AUC of 0.82 for predicting any stage of AKI and an AUC of 0.95 for predicting more severe forms (stage 2 or higher). Notably, the system was able to anticipate the onset of AKI before it was identified by conventional diagnostic criteria in nearly 90% of cases. These findings highlight the potential of continuous, data-driven surveillance in the early detection and management of postoperative renal complications [30].

Consequently, predictive models for AKI after cardiac surgery show increasing clinical relevance. While traditional methods offer moderate accuracy, dynamic tools using real-time perioperative and ICU data can detect AKI earlier and with greater precision. These systems may improve prevention and intervention efforts, particularly for severe cases. Further validation and integration into clinical workflows remain essential [29].

(d) Prediction of Major Postoperative Bleeding

One study analyzed the effectiveness of several computational models in estimating the risk of major bleeding following isolated coronary artery bypass grafting. Using data from 1045 patients, the authors compared multiple algorithms with conventional risk scores such as TRUST and WILL-BLEED. The conditional inference random forest model achieved the best performance, with an AUC of 0.831 in the test set. Other models, including stochastic gradient boosting and traditional random forest, also showed strong predictive capacity, with AUCs exceeding 0.81. In contrast, traditional scoring systems demonstrated markedly lower accuracy. These findings suggest that modern risk stratification models can offer more reliable identification of patients at increased risk for significant postoperative bleeding, potentially improving perioperative planning and patient safety [31].

AI in Surgical Education

Simulation-based training could become an integral element in the preparation of cardiac surgeons, offering a controlled and replicable environment to practice intricate procedures before they are performed on patients. From open-heart surgery to robotic valve interventions, the complexity of cardiac operations demands that trainees develop not only technical proficiency but also decision-making and spatial awareness under conditions that closely mimic the clinical setting. Simulation centers now routinely employ structured programs that define clear learning goals and use high-fidelity models, including synthetic, virtual, or hybrid simulators, to support progressive skill acquisition [32, 33].

One of the key limitations in surgical training lies in the availability of expert instructors who can deliver high-quality, individualized feedback. Traditional models of training depend on real-time, direct supervision, which is both resource-intensive and variable in its consistency. As a result, there is a growing interest in systems that can provide structured evaluation without continuous human oversight. In the context of robotic cardiac surgery, where technical performance can be quantified with high precision, automated systems have been developed to track metrics such as motion economy, instrument usage patterns, and task completion time. These platforms enable objective assessment and facilitate targeted feedback without requiring the constant presence of an expert surgeon [32–34].

Several studies have evaluated the effectiveness of such systems. One clinical trial compared performance outcomes among medical trainees receiving feedback from either a human instructor or an automated tutoring system. The results showed that those in the automated feedback group achieved higher procedural scores, with no significant difference in perceived cognitive load or emotional response between the groups. Therefore, these automated systems could be comparable to traditional instruction (or even better) in terms of skill acquisition, particularly when focused on quantifiable outcomes such as instrument handling or task precision [32, 34].

Despite these advancements, challenges remain. Many systems are developed for specific procedures and lack generalizability across different surgical contexts. Furthermore, the integration of such tools into national or international training curricula requires agreement on standard metrics, validation protocols, and credentialing frameworks. Nevertheless, the use of structured educational technologies, particularly in robotic and minimally invasive cardiac surgery, represents a critical step toward more scalable, equitable, and effective surgical training [32, 33].

Challenges and Perspectives for the Integration of AI in Cardiac Surgery

Despite the progress achieved in recent years, the implementation of artificial intelligence tools in cardiac surgery remains constrained by some limitations. One of the most important issues is the limited generalizability of current models. Many systems are developed using data from single centers or homogeneous populations, which restricts their applicability across diverse clinical environments. The variability in surgical techniques, patient characteristics, and institutional protocols often limits external validation, raising concerns about the reliability of AI-assisted tools in routine clinical decision-making [3, 35, 36].

Another significant barrier is the quality and structure of available clinical data. Algorithms rely on accurate, complete, and temporally consistent datasets to generate meaningful predictions. However, the real-world data used in clinical practice often suffer from missing variables, inconsistent documentation, and limited standardization. These flaws can introduce noise into predictive models, weakening their clinical relevance and potentially amplifying diagnostic or therapeutic errors [3, 37].

Ethical and legal challenges also complicate the path toward integration. Cardiac surgery involves high-stakes decisions, and the introduction of algorithm-based recommendations into perioperative workflows raises unresolved questions about responsibility in case of adverse outcomes. When an AI system contributes to a clinical error, it remains unclear whether liability rests with the physician, the institution, the software developers, or the data providers [3, 38].

Concerns regarding data privacy and security are also important. Most AI systems depend on large volumes of patient data, often integrated from multiple sources. Without robust encryption, governance, and institutional control, there is a risk that sensitive health information may be compromised, shared without consent, or misused for non-clinical purposes. The increasing involvement of private-sector companies in data handling raises additional concerns about proprietary ownership, long-term access, and regulatory oversight [3, 39].

Looking forward, the future development of intelligent surgical tools must prioritize transparency, interpretability, and clinician-in-the-loop systems. Enhancing the interpretability of predictive outputs will help build trust, allowing surgeons to understand and evaluate algorithmic suggestions in the context of patient-specific complexity. Prospective multicenter studies are also essential to test performance across varied environments and populations, ensuring that tools are robust and equitable [3].

Lastly, training the future surgical workforce in data science principles will be crucial. As machine-guided tools become more integrated into the operating room, the surgeon's role will evolve, not in opposition to technology, but in collaboration with it. Preparing trainees to critically assess, oversee, and collaborate with digital systems may prove just as important as traditional manual skills. Establishing formal curricula that include exposure to algorithmic limitations, bias recognition, and ethical standards may help ensure safe and effective implementation [3].

References

1. Miles TJ, Ghanta RK. Machine learning in cardiac surgery: a narrative review. J Thorac Dis. 2024;16(4):2644–53.

2. Hashimoto DA, et al. Artificial intelligence in surgery: promises and perils. Ann Surg. 2018;268(1):70–6.
3. Leivaditis V, et al. Artificial intelligence in cardiac surgery: transforming outcomes and shaping the future. Clin Pract. 2025;15(1):17.
4. Nedadur R, et al. The emerging and important role of artificial intelligence in cardiac surgery. Can J Cardiol. 2024;40(10):1865–79.
5. Roth GA, et al. Global burden of cardiovascular diseases and risk factors, 1990–2019: update from the GBD 2019 study. J Am Coll Cardiol. 2020;76(25):2982–3021.
6. Clough RA, et al. The effect of comorbid illness on mortality outcomes in cardiac surgery. Arch Surg. 2002;137(4):428–33.
7. Scrutinio D, Giannuzzi P. Comorbidity in patients undergoing coronary artery bypass graft surgery: impact on outcome and implications for cardiac rehabilitation. Eur J Cardiovasc Prev Rehabil. 2008;15(4):379–85.
8. Tolu-Akinnawo OZ, et al. Advancements in artificial intelligence in noninvasive cardiac imaging: a comprehensive review. Clin Cardiol. 2025;48(1):e70087.
9. Mohsin SN, et al. The role of artificial intelligence in prediction, risk stratification, and personalized treatment planning for congenital heart diseases. Cureus. 2023;15(8)
10. Mumtaz H, et al. The future of cardiothoracic surgery in artificial intelligence. Ann Med Surg. 2022;80:80.
11. Iftikhar M, et al. Artificial intelligence: revolutionizing robotic surgery. Ann Med Surg. 2024;86(9):5401–9.
12. Arjomandi Rad A, Hajzamani D, Sardari Nia P. Simulation-based training in cardiac surgery: a systematic review. Interdisciplinary Cardio Vasc Thoracic Surg. 2023;37(2):ivad079.
13. Cates CU, Gallagher AG. The future of simulation technologies for complex cardiovascular procedures. Eur Heart J. 2012;33(17):2127–34.
14. Ahmad A, et al. Equity and artificial intelligence in surgical care: a comprehensive review of current challenges and promising solutions. BULLET: Jurnal Multidisiplin Ilmu. 2023;2(2):443–55.
15. Allyn J, et al. A comparison of a machine learning model with EuroSCORE II in predicting mortality after elective cardiac surgery: a decision curve analysis. PLoS One. 2017;12(1):e0169772.
16. Nannini G, et al. A fully automated deep learning approach for coronary artery segmentation and comprehensive characterization. APL Bioeng. 2024;8(1):016103.
17. Baskaran L, et al. Automatic segmentation of multiple cardiovascular structures from cardiac computed tomography angiography images using deep learning. PLoS One. 2020;15(5):e0232573.
18. Fan Y, et al. Development of machine learning models for mortality risk prediction after cardiac surgery. Cardiovasc Diagn Ther. 2022;12(1):12–23.
19. Zhang C, et al. The integration of artificial intelligence in robotic surgery: a narrative review. Surgery. 2024;176(3):552–7.
20. Dias RD, et al. Using machine learning to predict perfusionists' critical decision-making during cardiac surgery. Comput Methods Biomech Biomed Eng Imaging Vis. 2022;10(3):308–12.
21. Liu S, et al. Machine learning models to predict red blood cell transfusion in patients undergoing mitral valve surgery. Ann Transl Med. 2021;9(7):530.
22. Wang Z, et al. Development and validation of a machine learning method to predict intraoperative red blood cell transfusions in cardiothoracic surgery. Sci Rep. 2022;12(1):1355.
23. Shi J, et al. Machine learning for prediction of acute kidney injury in patients diagnosed with sepsis in critical care. PLoS One. 2024;19(4):e0301014.
24. Guan C, et al. Interpretable machine learning model for new-onset atrial fibrillation prediction in critically ill patients: a multi-center study. Crit Care. 2024;28(1):349.
25. Khalpey Z, et al. Leveling up: a review of machine learning models in the cardiac ICU. Am J Med. 2023;136(10):979–84.
26. Zhong Z, et al. Machine learning prediction models for prognosis of critically ill patients after open-heart surgery. Sci Rep. 2021;11(1):3384.

27. Andrei A-C, et al. Machine learning-based prediction of new onset of atrial fibrillation after mitral valve surgery. Int J Arrhythm. 2024;25(1):18.
28. El-Sherbini AH, et al. Machine learning for predicting postoperative atrial fibrillation after cardiac surgery: a scoping review of current literature. Am J Cardiol. 2023;209:66–75.
29. Song Z, et al. Machine learning in predicting cardiac surgery-associated acute kidney injury: a systemic review and meta-analysis. Front Cardiovasc Med. 2022;9:2022.
30. Ryan CT, et al. Machine learning for dynamic and early prediction of acute kidney injury after cardiac surgery. J Thorac Cardiovasc Surg. 2023;166(6):e551–64.
31. Gao Y, et al. Machine learning algorithms to predict major bleeding after isolated coronary artery bypass grafting. Front Cardiovasc Med. 2022;9:881881.
32. Jarry C, et al. Surgical training scalability through AI-based innovations. Glob Surg Educ J Assoc Surg Educ. 2025;4(1):37.
33. Leon S, et al. Artificial intelligence and the education of future surgeons. Am J Surg. 2025;246:116257.
34. Fazlollahi AM, et al. Effect of artificial intelligence tutoring vs expert instruction on learning simulated surgical skills among medical students: a randomized clinical trial. JAMA Netw Open. 2022;5(2):e2149008.
35. Gulati G, et al. Generalizability of cardiovascular disease clinical prediction models: 158 independent external validations of 104 unique models. Circ Cardiovasc Qual Outcomes. 2022;15(4):e008487.
36. Lee SW, et al. Internal and external validation of machine learning models for predicting acute kidney injury following non-cardiac surgery using open datasets. J Pers Med. 2024;14(6)
37. Syed R, et al. Digital health data quality issues: systematic review. J Med Internet Res. 2023;25:e42615.
38. Blackman J, Veerapen R. On the practical, ethical, and legal necessity of clinical artificial intelligence explainability: an examination of key arguments. BMC Med Inform Decis Mak. 2025;25(1):111.
39. Kerasidou A, Kerasidou C. Data-driven research and healthcare: public trust, data governance and the NHS. BMC Med Ethics. 2023;24(1):51.

Index

G. Tinică, A. Burlacu (eds.), *Surgical, Hybrid and Minimally Invasive Structural Cardiac Interventions*, https://doi.org/10.1007/978-3-032-16676-0

GPSR Compliance

The European Union's (EU) General Product Safety Regulation (GPSR) is a set of rules that requires consumer products to be safe and our obligations to ensure this.

If you have any concerns about our products, you can contact us on ProductSafety@springernature.com

In case Publisher is established outside the EU, the EU authorized representative is:

Springer Nature Customer Service Center GmbH
Europaplatz 3
69115 Heidelberg, Germany

Batch number: 10732076

Printed by Printforce, the Netherlands